Health Care Ethics
An Introduction

Health Care Ethics
An Introduction

Edited by Donald VanDeVeer
and Tom Regan

Temple University Press · Philadelphia

R
724
H34
.
1987

Temple University Press,

Philadelphia 19122

Copyright © 1987

by Temple University.

All rights reserved

Published 1987

Printed in the United States of America

The paper used in this publication meets the

minimum requirements of American National Standard for

Information Sciences—Permanence of Paper for Printed

Library Materials, ANSI Z39.48-1984.

Library of Congress Cataloging-in-Publication Data

Health care ethics.

  Includes bibliographical references.

  1. Medical ethics.   2. Bioethics.   I. VanDeVeer,

Donald, 1939–   . II. Regan, Tom.   [DNLM:

1. Bioethics.   2. Ethics, Medical.   W 50 H4335]

R724.H34   1986   174'.2   85-22048

ISBN 0-87722-408-0

ISBN 0-87722-441-2 (pbk.)

For Ida Lena Askew
and Dallas Pratt, M.D.

Contents

Preface

A week seldom passes in which ethical perplexities and controversies related to health care matters are not put before the public eye. Only in the past decade, however, have good collections of essays in this field become available. Some of these have come to resemble miniencyclopedias with a bewildering array of excerpts of existing materials, materials frequently obscure to the student or layperson because they originally were written with other professionals in mind. In some cases, we believe, earlier explorations and analyses have been superseded, but this fact is not always reflected in available texts. We have sought to improve this situation by collecting entirely new essays, each comprehensive on its topic, by leading philosophers (and one health care professional). In areas that are intellectually challenging, and often resistant to analysis, it is no easy task to explore systematically and lucidly marshall the relevant arguments in the ongoing effort to arrive at reasonable solutions to the controversies that prevail. We have encouraged our essayists, all leading contributors in their fields, to write as clearly as possible, to avoid jargon, and not to presuppose (without explanation) theories, principles, terms or distinctions that would be unfamiliar to the student or layperson untutored in philosophy, ethical theory, or relevant areas of medicine or nursing. The result, we believe, is an exceptional degree of clarity in a series of careful, informed, frequently provocative, but accessible essays about the core issues in the ethics of health care.

Those who believe that chemistry and biology, for example, are complex, but that no serious effort is needed to explore the nonempirical dimensions of health care ethics—or to acquire the analytical and conceptual tools to do so—are, alas, in for a bit of a surprise. Indeed, if the only source of dispute in biomedical areas were over "what the facts are," it would be hard to understand why so many persistent, and divisive, controversies exist. The essays that follow should help lay to rest the myth that the possession of empirical knowledge (e.g., in medicine) is sufficient to solve the moral disputes surrounding certain medical issues or to render the possessor of such knowledge an expert "medical ethicist." In addition, as will also become clear, we should be wary of drawing conclusions about what we ought to do with regard to abortion, experimentation on human beings, or decision making for incompetent parties, without understanding the relevant empirical knowledge— whether derived from genetics, chemistry, law, psychology, statistics, or other disciplines. One important challenge for the specialist today is to appreciate adequately the relevance, substance, and strengths of other disciplines.

Instructors who use this volume may or may not wish to explore the essays in the order presented here. The book's rather extensive introduction will help acquaint the reader with the leading ethical approaches, both general and intermediate-level moral principles, and conceptions invoked by different theorists in approaching the specific quandaries that are the focus of the various chapters. The introduction also provides some indication of the arguments advanced for and against such basic principles. A further aim is to sensitize the reader or student to the diverse types of claims that are relevant to settling disputes, whether moral, empirical, or conceptual. Some who study health care ethics will bring empirical expertise from areas outside philosophy. Some will be skilled in the logical analysis of arguments. Others will not be familiar with the basic concepts of logic or have a clear sense of what sorts of virtues or vices an argument may exhibit. For those readers, the introduction briefly reviews the elements essential to the critical analysis of arguments. Depending on the makeup of a class using this text, instructors may choose to give much, little, or no emphasis to such matters. For some students, this review will serve as a succinct refresher.

No collection of essays can satisfy all interests. Indeed, space considerations have forced us to exclude certain important matters. For example, discussion of natural law theory and the doctrine of double effect is omitted from an already ample introduction (instructors might want to assign the latter in segments). In addition, eyecatching new therapies or techniques—such as artificial heart implants, cross-species organ transplants, frozen embryos, and genetic intervention to correct defects—are not explored. Similarly, the current problem of AIDS (acquired immune deficiency syndrome) is not directly addressed in the following essays, but controversies over AIDS frequently focus on personal responsibility for illness (see Wikler's essay), consent to treatment (see Brock's essay), or what is owed AIDS victims (see Daniels' essay on justice and health-care.) Thus, the fundamental questions and principles addressed here have important bearings on a wider range of ethical issues in health care than those directly addressed herein.

Many instructors, however, will find it useful to supplement this book with additional readings. Indeed, it is, we believe, a significant advantage that *Health Care Ethics* is comparatively "lean and wiry." Thus, it can function as a core text to be complemented by articles or narrowly focused monographs of special interest to the class and/or the instructor. For example, some instructors, espe-cially those accustomed to a legal or medical orientation, may wish to focus on specific cases. Several new books are now available whose sole aim is to provide a useful collection of cases.[1]

We are much indebted to Dan Brock, Dan Wikler, and Martin Ben-jamin for their helpful suggestions regarding (other) potential con-tributors. We also wish to acknowledge the first-rate efforts and the patience of our contributors, both visible and invisible, who endured our editorial comments, suggestions, delays, more delays, and a sea of correspondence.

We add that we have, as editors, chosen not to impose on our con-tributors a uniformity of style with respect to the use of gender tied words, e.g., pronouns. Unless the context suggests otherwise, refer-ence to 'he' normally can be understood to mean 'he or she.' The same is true of occurrences of 'she.'

We wish to thank Jane Cullen and Jennifer French of Temple Uni-versity Press for their generous assistance. We also are much in-debted to Maria Bartolini for her assistance in correspondence, and to Patricia Spiller for her help with the manuscript. Finally, without the patience, responsiveness, and excellent help of two world-class professionals, Ruth Boone and Ann Rives, *Health Care Ethics: An Introduction* would have remained a gleam in our editorial eyes.[2]

Notes

1. For example, see Robert M. Veatch, *Case Studies in Medical Ethics* (Cambridge: Harvard University Press, 1977). See also Thomas A. Shannon and Jo Ann Manfra, eds., *Law and Bioethics* (Ramsey, N.J.: Paulist Press, 1982).

2. An earlier, pre-natal title of this volume was *Border Crossings*. Prior to actual publication, it is worth noting, some references in the philosophical literature to *Border Crossings* have appeared. Generally, material thus cited will be found in this volume.

Health Care Ethics
An Introduction

Introduction

Donald VanDeVeer

The Phenomenon of Health Care Ethics

A few decades ago, and to an extent today, the term *medical ethics* called to mind a less than intriguing set of questions about whether physicians overcharged patients, paid their taxes, remained sober on the job, were unduly ostentatious, or, if male, were properly chaperoned when providing gynecological services for female patients. Such delimited concerns fail to suggest why the past decade has given rise to the increasing number of new journals devoted to biomedical or health care ethics, the rapid increase in undergraduate and graduate courses in the area, the proliferation of new texts and media documentaries, and a vigorous, ongoing inquiry and interchange among persons professionally trained in, for example, medicine, psychology, biology, law, philosophy, economics, nursing, and religion—as well as a heightened awareness and interest on the part of the general public. The term "health care ethics" is now construed to refer to a diverse array of pressing issues that are perplexing, recalcitrant, and controversial. Their importance extends far beyond those narrow concerns mentioned earlier. Many of the issues, but not all, now concern matters of life and death, of suffering and healing, and of liberty and constraint.

Few literate adults today are entirely unacquainted with, or have not felt some puzzlement about, current dilemmas in health care ethics. These include such questions as whether it is acceptable to abort human fetuses, to kill (or allow to die) "defective" (e.g., Tay-Sachs) infants, to withdraw life support systems from comatose patients, to have compulsory screening programs for populations that commonly suffer from significant genetic defects (or are members of groups at high risk for getting AIDS), to deceive patients "for their own good," to perform psychosurgery on involuntary, violence-prone, subjects, to engage in medical experimentation on children or

3

(consenting or unconsenting) prisoners, or to distribute health care on the basis of the willingness and ability to pay of the potential recipients. Such issues, among others, are noteworthy because of their drama, their urgency, and their unsettling nature; they resist glib or simple solutions. They are, understandably, matters about which reasonable and informed persons of good will often disagree. In that respect they differ sharply from possible but unlikely debates about the morality of, or whether to legalize, rape, child abuse, terrorism, or whether a humane society should allow the enslavement of those captured in wars. Although some moral questions may surround these acts, we can still take note of the *striking moral consensus* about such issues compared with the *persistent disagreements* regarding many of the questions of health care ethics. A point for further reflection as we proceed concerns how there can be widespread consensus on a variety of social issues and yet residual dispute over others. Searching for the *principled grounds* of our shared moral judgments may provide a coherent basis for resolving some of the persistent disagreements to be explored—or at least *narrow the range of reasonable controversy.*

In any attempt to think clearly about any rather complex set of issues, it is helpful to be aware of of the relevant distinctions, categories, theoretical viewpoints, and tools of inquiry of previous investigators. This introduction can hardly summarize all that is relevant to the investigation of the problems of biomedical ethics. Still, what we can do here is to identify basic questions, define relevant concepts, explain some tools of philosophical investigation, and at least acquaint the reader with the general features of the leading ethical theories. That much is essential for a thoughtful, critical exploration of the intellectually challenging matters that are the focus of this book's essays.

Empirical, Evaluative, and Conceptual Questions

It is a philosophical commonplace that certain claims or questions are either *empirical, evaluative,* or *conceptual.* Some problems are said to raise questions of all three types. We need to be clear about what is meant by such terminology. Although the categories are not entirely uncontroversial, we will take note of the standard view. *Empirical claims* are claims about what, as a matter of contingent fact, is, was, or will be the case. Examples include:

1. Maria is pregnant.
2. A nuclear war will occur in 1994.
3. Nip stole Tuck's car.
4. Carl was passive-aggressive at the staff meeting.

Notice that in labeling some claims as empirical we have made no commitment as to their truth or falsity.[1] Generally it is possible to settle the truth or falsity of empirical claims by obtaining relevant evidence and, perhaps, making appropriate inferences. Of course, the degree of difficulty varies. Consider the sort of evidence or experience we would need to determine the truth or falsity of the following:

1. Tracy is five feet tall.
2. Tracy is a Down's syndrome person.
3. Dinosaurs descended from birds.
4. The world was created, fossils and all, ten minutes ago.
5. In my former life, I was a cockroach.

We might agree that there is no way to conclusively verify or falsify some of these claims (such as number 4). Still, they are all, given our definition, empirical claims. Thus, we can distinguish the further question of their belief-worthiness as a separate, *epistemological*, issue.[2] Perhaps if we were or could be in the appropriate situation, we could know, or justifiably believe, the truth or falsity of any of these claims. If so, we might say that such claims were falsifiable in principle or verifiable in principle by observation or what is inferrable from what we know by observation. Indeed, some philosophers have defined 'empirical claim' as any claim having just such a property. However, our definition does not tie the definition of 'empirical claim' to a particular proviso concerning *how* the truth or falsity of such a claim is to be ascertained.

A further point is worth noting. We cannot say that a statement is an empirical claim simply because it employs as its main or sole verb "is", "was", or "will be". Some of the following claims have that characteristic, but we shall classify them all as evaluative claims:

1. Beethoven's Fifth Symphony is sublime.
2. Pleasure is good.
3. Hitler was evil.
4. Involuntary euthanasia is wrong.
5. Limited experimentation on fetuses is permissible.

Why are these evaluative claims? How is 'evaluative claim' to be defined? Although a precise, fully adequate definition is not easy to come by, this fact need not unduly deter us (consider the difficulty of adequately defining 'law,' 'medicine,' 'science,' 'nursing,' 'illness,' or 'game'). A rough but useful definition of 'evaluative claim' is 'a claim about *what is good or bad or what ought or ought not to be the case*' (including what ought or ought not be done). Using this definition, we can see that the above statements are evaluative in nature. Some claims are *purely evaluative* (numbers 2 and 4), and some are *purely empirical* ("Tracy is five feet tall"). Some claims seem both to convey empirical information and to proffer an evaluation:

1. American slavery was thoroughly racist.
2. Professor Puck exploits his graduate students.
3. The Nazis murdered millions of Jews.

The modes of establishing or refuting empirical claims (by gathering empirical evidence and related theorizing) seem to differ significantly from the accepted modes of defending or subverting evaluative claims (we will discuss this shortly). Thus, it is important to be clear about what sort of claim we are considering—whether it is proposed by others or ourselves. If we fail to do this, we are likely to bark up the wrong tree. In other words, we may attempt to resolve a dispute or answer a question by gathering empirical data when that effort is either irrelevant or not sufficient. For example, from the fact that

1. In Toomany County it is standard medical practice to sterilize poor women in their late thirties with four or more children.

It does not follow that

2. Such women ought to be sterilized (or that it is permissible to do so).

any more than   b. We ought to have wars.

follows from   a. Wars have always been with us.

The inferences from (1) to (2) and from (a) to (b) are rather transparently *invalid* ones; that is, it is not necessarily the case that: if the premises are true the conclusion must be true. Invalid arguments such as these fail to provide the most compelling defense of their conclusions. In general, it is not obvious that one can ever adequately defend an evaluative proposal by appealing to purely empirical premises (even if those premises are true). The failure to note the move from purely empirical claims to evaluative ones may stem from a failure to distinguish empirical from evaluative (or normative) claims.

How are ethical claims related to evaluative claims? Given our broad construal of 'evaluative claim' we can distinguish among different sorts of evaluative claims. Roughly, some evaluative claims concern whether acts ought or ought not be done—or whether they are permissible or not. These evaluative claims are often labeled ethical, moral, or sometimes normative. The terminology here is not completely standardized in the literature, and one often needs to pay close attention to context to discern what a writer means by such terms. Some writers use 'ethical' and 'evaluative' interchangeably; some do likewise with 'normative' and 'evaluative.' Given our characterization of 'moral' or 'ethical,' there are some evaluative claims that are not moral (or ethical) claims. Evaluative claims about the nature of certain objects are more aptly labeled aesthetic claims or judgments, such as:

1. Beethoven's Fifth Symphony is sublime.
2. That's a beautiful sunset.
3. Her house is a paradigm of tackiness.

More important for our purposes (since we shall not focus on the aesthetic qualities of biomedical practices) is the distinction between moral claims about acts and evaluative claims about states of affairs. As examples of the latter, consider the following:

1. Health is good.
2. Sickness is bad.
3. Pleasure is good.
4. Pain is bad.
5. Life is good.
6. Autonomy is desirable.
7. Pleasure is bad.

Many people would find claims 1 through 6 plausible, but deny 7. Claim 7 is included here to emphasize the point that we are focusing on types of claims and not on their plausibility—which is another matter.

The distinction between evaluative claims about states of affairs on the one hand and moral claims about acts on the other is crucial to understanding much ethical theorizing and the influential theory

of utilitarianism (discussed later) in particular. Notice that we may
agree with some evaluative claim about a state of affairs but reasonably deny, or at least doubt, that much follows with regard to what
moral agents (those beings capable of acting voluntarily and for conscious reasons) ought or ought not to do—or what it is permissible
for them to do. For example, suppose we agree with claim 5, that life
is good, or a variant, that human life is good. It does not obviously
follow that we should do whatever will maximize the number of humans or that we should never take human life (reflect here, perhaps,
on your moral views about killing in self-defense—or about the
heroic self-sacrifice of soldiers who jump on grenades). In short,
evaluative claims about states of affairs (sometimes identified as
nonmoral evaluative judgments) do not obviously entail moral
claims, claims about which acts are either permissible or a matter of
duty. The relation of the former claims to the latter (sometimes referred to as matters of right or wrong) is a question deserving further
thought and attention. Whether we should always promote or prolong human life because human life is good, whether we should always relieve pain because pain is bad, whether we should always
promote health because health is good are all issues involving complex considerations.

Indeed, we may be accused of begging important questions, or at
least bypassing them, if we argue in the ways mentioned in the preceding sentence since it is not obvious that: human life is always, or
necessarily, good; that pain is always, or necessarily, bad; or that
health is always, or necessarily, a good.[3] Whether these objections
are plausible we leave open, but at least part of a critical reflection
on such matters would take into account the standardly employed
distinction between *intrinsically* good (or bad) states of affairs and
extrinsically (or instrumentally) good (or bad) states of affairs or objects. Some things are said to be good simply because they constitute effective means to some further end that is thought good or desirable (e.g., a good drug, a good scalpel, or a good stereo). Such
things are, at least, extrinsically good. Are any things or states of affairs good for their own sake? Alternatively put, is there any intrinsic, nonmoral, good? A plausible answer here is that pleasure is such
a good. This classic view (or the stronger claim that pleasure *and
pleasure alone* is intrinsically good) is often referred to as the hedonistic theory of the good (not to be confused with the popular use of
'hedonistic' to describe certain motives). Whether hedonism, so understood, is a plausible view is a matter of some dispute. The British

philosopher G. E. Moore held the view that certain types of states of affairs are intrinsically good: pleasure, friendship, and the existence of beauiful objects. Hedonistic opponents of Moore might argue that the latter matters are only extrinsically good—that is, they are good only as a means to pleasure. The intrinsic good/extrinsic good distinction is of some relevance here for at least two reasons. As noted, it is necessary to understand the influential theory of utilitarianism (see our later discussion)—a theory that in most versions presupposes the acceptability of the hedonistic theory of the good. Second, when one contemplates the aims of medicine, one can hardly avoid reflecting on whether, for example, health or the prolongation of life are nonmoral goods and, if so, whether they are intrinsic goods. Further, even if they are, are there other, competing intrinsic goods? And is it morally permissible or obligatory (note the shift here to a focus on acts or practices) to promote health or the prolongation of life at the expense of other goods (such as individual autonomy)?

A further comment is in order regarding our more basic distinction between evaluative and empirical claims. The examples of evaluative claims set out so far have been examples of rather explicitly evaluative claims (e.g., pleasure is good). However, many evaluative claims are not couched in explicitly evaluative language. Perhaps out of a desire to avoid the appearance of "moralizing" or out of a desire to appear to be operating within a purely scientific framework (making only descriptive empirical judgments?), many persons, professional scientists and others, tend to avoid explicitly moral or evaluative language (involving, e.g., 'right,' 'wrong,' 'duty,' 'obligation,' 'permissible,' 'just,' 'unjust,' 'good,' 'bad,' 'morally justifiable'). Still, it is often clear (context may make it so) that moral claims about actions (recall our definition) are being made—that is, claims about what ought or ought not to be done, or what is permissible or not. Sometimes the evaluation is thinly veiled; sometimes it is left almost entirely tacit even though the message is quite clear. Consider these remarks:

1. Triage is a workable policy.
2. Radical mastectomies are old-fashioned.
3. An appendectomy is contraindicated.
4. Only a physician trained prior to 1960 would do that.
5. A CAT scanner at every county hospital is excessive.
6. Disclosing that information is most unprofessional.
7. Capitalism is the by-product of a bourgeois mentality.

Each of these remarks contains some evaluation about what should be done. There is no suggestion here that evaluative claims ought to be avoided (itself an evaluative claim!) but only that it is important to recognize when we, or others, make such claims. This sort of conceptual clarity is vital if we are to know what is at issue and to assess appropriately the issue at hand.

Let us pursue this matter of conceptual clarity a bit further. There are various ways in which we can be conceptually confused or in which an issue deserves to be described as a conceptually problematic one. We already have observed the occasional failure to distinguish empirical from evaluative claims or, similarly, to infer invalidly moral conclusions from purely empirical premises. Many philosophers (myself included) regard one frequently espoused view about the abortion dispute as a prime example of conceptual confusion. I have in mind the tendency to believe that the central issue in that dispute is whether terminating a fetus or embryo constitutes the taking of a life. More popularly, the question is expressed as "When does life begin?" This question then is assumed to be a purely empirical (or medical) issue, and empirical experts (e.g., neonatologists, embryologists) are called in to answer it. What should be clearer is that the fetuses, embryos, or zygotes being considered evidently are alive in one perfectly straightforward sense—namely, they exhibit continued cell functioning. Without question they are all living biological organisms. From conception forward there is a life; hence, there is no puzzle whatsoever about whether a life has begun.

We come closer to one important source of the dispute when we more carefully pose the question of whether, say, at conception a human life has begun or, even more clearly, whether the zygote is a human being. But determining whether the zygote or embryo generated by members of Homo Sapiens *is a human being* is not at all like determining whether, for example, the small biological organism on my deck is a human being. Finding out that the latter organism is or is not a human being may require only a simple empirical investigation. We look and discover that it is a squirrel. Remedying our initial ignorance about the empirical properties of the organism is all that needs to be done—given our knowledge of the criteria for the correct application of the term 'squirrel'—in order to properly classify the organism. The contrast between this case and the dispute over whether the zygote is a human being is striking. This is the case because empirical experts and others who agree as to what empirical traits are possessed by the zygote or fetus may disagree about whether it is a human being. All of this suggests that this dispute does not have its source in (or only in) contrary *empirical* beliefs (as might well be the case if you claim that Washington, D.C., is west of New York City and I claim that it is east). The dispute about the zygote is, rather, a *conceptual* one—namely, does this entity (about whose empirical features we may fully agree) count as a human being or not. To resolve that issue, if we can, requires not new facts about fetuses or zygotes but rather clarity about the criteria for correctly calling an entity a human being. We need, in some sense, to be clear about the boundaries of the concept. Since the term *human being* is not a technical term (such as *meter, Goldbach's Theorem, Godel's proof, regression analysis, Heimlich maneuver, algorithm, Hollandaise sauce,* or *starboard tack*), there is little reason to assume that those empirically knowledgable about fetal development have any claim to unique conceptual expertise in deciding the conceptual question. For this reason testimony by empirical experts, though relevant for many purposes, is not decisive with regard to the conceptual issue. For example, suppose someone were to argue that:

1. A human fetus counts as a human being if it exhibits brain functioning.
2. Fetus X exhibits brain functioning.
3. Fetus X is a human being.

To apply our earlier point, an embryologist may be expert with regard to deciding the truth of the second statement, but not the first. Two points are worth emphasizing here. First, deciding empirical questions may be crucial to deciding the acceptability of certain claims, such as number 3. But second, this fact should not seduce us into thinking that the above argument is a purely scientific or a purely medical matter.

Whether the conceptual question can be resolved and, if so, precisely how are further matters. One popular view is "You pay your money and take your choice." That is, conceptual disputes are not rationally soluble. But such a view is not obviously true. To the contrary, we commonly suppose that conceptual mistakes can be made; correlatively, one can be conceptually correct. I am mistaken if I think that four is (counts as) a prime number, and I am correct if I think that malarial plasmodium is (counts as) a microscopic organism. Whether a given conceptual qustion is rationally resolvable must be regarded as an open question before the relevant arguments are examined.

As we shall see, many disputes in health care ethics seem to derive from lack of conceptual clarity or downright conceptual disagreement. Consider these issues. Is alcoholism an illness or a disease? What counts as mental illness? Are judgments of illness evaluative? Is PMS (premenstrual syndrome) an illness? Is homosexuality? Is promoting human health logically equivalent to promoting human well-being?[4] If so, and if medicine's aim is to promote health, may not publicly provided sources of sexual satisfaction be a proper aim of medicine? If not, why not? Is death an evil? Are late-stage fetuses persons? Are irreversibly comatose human beings persons? If placebo use has an acceptable role in medicine, is not faith healing a placebo as well? What sickness or disability is self-induced? What counts as informed consent? The contention that surrounds most or all of these questions is not resolvable simply by getting the facts straight. Typically such disputes involve conceptual and/or evaluative disagreements of a more or less recalcitrant sort—a prime reason why they are often regarded as philosophical. Labels aside, how we decide such matters directly affects important practical policy questions, such as who does or who does not receive health care, who lives and who dies, and who should decide such important issues.

Tools for Unraveling and Assessing Arguments

Some claims are obviously true, some obviously false, and comparatively noncontroversial. Those that are of interest usually lack these traits. As such they tend to be controversial and, thus, demand support or defense. This point is, of course, a general one and does not uniquely apply to philosophical, empirical, or evaluative claims. When we give reasons in support of claims, we set forth, perspicuously or not, arguments. Hence, the assessment of controversial claims (beliefs, proposals) requires assessing arguments. Achieving a reasoned and critically held view about the issues central to biomedical ethics, then, calls for the analysis of arguments. The distinctions in the previous section are one dimension of pursuing this goal; after all, we must be clear about what is being claimed, what type of claim we are confronting (or proposing), and what sorts of considerations are relevant to its reasoned assessment. There are further considerations, distinctions, and strategies for assessing arguments that are important for a critical exploration of the issues later discussed. Here we shall set forth some of the basic tools for assessing arguments.

As philosophers, logicians, and mathematicians use the term *argument*, it does not refer to a family feud. Rather, it denotes a *set of statements* in which one statement is put forward as (or may be construed to be) the main contention whose truth or reasonableness is in question, and in which the remaining claims purportedly provide support for (or a good reason for concluding) the truth or reasonableness of the main contention. The main contention is labeled the *conclusion* and the supporting statements *premises.* An argument can have one premise or many. The point of giving an argument is to establish the truth of some nonobvious claim (nonobvious to others or oneself). If the claim were obvious (e.g., there are trees, most people have a nose), there would be little point in appealing to other claims for support. Typically we resort to setting forth arguments only when a claim is controversial to some degree. Hence, we in effect say, "You should accept our claim because you accept these premises."

Of course, if the premises are even more controversial than the claim, we may not get anywhere since new, equally problematic, questions may arise. Providing arguments, then, is a mode of conflict resolution. The conflict, it should not be forgotten, need not be interpersonal; it may be intrapersonal. I may be undecided about whether some claim is belief-worthy, such as "Nuclear war is unlikely," "The butler did it," "Philosophers are intellectually hostile," or "Surgeons tend to be macho types." Not all consideration of argument is oriented toward persuading others; we may simply aim to find the truth for ourselves.

Basically, an explicit argument can have three sorts of defects. Shortly, we shall identify these, but first it deserves mention that we shall be hard put to search for these defects, or contrasting virtues, in an argument unless we have clearly identified precisely what the argument is (again, either one with which we are confronted or one we are formulating ourselves). Much writing, both academic and popular, suffers from inexplicit and imprecise argument.[5] For example, speeches and editorials often involve *enthymematic* argument in which a premise (essential to the plausibility of the argument) or the conclusion is omitted and is, perhaps, only implied. Consider the following:

1. Fetuses are not persons.
2. Abortion is permissible.

This argument may presuppose that aborting nonpersons is permissible (or some analogous premise, such as only persons have a right to life), at least if the conclusion is to follow from the premises. We will examine the notion of "following from" shortly. If the argument does rely on a missing premise, the assessor of it can only conjecture about just what is missing. Still, we may be able to patch up or complete the argument; at least we ought to consider the most plausible possibilities, a step that goes beyond the rather unedifying complaint that the argument is incompletely stated or that the conclusion does not follow. Another barrier to identifying the argument (an essential precondition of assessing it) is the fact that the constituents of an argument often are scattered amidst an array of other remarks, comments often added to illustrate, elaborate, arouse, or perhaps even deflect attention from dubious assumptions. Sometimes arguments must be extracted from a bed of surrounding, less essential, material. The main point here is simply that to critically analyze an argument we must first identify it, and this may be no easy task.

FEATURES OF ARGUMENTS

Aside from turgid prose or questionable grammar, there are three sorts of features an argument may have in virtue of which it can fail to achieve its primary purpose—namely, establishing the truth or reasonableness of the conclusion. Two concern, the relation between the premises of the argument and the conclusion. The other concerns the truth-value (truth or falsity) of the premises separately considered. What we will see is, in part, intuitively familiar, but it is useful to have a common terminology in order to designate consciously and precisely the particular successes or failures of an argument. Some arguments have the property that if their premises are true, the conclusion must be true. Philosophers label all and only such arguments *valid arguments*. In such arguments it is not logically possible for the premises to be true and the conclusion to be false. Consider these arguments:

A. 1. Whoever wrote *Tinker, Tailor, Solier, Spy* is a clever person.
    2. John le Carré wrote *Tinker, Tailor, Soldier, Spy.*
so 3. John le Carré is a clever person.

B. 1. Whoever discovered the structure of DNA was a clever person.
    2. Alfred Einstein did not discover the structure of DNA.
so 3. Alfred Einstein was not a clever person.

Whatever one might wish to say about the truth or falsity of the six sentences in those two arguments, we note that A and B differ in the following respect. In A if the premises are true, the conclusion must also be true, and B lacks that property. We may agree that argument B has true premises and a false conclusion, but this just happens to be the case; invalid arguments are not by definition like that. Consider this argument:

C. 1. If Johns Hopkins University is in Baltimore, then it is in Maryland.
    2. Johns Hopkins University is in Maryland.
so 3. Johns Hopkins University is in Baltimore.

Argument C contains only true statements; still, it is invalid because statement 3 does not logically follow from 1 and 2. Alternatively, we may say that the joint truth of 1 and 2 does not guarantee the truth of 3; it is logically possible for 1 and 2 to be true and 3 to be false. The argument is invalid, and we define an *invalid argument* as any argument that is not valid. In that respect, contrast A. Succinctly put, a valid argument can have any combination of true and false statements except one: all true premises and a false conclusion. The exclusion of this possibility is precisely what makes valid arguments desirable ones for in such arguments we will never start out well (with all true premises) and end up badly (with a false conclusion). Hence, valid arguments provide us with a certain assurance that invalid arguments do not provide. However, this assurance is a limited one. We may start off badly (e.g., with one or more false premises), and, if so, the validity of the argument (if it is valid) will not guarantee that the conclusion is true. Indeed, a valid argument need not have, but can have, all false statements, such as the following:

D. 1. Two is greater than four.
    2. Four is greater than six.
so 3. Two is greater than six.

Although we cannot sufficiently elaborate here on this pregnant point, the logical structure of some arguments guarantees their validity; that is, it is impossible to have *both* all true premises and a false conclusion. But any other combination of truth-values is possible in a valid argument. If our argument is valid, it cannot begin with true premises and end with a false conclusion, but validity is also compatible with starting badly and winding up badly.[6]

If along with validity an argument has one further trait—that of having all true premises—we approach the best form of argument. If an argument has all true premises *and* is valid (recall our definition), it must have a true conclusion. All and only arguments with *both* of those traits are labeled *sound arguments.* If we can identify or formulate a sound argument for a claim, we have established its truth beyond rational dispute. An *unsound argument* is defined as an argument that is not sound. Note that an argument can be unsound because it has one or more false premises, it is invalid, or both. The following is an evidently sound argument:

E. 1. Six is greater than four.
    2. Four is greater than two.
so 3. Six is greater than two.

More typically, even if the validity of an argument is beyond dispute, there may be disagreement about the acceptability of one or more of the premises. In that respect, consider the following:

F. 1. In most cases of voluntary active euthanasia, an innocent person is killed.
    2. It is always wrong to kill an innocent person.
so 3. Most cases of voluntary euthanasia are wrong.

The argument is valid, but is it sound? Perhaps 2 is true, but it is not uncontroversial. A defender of this argument would need to defend 2 against all objections or set forth another argument, desirably a sound one, in which 2 were the conclusion. If the latter can be done, 2 would have to be true. Controversy over the further argument can arise as well, and the reader may sense the possibility of more and more defenses and further questions. That is a possibility, but there is no reason to assume at the outset that some compelling, dispute-resolving, argument will not be found—or even that the initial argument will fail to be of that sort.

A critic of statement 2 might well seek a *counterexample* to it. To illustrate the notion of a counterexample, let us consider another hypothetical claim. Universal generalizations, statements of the form "All S are P" (where S and P stand for terms denoting sets of objects), exhibit an interesting epistemological asymmetry. This last remark calls for some explication. Suppose a premise in an argument is that all gorillas are vegetarians. The burden on the defender of this strong claim (note what it precludes if true) is heavy in terms of giving reasons or evidence for accepting it. In contrast the skeptic need only show that there is or was at least one nonvegetarian gorilla. The latter would be a decisive counterexample to the universal generalization. More medically oriented examples of universal generalizations are that all extended periods of dying exhibit a stage of denial and anger, or that all surgery is risky. To return to the argu-

ment about euthanasia (F), a critic might focus on seemingly justified acts of killing in self-defense in which an innocent party is
killed.[7] This may not be a decisive counterexample, but it generates
some reasonable doubt about statement 2, independent of what one
thinks about statement 3.

At this point, we must not lose sight of the forest for looking at
the trees. We have noted two major defects an argument can have: it
may be invalid (and thus fail to ensure that if we start with true
statements we will "move" to a true conclusion), and it may have
one or more false premises (if so, we cannot be sure that the conclusion is true even if the argument is valid). A sound argument, by definition, avoids both of these pitfalls. Still, both sound and unsound
arguments can have a third defect. They can *beg the question* by assuming as a premise (tacitly or explicitly) what is concluded; if so,
the argument will fail to provide independent reasons for accepting
the conclusion. Consider the following:

G. 1. All serious defenses of non-Freudian theories are marred
        by clear indications of Oedipal fixations.
so 2. No such critiques of Freudian theory deserve serious
        consideration.
H. 1. It is wrong to engage in prostitution.
since 2. It is self-demeaning to function as a prostitute,
        and self-demeaning by virture of the fact that
        prostitution is an immoral activity.

Even if an argument is sound, such as H, it may fail to do what we
expect of arguments. Anyone who had doubts about the conclusion
would (or ought to) have similar doubts about the premise. Thus, it
fails to provide independent support for the conclusion. Even sound
arguments, then, can be defective. Our limited methodological ex-
cursion allows us to conclude, at this point, that the best form of argument is a sound argument that avoids begging the question.[8]

Our discussion thus far also allows us to recognize the ambiguity and considerable imprecision that typically are involved when
we speak simply of "good" and "bad" arguments. One might be
tempted to assume that a reasonable person would rely only on a
certain type of sound argument. If so, any invalid (and, hence, unsound) argument (even one with all true premises) should be ignored
or avoided. However, this would be a mistake. If we reflect on our
reasons for a wide variety of acts and decisions, it is clear that many
seem perfectly reasonable, yet when expressly cast in the form of an
argument are not valid. The point, vaguely put, is that not all invalid

arguments are bad or, at least, are ones to be dismissed by reasonable persons. Let us see why. Consider this example:

I.   1. On all previous occasions when I have turned on the ignition in a car, it has not exploded.

so   2. The next time I turn on the ignition in a car it will not explode.

Assume 1 is true; even so, the argument is invalid. Even if 1 is true, the next time may result in an explosion (i.e., 2 may be false). Why should we believe 2? The answer, in brief, is that the truth of 1 provides a rather compelling reason to accept 2 even if the argument is not a sound one. Some invalid arguments have the following trait: the truth of the premises renders highly probable the truth of the conclusion (even though it is logically possible that: the premises are true and the conclusion false). Although the term is not completely standardized, such arguments normally are labeled *strong arguments* (notice that, like 'valid,' or 'sound,' 'strong,' is assigned a technical sense here). The distinction between valid and invalid arguments focuses on what is logically possible. The distinction among invalid arguments between those that are strong and those that are not (*weak arguments*) requires making probability judgments. Thus, a weak argument is by definition any argument that is invalid *and* is one in which the truth of the premises does not render highly probable the truth of the conclusion. The following is a weak argument:

J.   1. Last week when I dreamt that lightning would strike in my yard, it did.

so   2. The next time that I dream that lightning will strike, it will.

Although I and J are rather clear examples of strong and weak arguments, determining whether an argument is strong or weak is complicated by the difficulty of making probability judgments. A more basic point here is that rationality is not incompatible with reliance on strong arguments and, hence, some invalid arguments. Since our definition of a strong argument leaves open the question of whether it has all true premises, a moment's reeflection makes it clear that strong arguments that are belief-worthy also have the feature that their premises are all true. Consider this argument:

K.   1. Ninety-eight percent of all diseases of type T can be cured with drug D.

       2. Maria has a disease of type T.

so   3. Maria's disease can be cured with drug D.

Although K is a strong argument, whether K reasonably supports 3 also depends on the truth of 1 and 2.

CONSISTENCY

Generally speaking, examining the logical form or structure of an argument will be a means only to determining what sort of relationship obtains between the premises and the argument's conclusion—the sort denoted by "valid," "invalid," "strong," or "weak." In short, classifying the sort of relation that obtains between premises and conclusion typically does not yield an answer to the further question of whether the premises are all true. As noted, what sort of inquiry is relevant to answering that question will depend on the type of claim we find in a particular premise—for example, empirical, evaluative, or, perhaps, a tautological one (such as all bachelors are male, prime numbers are evenly divisible only by themselves or one, or not everyone now is taller than the current average height). There is a special case, however, in which formal examination alone allows us to conclude that at least one premise is false, and that is the case in which the premises are logically inconsistent. A logically inconsistent set of statements is, by definition, a set of statements that cannot all be true. The set may be a set of premises, but it need not be. Here are three inconsistent sets:

Set 1   1. X is greater than Y.
        2. Y is greater than X.
Set 2   1. Nothing should impede the search for scientific
           knowledge.
        2. It is unqualifiedly wrong to test new skin care ointments
           on animals.
        3. Testing new skin care ointments on animals yields
           scientific knowledge.
Set 3   1. Homosexuality is solely a by-product of genetic factors.
        2. Homosexuality is solely a by-product of socialization.

Inspection reveals the inconsistency of each set. But note that to so conclude we need not know, for example, the truth-values of statements 1 and 2, separately considered, in set 1. Further, we might believe in set 3 that 1 and 2 are both false. An inconsistent set of statements can have any combination of true and false statements *except one*; by definition an inconsistent set is one in which it *cannot* be the case (not merely: *is* not the case) that all its members are true.

Nevertheless, note that a set with all false members, or a mixture of true and false statements, need not be inconsistent, but if a set is inconsistent it must have one of these combinations.

Why is inconsistency an interesting and important property? Perhaps the answer is obvious. First, if we can discern inconsistency in the premises of someone's argument (alas, it may be our own), we will know that at least one of the premises is false. If the argument is our own, we have started badly; indeed, our argument is unsound.[9] We can demonstrate the unsoundness of an argument if we can show that its premises are inconsistent. More generally, and aside from a focus on a specific argument, it would seem that a rational person would generally want to have all true beliefs; for all of them to be true, they at least must be consistent. Similarly, it is desirable that all the assumptions in a theory (empirical or ethical) be true. Therefore, achieving consistency seems to be a necessary condition of the adequacy of any theory. One reasonable standard for assessing any theory, then, is that at a bare minimum it be consistent. In reflecting on the ethical theories discussed later, it is worth considering whether they are consistent—as well as whether they possess other traits desirable in a theory (e.g., comprehensiveness, reasonable precision, intuitive plausibility, and, other things being equal, simplicity).

Dilemmas and Ethical Dilemmas

In discussions of biomedical ethics one often hears talk of "ethical dilemmas." Nevertheless, a certain gap exists between what logicians or philosophers often mean when they speak of "dilemmas" and what is referred to as an ethical dilemma. A brief comment may be useful if only to demystify somewhat the notion of an ethical dilemma. One loose and popular meaning of 'dilemma' denotes a difficult choice between two or more alternatives. Such a choice may be a purely prudential matter, such as deciding whether to purchase a house or to rent. In contrast, the term 'ethical dilemma' often denotes a situation in which all the alternatives seem morally problematic (e.g., each may seem to involve a *presumptively wrong* act). A physician, for example, may be hard put to decide between revealing a disturbing diagnosis to a patient whose health is precarious (and who may be prone to react in a bizarre or self-destructive manner) and withholding the diagnosis. Here the situation may be viewed as morally troublesome since revealing the diagnosis may violate the Hippocratic dictum to do no harm, and keeping silent may violate the principle "respect the autonomy of the patient," or "tell the truth." Deciding what to do depends, at least in part, on ascertaining whether the principles mentioned are merely presumptive, whether one should take precedence over the other, or, more generally, which (if either) is well supported by the most reasonable ethical theory one can identify.

Most, if not all, of the morally "hard cases" in health care ethics have the sort of dilemmatic feature characterized. For this reason they are intellectually challenging and force us to assess or reassess the defensibility of moral principles widely accepted in other contexts, or traditionally thought acceptable in health care.

There are similarities between the situations that involve a moral dilemma and what elsewhere (e.g., in logic) is called a dilemma. In the latter context, 'dilemma' refers to a range of arguments of a certain form, typically ones that involve two conditional premises (of the form: if p, then q) and a disjunctive premise (of the form p or s). An example will be given shortly. A further feature typically is that the proponent of the argument arrives at a conclusion (sometimes a disjunctive one) that is unpalatable for some actual or hypothetical opponent. Compare these dilemmas:

L.   1. If the United States continues to build its nuclear arsenal, nuclear war will become more probable.
2. If the United States does not continue to build its nuclear arsenal, it will become defenseless among the superpowers.
3. Either the United States will continue to build its nuclear arsenal or it does not.

so 4. Either nuclear war will become more probable or the United States will become defenseless among the superpowers.

M. 1. If you marry Tex, you will be economically wealthy but emotionally poor.
2. If you marry Rex, you will be economically poor but emotionally wealthy.
3. Either you marry Tex or you marry Rex.

so 4. You will either be economically wealthy but emotionally poor, or you will be economically poor but emotionally wealthy.

Arguments L and M are both valid; so one strategy for avoiding acceptance of the conclusion is not viable (i.e., accepting the premises but denying that the conclusion logically follows). Two other strategies, abstractly speaking, are possible in criticizing a dilemma: (1)

denying one of the "horns" of the dilemma (i.e., one of the conditional premises) or (2) slipping between the horns, i.e., denying the disjunction (e.g., rejecting the third premise in argument M).[10] Some defenders of an increase in nuclear weaponry take the former tack by arguing that statement 1 of argument L is implausible. That issue, of course, leads to the introduction of further arguments requiring assessment. Notice that we cannot slip between the horns in L, because the two alternatives (continuing to build nuclear weapons or not) are *jointly exhaustive*; there is no third alternative. Such a tactic is possible (whether or not plausible) with regard to M.

Various moral dilemmas, with some effort, often can be cast in the form of an explicit dilemmatic argument, such as:

N. 1. If scientists do not perform painful or lethal experiments on primates, we will fail to meet our obligations to relieve pervasive human misery.
    2. If scientists do perform painful and lethal experiments on primates, they will cause unjustified suffering on the part of innocent, sentient, creatures.[11]
    3. Either scientists perform such experiments or they do not.
so 4. Either we will fail to meet our obligations to relieve pervasive human misery, or scientists will cause unjustified suffering on the part of innocent, sentient, creatures.

One approach to this dilemma is set out in a later essay by Tom Regan (see chapter VI). A more general point worth stressing here is that it is often useful to reformulate certain moral dilemmas (often alluded to in a vague manner) in the form of an explicit argument. Doing so may make clearer the difficulty of choosing between alternatives, the principles at stake, and (given our earlier remarks) some notion of the logically possible strategies one can pursue in trying to make some analytic advance toward resolving a problem. Genuine dilemmas do involve difficult questions; nonetheless, there is no reason to assume at the outset of inquiry that such questions are ultimately inscrutable or impervious to rational resolution.

Ethical Theorizing

Regarding ethical questions and claims, it is useful to recognize a rough distinction that can be made among different levels of generality an ethical claim may exhibit. Some claims are highly individuated or particular, such as:

Roland's lying on his application to Harvard Medical School was unfair.

Other moral claims make a judgment about a range of cases, such as:

Sterilizing poor women with four or more children and who have not consented to such a procedure is not permissible.

Some are even more general:

It is always wrong to kill an innocent person.

Some mention no particular type of act (such as killing, lying, or torturing) and are highly generic:

Never treat a person as a mere means.

We should do whatever brings about the greatest balance of happiness over pain.

Do no harm.

Evaluative claims about types of acts are understandably labeled ethical or moral principles. Often it is clear that comparatively specific moral claims are defended by appeal to more general principles; the defense may be cast in the form of an explicit argument, such as:

O.   3. It is justifiable to quarantine persons with serious, contagious, diseases.
since 1. Such persons constitute an unprovoked, serious threat to others.
and   2. It is right coercively to intervene to protect innocent parties from an unprovoked, serious threat posed by others.

Here the comparatively specific normative judgment (3) is defended, in part, by an appeal to (2), a moral principle of some generality. In short, moral principles often enter as premises in arguments purporting to justify specific moral claims. Whether the defense succeeds depends in part on whether the argument is valid. Hence, our tools for assessing arguments are directly relevant to assessing the adequacy of moral judgments or particular defenses of such judgments.[12]

A further point about the notion of a moral principle deserves our attention. Specifically, the term 'moral' is ambiguous. Sometimes the term 'moral' itself has a positive evaluative meaning, as in "Joe is a moral person." Here 'moral' is contrary to 'immoral,' and 'moral' here may be used to mean something like 'praiseworthy.' If that were the case in "moral principle," the suggestion would be that a principle could be, or is, praiseworthy, but that is bizarre since principles are not fit subjects of (moral) praise any more than rocks. Rather, the word *moral* in "moral principle" merely describes or categorizes the principle as being of a certain type. A related point arises here. We hear references to moral principles (or questions) and economic, medical, religious, or political principles (or questions). Are these mutually exclusive categories? Is it conceptually coherent to think that there are, distinctly, a medical point of view, a moral point of view, and a political point of view? Is "We should have a policy promoting limited experimentation on human fetuses" a *medical* or a *moral* claim? This last question deserves further reflection, and one might reflect on the interpretation we have assigned to "moral claim" and the role of empirical claims as premises in arguments defending specific moral judgments.

Let us return more directly to our concern with what is involved in theoretical ethics. It is one thing, of course, simply to make or state moral judgments. It is another to seek to defend them rationally. As noted, a defense will, or can, take the form of an argument. If so, particular moral judgments may be defended by invoking more general moral claims about types of acts; these claims are usually labeled moral principles. If the particular judgment validly follows from the premises, one source of failure in the purported justification is avoided. As noted earlier, however, the principle invoked (or other premises) may not be beyond dispute. Consider this argument:

P.   3. Amos's killing his seventy-five-year-old terminally ill,
            intensely suffering brother with a rifle was right.
since   1. It is right to minimize human suffering.
and   2. Amos's brother's suffering was minimized by Amos's
            killing him with a rifle.

The conclusion 3 is not uncontroversial, but the argument is an alleged justification of it. Although 1 seems benign and well intended, is it a principle by which we should live? Is it a basic or derivative principle in any rationally acceptable ethical theory? If we want to have a defensible theory, we cannot avoid critical reflection on this matter. We may be hard put to think of an objection to 1, but that may be true simply because we are not very good at the task or we are too lazy. In any case, consider this argument:

Q.   1. It is right to minimize human suffering.
     2. Creating and detonating a bomb that would kill instantly
        and painlessly and was of sufficient effectiveness to de-
        stroy all human life would minimize human suffering
        (there *never* would be any more suffering).
so   3. It is right to create and detonate such a bomb.

Argument Q is instructive. First, it is valid, but few would find the
conclusion plausible. But if the conclusion is false, one of the premises *must* be false (recall that in a valid argument, it is *impossible* to
have *both* all true premises *and* a false conclusion). In short, it is
tempting to regard Q as unsound, and unsound because 1 is false.
But if so, we must regard P as unsound since 1 appears in it as a
premise as well (statement 2). If so, P fails as a successful justification of its conclusion. Our discussion of P and Q, then, illustrates
one facet of critical ethical theorizing. Such investigation is often
subtle and difficult; still, if we are to identify principles that deserve
our reliance in public and private conduct, we must ferret out those
that can withstand rational scrutiny. If we do not, we shall not only
be naive; we shall also, in all likelihood, do or support (even if inadvertently) what is unjust. If we can be sure of what is just or right,
we may lack the will to do it. Conversely, we may have the will, but
that by itself will not resolve our ethical perplexities. Settling them,
or at least helping us avoid rationally defective views, is one aim of
ethical theory.

Before we turn to an overview of the leading ethical approaches,
we shall briefly survey various generally accepted criteria for assessing the adequacy of a proposed ethical theory. By now many of
these criteria will seem familiar. At certain points the criteria are
identical with, or similar to, criteria standardly presupposed as a basis for adjudicating among competing scientific theories.

As noted earlier, *consistency* is desirable in any set of assumptions. However we are to define 'theory,' a theory is at least a set of
assumptions. If a set of theoretical assumptions is inconsistent, at
least one is false. Further, any claim whatsoever will validly follow
from it. Inconsistency in a theory is seldom blatant, and a certain
amount of detective work may be required to discern it or demonstrate it.

It is also desirable that a theory be *comprehensive*. One might try
to formulate an ethical theory concerning when, if at all, it is permissible to kill human beings who are capable of rational choice. As
plausible as such a theory might be, it would fail to address other

perplexities about killing. Examples concern the killing of fetuses, animals, or comatose human beings, as well as the destruction of other forms of life. Hence, the theory's scope would be limited. To the extent that the scope of a theory is limited, it will fail to yield guidance on questions it does not address, and questions will arise about whether the limited theory "fits in" with a more comprehensive theory (and, if so, how). Theory building, of course, often proceeds successfully through the formulation of limited theories and the gradual construction of more broad-ranging ones. Given the obstacles to constructing broad-ranging theories in, say, ethics, physics, or biology, the wiser course often is to start small.

A somewhat more controversial criterion is that a theory be compatible with certain seemingly self-evident convictions of virtually all competent persons. In the sciences, for example, if a new theory implied that no human being could live to be more than 100 years old, that would count against the theory—given the well-documented evidence to the contrary. As a counterpart in ethics, recall argument Q. The claim that it is right to create and detonate the aforementioned bomb seems so evidently unjustified that we would regard such an implication as decisive against any set of assumptions that entails it. Some utilitarians (and others), however, look with suspicion or disdain on "appeals to moral intuitions."[13] One not unreasonable point they stress is that our moral intuitions (or, possibly, "pretheoretical convictions") may be mere prejudices (many people have, at one time or another, thought it obvious that women should be treated as inferior, that Jews are vermin, that those who curse God should be drawn and quartered, or that slavery is right and in the natural order of things). No interesting theory could be compatible with all moral intuitions; still, it does not follow that there are no lower level, limited-scope convictions with which an ethical theory must be compatible. Possible examples are that we must respect individual moral agents, that suffering in itself is bad, that in the absence of a relevant difference individuals ought not be treated unequally, or that if an act causes the death of a rational agent that is a morally relevant aspect of an action.

Bertrand Russell once said that common sense leads to physics but physics leads to the denial of common sense. A provocative point, but not one that is obviously true unless further qualified (physics is incompatible only with some commonsense convictions). It is not clear that there would be any reasonable basis for adequately discriminating among, say, consistent, equally comprehensive theories (in physics or elsewhere) unless we insist that theories match up with certain fundamental pretheoretical convictions that withstand elementary scrutiny. In this regard it is worth observing (to anticipate our discussion of utilitarianism) that utilitarians often defend their theory not by eschewing all moral intuitions but by denying that their theory is counterintuitive in the ways in which some critics maintain. To do that, however, is to take moral intuitions with some seriousness. Those who regard compatibility with deep moral intuitions as a necessary condition for a satisfactory ethical theory need not, we also observe, presuppose that human beings have some moral "sixth sense," special faculty, or conscience that renders its possessors infallible in their moral judgment.

Other features thought desirable in an ethical theory are that it be reasonably *precise* and that it be *empirically realistic.* Some principles do not seem readily to yield moral implications that are sufficiently clear to guide us. For example, it is not obvious what would be involved in adhering to the Kantian dictum "Never treat a person as a mere means," or other principles such as "Love God and do as you please," or "Do not do unto others what you would not have them do unto you." Is lying to a patient for his own good treating him as a mere means? Does doing so violate the canon of the Golden Rule? Or "do no harm"?

Why must an evaluative theory be empirically realistic? The answer lies in the fact that any full-blown ethic will involve empirical presuppositions—about what sorts of things exist, what sorts of beings are capable of voluntary choice, what is beyond the capacity of moral agents, and so on. Such presuppositions are often referred to by such august labels as a "theory of man" or a "theory of human nature." It seems evident that any ethic that presupposed, in a fundamental way, a false picture of human life or the world in general would be defective. For example, if some human beings suffer from irresistible compulsions, any theory about personal responsibility that ignored such a fact would be less plausible. Similarly, any ethical theory that presupposed the existence of God (e.g., the Divine Command Theory, which equates what is right with what God commands) must be judged defective if the assumption of God's existence is false.

Briefly, we have outlined the main, generally agreed upon, standards for assessing competing ethical viewpoints. The reader may wish to consider whether they seem to be appropriate criteria. If they are, they are worth bearing in mind as we consider the leading ethical theories, and, later, the applications of such theories to bio-medical disputes—or, indeed, attacks upon the employment of such theories or related principles.

Ethical Theories

UNDERSTANDING UTILITARIANISM

Historically, the most well-known advocates of the utilitarian theory were the late eighteenth- and early nineteenth-century British philosophers Jeremy Bentham and John Stuart Mill. This theory, or various contemporary variants, has exercised considerable influence over the decades. The theory purports to answer the question "What ought we to do?" As noted earlier, utilitarianism in its classical version supposes that there is one type of state of affairs that is intrinsically good; this nonmoral good is pleasure or satisfaction ('satisfaction' is perhaps the preferable term since Bentham and especially Mill were referring to a kind of contentment, broadly understood, and not merely pleasurable sensations). If this hedonistic assumption (recall our earlier definition of hedonism) of the good is reasonable, and we focus on the question of what acts we should do, it is tempting to think that we ought to promote as much good as possible. If we use 'utility' to stand for this good, we obtain a familiar statement of the utilitarian principle: we should maximize utility. Two qualifications, however, are usually made. First, many acts that produce utility also promote disutility (dissatisfaction, or what is intrinsically bad). Suppose we could measure utility and disutility in cardinal units; the utility of an act, then, would involve a certain number of hedons (units of pleasure) and any disutility a certain number of dolours (units of pain or dissatisfaction). Hence, a given act of surgery might involve 1,000 hedons and 300 dolours, yielding a net balance of 700 hedons. The utilitarian view is better stated as: *maximize net utility* (often the formulation is to maximize the greatest balance of pleasure over pain). We cannot always produce unadulterated utility. There may be circumstances in which a moral agent can perform more than one act that will result in, say, 1,000 hedons on balance. Suppose this is true of both act X and act Y; no other act is possible for the agent that will produce as much net utility. If so, the principle of maximizing net utility will not guide the agent as to whether to do X or Y. The utilitarian response here is that either act is satisfactory, and the central principle is modified to mean: *we ought to perform an act that will produce at least as much net utility as would any other act.* This is what is meant by the principle of utility, or PU.[14] PU is understood not merely as a criterion of what it is *permissible* to do, but as a criterion of what is *obligatory,* or a matter of duty, for all moral agents.

PU is frequently misinterpreted to mean that we should do whatever pleases the majority (a tempting reading of the classic formulation of "promote the greatest happiness for the greatest number"). Suppose we consider distributing a limited drug supply, in equal amounts, among persons A, B, C, and D, and that doing so would benefit A, B, C, but not D (she needs all of the drug to receive any benefit ('benefit' gets cashed in terms of utility, of course). Further, no other utilities or disutilities will result from distributing the drug evenly. Such an act would benefit the majority. We might think that this is unfair to D, and in general we might believe that it is not right always to do what benefits or pleases the majority (Mill himself denounced a tyranny of the majority and, relatedly, opposed racism and sexism). This reasonable objection, however, misses the mark if aimed at PU. If the utility of giving all the drug to D outweighs the sum of the disutilities of withholding the drug to A, B, and C (and no other utilities or disutilities are involved), PU requires giving it all to D since that is what woud maximize total net utility. In short, PU requires maximizing net aggregate utility (the sum of the individual utilities or disutilities) by our actions; doing so may or may not result in a net utility for the majority.

An understanding of the utilitarian approach calls for reflection on further dimensions of the theory. First, note that the utilitarian view makes an assumption about whose well-being is morally relevant—that is what counts in deciding what we ought to do. Typically, the supposition is any being capable of experiencing pleasure or pain (i.e., any sentient creature). Although the familiar focus of ethical theory is on people, Mill and Bentham thought many animals were sentient. Hence, such beings, in contemporary terms, have *moral standing* or are members in the *moral community.* Which beings have moral standing is a question that has historically been ignored but in recent years has received closer attention due to its relevance to our dealings with (a) human fetuses, (b) sentient animals, and (c) comatose humans. One could consistently accept the sentience criterion without being swayed by utilitarianism. The issue of moral standing is evidently central to many questions of biomedical ethics.

Second, note the fundamental point that utilitarianism is forward-looking and a purely *consequentialist theory.* What makes an act right is that it promotes a certain type of consequence; in deciding what is right we must focus on the consequences of our acts. Whether, for example, we should keep a promise (a past act) is not settled solely by the fact that we made a sincere promise. We must consider whether keeping that promise will, at least as much as any alternative act, maximize net utility. It may be obvious that this focus on consequences (some critics pejoratively characterize it as "mere expediency") is one source of contention.

The contention is related to a third feature worth comment. As noted, utilitarianism seems commonsensical in one respect: we should maximize the amount of net good in the world. What seems more natural or a loftier goal? Still, utilitarianism implies (at least the version we are considering) that traditional moral rules are not fundamental and are, at best, rules of thumb. Let us see why. There may be occasions in which we could maximize net utility by lying, breaking promises, stealing, killing innocent nonconsenting persons, or even torturing. If so, on PU, such acts are not merely permissible, they are obligatory. If a conflict exists between PU and traditional moral rules, then the utilitarian view would cast off the traditional rules. In this way utilitarianism is a somewhat anticommonsensical position, perhaps even a radical one. Whether this result is undesirable we leave open; after all, perhaps traditional morality (vaguely characterized here) rationally cannot stand up to scrutiny or stand up as well as utilitarianism.

A fourth feature concerns the importance of empirical questions to determining what is right. If the latter is a function of the consequences of our actions, we must determine what those consequences are; we must be able to predict if we are to apply PU rationally. In other words we cannot know a priori, or prior to answering empirical questions, whether a certain act will be (or even is, or was) right. We cannot reasonably say, unqualifiedly, that "all acts of type T are wrong."[15] To do so, we must reasonably believe that doing an act of that type in fact will fail to yield maximum utility. Thus, traditional rules are at best rules of thumb for those who cannot calculate utilities well or who lack relevant information. However, a utilitarian may take the view that children should be taught traditional rules since, although reliance on them will not always maximize utility, such reliance is more likely to have that result than the alternative.

A fifth feature of utilitarianism concerns its time frame. In the utilitarian view, we cannot justifiably consider the utilities only of members of the current generation. The long-term utility consequences of our acts are morally relevant, even if we are hard put to ascertain what they are. If generating nuclear wastes now, for example, will produce significant disutilities for yet unborn or unconceived generations, that is an important fact in assessing the morality of current policies of nuclear development. In this respect utilitarian theory diverges from certain ethical views that allow the existence of duties only with regard to existing human beings (perhaps on the view that duties between persons arises only as a result of bilateral agreements between such parties).

The nonethnocentric nature of utilitarian theory is manifested further by another feature of the theory—namely, a certain *egalitarian* dimension. A common criticism of utilitarianism is that it sanctions radically inegalitarian acts and policies, (i.e., ones generating an inequitable distribution of benefits or burdens). For example, it is claimed that what may maximize total net utility (considering the utilities and disutilities of all those affected by the act) is performing nontherapeutic medical experiments (to find a cure for, say, AIDS) on a small minority of persons who do not consent. But, critics assert, this would be an outrageous injustice. We leave open here the plausibility of this important objection. But why, then, suggest that utilitarianism has an egalitarian dimension? Utilitarians generally insist that *equal amounts of utility* (or disutility) *must be counted equally* when one is calculating the total utility of a policy—regardless of the identity of the possessors. That is, the fact that a subject of utility is black, white, male, female, Greek or Jew, Russian or American is not a reason in itself to weight heavily or discount the subject's utility (or disutility). At the stage of calculating utilities, then, the theory seems notably egalitarian and impartial. Whether the theory, in the end, sanctions intolerable inegalitarian treatment of persons is another issue.

ASSESSING UTILITARIANISM

A thorough assessment of utilitarianism is beyond our purview here. We will, however, succinctly review some of the attractions as well as objections to the theory. Among its desirable features are, apparently, its (1) recognition of the relevance of the consequences of actions, (2) its impartial egalitarian dimension, (3) its comprehensiveness, (4) its comparative simplicity (it has a single fundamental principle), (5) its consistency, and (6) its avoidance of rigid adherence to simple traditional rules when following them has counterintuitive results. For example, must we tell the truth to the Nazi who asks if any Jews are in our attic. Utilitarianism also seems to entail a seemingly reasonable form of moral relativism since, on this view, the rightness of *different performances* of a certain type of act will vary in moral value (right or wrong) depending on the consequences of their performance. It may be wrong to lie to your business partner (if doing so fails to maximize total utility) but right to lie to the Nazi in our example (if doing so would maximize utility).

We will note here only four types of criticism of the theory; they concern (1) the measurement of utility, (2) supererogatory acts, (3) counterintuitive implications, and (4) whether all utilities have moral weight. Critics claim that it is either conceptually incoherent to talk of measuring units of utility (e.g., hedons) or, if it is coherent, that it is practically impossible to do so. If either point is correct, it is impossible for nonomniscient moral agents to implement the theory. We leave the question open. A second objection is that the theory is too rigorous; it implies that we constantly must be calculating what will maximize utility, that there is no "time off" from engaging in beneficent (utility-promoting) works. The theory, critics say, leaves too little room for a range of activity in which certain choices are morally optional. Rather, it is claimed that the actual demands of morality are not so burdensome; we need not always be doing good even if it is true that we must avoid wronging others whatever we do. On this view many acts are morally optional. Some are supererogatory (i.e., permissible but beyond what duty requires). For example, if we donate a kidney to another, that may be praiseworthy, but if we do not, we may do no wrong, even if doing so would maximize net utility. Thus, what maximizes utility is not necessarily equivalent to acting rightly, and failing to maximize utility need not be acting wrongly.

Many critics of utilitarianism believe that the most serious objection to the theory is that it sanctions, as right, actions that are profoundly wrong. Often the wrong is construed to be one of injustice. Suppose a group of medical professionals could take a friendless, economically parasitic seventy-year-old man and, by transplanting various of his bodily parts (kidneys, liver, heart, skin), produce enormous benefits to others in dire need of such parts. Further, assume the person at the outset could be put asleep without generating any anxiety, anesthetized (to prevent pain), and that he would die soon in any event. If word of such an activity could be kept secret, it is plausible that the *sum* of the utilities produced for others would far outweigh any disutilities to the man. If so, the act would maximize aggregate net utility. Critics claim, however, that such an act would be a heinous injustice. The more general point is made that utilitarianism focuses only on the total quantity of aggregate utility producible by an act and ignores the question of how benefits (or burdens) are to be distributed (except insofar as how that, as a matter of contingent fact, will affect the quantity of net utility produced). Any adequate ethical theory, it is claimed, must involve principles of fair or just distribution of benefits and burdens—whether those be liberties, opportunities, wealth, income, or punishment. Such is an example of the general type of objection: that utilitarianism sanctions morally counterintuitive results.

It is worth noting briefly that utilitarians have open to them one of three logically possible responses to this type of objection. First, they can concede that the principle of utility fails as a criterion of right action. Second, they can deny that the apparent implication of utilitarianism is morally counterintuitive or allege that, if it is, that is too bad for our intuitions. Third, they can insist that utilities have been incorrectly calculated and that, for example, in a case such as the seventy-year-old man the procedure would not maximize net utility—since secrets leak out, fear is generated, guilt of the agents must be considered, the foregone utility of the seventy-year-old may have been weighted inadequately, and so on. Utilitarian responses typically take the second or third tack; the first, of course, is not a defense, but surrender.

We should add that many contemporary utilitarians have tried to develop variant versions of this theory and, thus, concede the inadequacy of the classical view. One type of maneuver is to defend a version of *rule-utilitarianism* (RU). Here it is claimed, roughly, that the obligatoriness of particular acts is to be decided by whether they accord with a certain set of ideal moral rules; in turn the ideal rules are to be identified by ascertaining which set of rules if generally followed (or if invariantly followed, or generally accepted) would result in maximizing net utility. With this view (there are variants), PU is directly invoked to justify not particular acts but rules, and the rules in turn are employed to determine the justification of particular acts; there is, then, a two-step procedure. It may be argued, then, that if a complex rule like "Do not painlessly dismember and terminate friendless persons over sixty-five who will die soon anyway even if doing so can generate substantial benefits for others" were accepted or followed, doing so would maximize utility. If so, RU would prohibit the gruesome procedure mentioned. Hence, RU may avoid seriously counterintuitive implications. We cannot here explore RU fully. We will note only that questions arise as to (1) whether RU, in any version, is actually equivalent to the classical view, (2) if it is not equivalent, whether it avoids counterintuitive results, and (3) whether notions such as "is generally accepted by society" can be coherently and plausibly analyzed. In passing, one might note regarding some rules that if they were followed, utility might be maximized, but it may be true that they are not and will not be followed; if so, following them in the real world may not maximize utility.[16]

A fourth objection to utilitarianism concerns the fact that it allows some utilities morally to count toward determining the rightness or wrongness of an act. For example, if a child molester derives considerable utility from his or her acts, that has positive weight in determining the morality of such acts. It, then, is conceivable that such an ill-gotten gain may tip the balance toward the act's maximizing aggregate utility. Such a view is troublesome, to say the least. Why should we think that such satisfactions count at all in determining the morality of the act? To make this point is to suggest that either pleasure is not necessarily an intrinsic good or that not all intrinsic goods have moral weight. If, however, that is true, it seems that classical utilitarianism is fundamentally misconceived.

KANT'S THEORY

Another historically influential ethical theory was developed by the eighteenth-century German (Prussian) philosopher, Immanuel Kant. His theory is an example of what are often called *deontological* or *nonconsequentialist* theories. 'Deontological' derives from the Greek 'deontos' (transliterated), meaning 'duty.' Saying that Kant's ethic is an "ethics of duty" seems to say little. Is not utilitarianism an ethic of duty as well? The term 'nonconsequentialist' is somewhat more descriptive. It refers to any ethical theory that implies or supposes that the rightness or wrongness of an act is not solely a function of its consequences satisfying certain conditions (sometimes, it is used to mean that it is *not at all* a function of those consequences). One basic assumption of this sort of approach is that there are moral constraints on what we may do quite apart from whether or not an act produces good consequences (somehow calculated). Part of the attraction of Kant's view and other nonconsequentialist theories (e.g., theories whose central explicit suppositions concern rights) is the set of difficulties confronting utili-tarianism and other consequentialist views (e.g., ethical egoism, an approach that we do not explore here).

Kant argued that moral agents have an unqualified duty to obey the Categorical Imperative. The Imperative is stated in several ways by Kant, formulations that are not obviously equivalent to one an-other. Here, we shall focus only on two formulations, which we shall label the Universalizability Principle (UP) and the Mere Means Principle (MP).[17] A statement of UP is:

> Act only on those maxims that you can consistently will to be a universal law (a rule actually guiding the decisions of all moral agents).

A statement of MP is:

> Never treat a person as a mere means.

According to Kant an act has *moral worth* only if the agent acts *for the sake of duty* but not if his or her act merely happens to be in ac-cord with the Categorical Imperative. However, our focus here only concerns whether the Imperative, considering its construal as either UP or MP, is an adequate criterion of right action—not with the praiseworthiness of the agent.

One of the attractions of UP is that it seems to embody a certain impartiality: we should treat others only according to principles (rules, prescriptions) by which we are willing to be treated. No spe-cial exemptions for ourselves are permissible. Thus, we might be tempted to lie to others when it is convenient to do so. But then, in Kant's view, we must ask, as rational agents, whether we are willing that all agents act according to the maxim "Lie when it is conve-nient to do so." According to Kant, following such a rule may not merely have bad consequences; no agent rationally could will that everyone follow such a maxim. We would not want others to act on such a principle, and, hence, cannot will that everyone do so. Thus, so willing would involve a kind of "contradiction of the will." That is something we can know, he alleged, independently of ascer-taining the actual consequences of following such a maxim. Kant reaches a similar conclusion about the maxim "Do not help those in distress unless it is convenient to do so." Thus, in Kant's view, UP provides a means of testing the adequacy of any moral maxim em-bodied in an actual or prospective act in which an agent might en-gage.

Consider MP. On the face of it, testing maxims by ascertaining whether they violate MP would yield the same results. To lie to others when we find it convenient seems to treat them as mere objects—purely as a means to our own ends. If it is convenient, one lets a tree grow in the yard; if not, one cuts it down. The desideratum is one's own purposes, not the well-being of the tree. Similarly, lying to, killing, stealing from, and breaking promises to others all seem to treat others as a mere means to our own ends and, hence, violates MP. It is usually noted that Kant's dictum does not prohibit using people as a means in one sense. For example, when we hire persons, or they consent to help us in a project, we do not treat them as mere means. In such cases we need not deny their independent worth as rational agents; we do not treat them as if they were not autonomous centers of choice and will. These points are of evident relevance in thinking about the later essays on informed consent and experimentation. Both UP and MP seem to place a moral constraint on what we may do to rational agents even if we could produce substantial utility by going ahead. Kant's theory, as well as various rights theories, seem to insist that for certain otherwise desirable goals (e.g., promoting aggregate happiness or welfare) we morally cannot get there from here. Such an idea is a fundamental one and one that exercises a continued, powerful, attraction to those who give hard thought to the ethical perplexities that confront us.

Again we can only identify briefly a few of the objections to and questions regarding Kant's view. Are UP and MP really equivalent to each other? How are we to identify "the maxim of our act"? After all, a given act may have multiple true descriptions (e.g., "having fun," "doing what is convenient," "torturing Grandma," "sawing off a body part," "entertaining others," or, maybe, "maximizing net utility"). Suppose I am not willing to universalize "Lie when it is convenient to do so" but I am willing to universalize "Lie to VanDeVeer's mortal enemies when VanDeVeer finds it convenient to do so." Does the latter maxim pass Kant's test? Further, with regard to MP or UP, is acting in accord with either UP or MP supposed to be a necessary condition of doing what is right, a sufficient condition, or both?

A further point with regard to MP bears mentioning. Suppose Theresa likes to have sexual relations with Lothar and likes it only when Lothar consents. Still, she cares about Lothar's preferences, pleasure, and well-being only insofar as it affects her prospective sexual satisfaction.[18] Further, Lothar's attitude toward Theresa is precisely parallel to hers. Also, they are mutually aware of each other's attitudes. Are they using each other as a mere means? They obviously are not "exploiting" (a weasel-word) each other in many of the ways that 'exploitation' calls to mind (e.g., rape, lying, depriving, physically abusing, and so on). What are the precise criteria for determining when people are used as a mere means? Can people consent to exploitation? If so, is the exploitation wrong? What is exploitation, anyway?

Even though we note some serious puzzles about Kant's approach, his central idea is attractive and there may be plausible answers to our questions—within Kant's theory, or perhaps in a revised version of it. If Kant's theory is mistaken, or if utilitarians are mistaken, the mistakes and inadequacies are instructive ones. We profit from grappling with their seductive theories.

RIGHTS THEORIES

If we believe, quite minimally, that there are some constraints on what we can do to people, we might express such a point by saying that we have certain duties toward others, possibly negative ones to refrain from doing certain things to them (e.g., causing pain to them) or positive ones (e.g., providing health care). Alternatively, we may believe that people (and perhaps some animals as well) have certain *rights*, possibly negative ones (e.g., not to be caused to suffer by moral agents) or positive ones (e.g., to be told the truth, that promises be kept, or that health care be provided). For some, to say that persons have rights is only another way of saying that persons are owed certain duties. If this is true, perhaps any theory employing the notion of rights is equivalent to some theory couched solely in terms of duties, and there may be no distinct theory of rights. Others maintain that we have a duty not to kill, for example, because others have a right not to be killed. The suggestion is that rights are somehow more basic, and that duties (at least some) are derivative. How to understand 'because' (above) is an intriguing and open question.

In any case, there are various rights theorists and rights theories, and we cannot here point to single well-developed theory of rights that is as historically influential as utilitarianism or Kantian theory. Still, it cannot go unobserved that the writings of Thomas Hobbes, John Locke, Thomas Paine, and others exercised a great influence on the Founding Fathers in the United States and on subsequent political, legal, and especially constitutional, developments in the American tradition (regarding "inalienable human rights," "right to life, liberty, and the pursuit of happiness," the Bill of Rights).

Discussion of rights has tended to focus on debates over particular rights (such as the right to life, to privacy, to procreate, or to determine the destiny of one's body); as noted, there is no full-blown, integrated, theory of rights that can be our focus here. Any such theory, however, would have to answer certain questions. We shall survey some of them and review some proposed answers.

First, what does it mean to say that "A has a right to X"? One answer we have noted: other moral agents have a duty to allow A to do X (if X is an act A may wish to do, such as speaking freely), or to be X (if X is a state, such as being alive), or to receive X (if X stands in place for, say, being nurtured). When X stands for an act that A may wish to do, one perhaps plausible analysis of "A has a right to do X" is:

1. It is permissible for A to do X or to refrain.

and 2. It is not permissible for others to interfere with A's choice.

What is meant by saying that A has a right to do X will affect our answer to another question: Are rights and duties always correlative? In other words, is it true that for every right there is a corresponding duty on the part of others, and for every duty there is a corresponding right?

The precise interpretation of rights claims is, perhaps, less controversial than another question: What sorts of beings (or things) logically can have rights? One can imagine quite tolerant answers (e.g., anything that exists, whether a redwood tree, a cloud, or the ecosystem) or even things that do not now but will exist (e.g., future generations of persons, animals, or redwood trees). One plausible, but more restrictive view, is that for something to have any rights at all it logically must be capable of experiencing satisfactions or dissatisfactions (i.e., it must be sentient). Here it may be noted that the debate over what has moral standing may be equivalent to, parallel to, or involve, the question about what sorts of things can have rights. Those who take the latter view deny that it makes sense to attribute rights to rocks, plants, nonsentient animals, or comatose human beings (and, probably, deny that "Life is sacred" or "of infinite value" is a coherent statement). An even more restrictive criterion, so it appears, is that something cannot logically have a right unless it is consciously aware of itself as a continuing being over time and has future-oriented preferences (perhaps, not all [or any?] sentient animals or neonatal humans satisfy this criterion).

If it is allowed, for example, that to be a bearer of rights a being must be sentient, do sentient beings have rights? That is, is possession of sentience (or pick another apparently logically *necessary* condition for having rights; we have not tried to settle the matter) a *sufficient* condition for actually having rights? This question calls attention to a third important issue: What are plausible grounds for attributing rights to certain individuals? Here one might claim that, for example, being sentient is not only logically necessary but sufficient as well. This answer competes with other proposed criteria, such as being created by God, being capable of rational choice, being a member of the human race, or possessing the potential for rational choice. If we believe that the possession or absence of moral rights (quite aside from the exigencies of what, at a particular time and place, is a bearer of legal rights) is decisive or important in deciding what we may, or must, do with regard to certain beings, it is crucial that we reasonably decide who or what has rights (and *which* rights are possessed). Hence, we must have defensible grounds for recognizing rights or refusing to recognize rights. The bearings of these fundamental questions on our thinking (and acting) about abortion, euthanasia of defective neonates, euthanasia of irreversibily comatose human beings, or experimentation on sentient animals should be obvious. In any event, later essays in this book will delve into these matters more deeply than we can in our brief discussion here.

Even if these questions could be answered adequately, much would remain to be done. A rights theory also must tell us precisely what sorts of rights bearers have. It is widely held, for example, that people (for starters) have a right to life. Even if the extension of 'people' were perfectly clear, there are some questions about what is meant by a 'right to life.' Note that this is a further question even if we have some agreement at a more general level regarding how to understand sentences of the form "A has a right to X." Discussion in recent years has made clear the ambiguity of, for example, 'right to life' among, at least, these interpretations:

1. A has a right not to be killed.
2. A has a right to be supplied with those things necessary for continued life.
3. A has the rights mentioned in both 1 and 2.
4. A has a right not to be killed unjustly.
5. A has a right to defend A against threats to A's life.
6. A has a right to defend A against unjust threats to A's life.
7. A has a right not to have A's personal identity eliminated.[19]

One can imagine other construals of the right to life. We need not see all these proposals as equally plausible. What the implications are of recognizing a right to life will depend on what is meant by the key phrase; a similar point is true for: a right to autonomy, and so on. Settling such matters is crucial to determining what will count as an *infringement of the right.*[20]

If we could achieve clarity about that, we would need to ascertain whether the right were *absolute* or *presumptive.* 'Absolute' is used in various ways; a standard construal of 'absolute right' is 'a right it is always wrong to infringe.' A 'presumptive right' is construed to mean 'a right such that it is wrong to infringe it in the absence of other weightier, and contrary, morally relevant considerations.' It is plausible to believe that if I promise to meet you for lunch, you have a right to my showing up. However, it may not be wrong for me not to show up if my not doing so is the only way to avoid an assassin bent on terminating me. Some rights, then, seem merely presumptive. Still, it is not obvious that no rights are absolute. For example, a plausible case may be made that the right not to be killed unjustly is an absolute right. In passing, we note that if a right is said to be merely presumptive, we need to know what would justify our going ahead and infringing it. Possible answers: it conflicts with other more stringent rights, or by infringing it we can produce substantial utility.

If something has a right to life and it is not absolute, we cannot conclude further argument that if the right is infringed the infringement is unqualifiedly wrong. Thus, if fetuses possess a nonabsolute right to life, killing them may not be wrong (rather, there may be a *justified infringement*). Alternatively, if it is allowed that fetuses have an absolute right to life construed along the lines of the right not to be killed unjustly, it may be argued that a particular abortion is not wrong since (if the case can be made) the killing was just, i.e., a just killing of A does not infringe A's right not to be killed unjustly. Instead, a defender of abortion who is committed to a rights theory may deny that fetuses have rights (recall our discussion of the grounds for attributing rights and what sorts of things can have rights); one might call this the *no right to infringe argument.* These are some of the subtle strategies for defending various moral judgments when disputes over rights arise. In sum, we have identified three: (1) arguing that a right bearer did have a right infringed, but justifiably; (2) that a right bearer had a relevant right but, on proper construal, it was not infringed; or (3) that, in fact, the being in question lacked the alleged right.

The reader may sense the tension between utilitarianism and rights theories. It is also evident that there is a certain amiability between Kant's emphasis on never treating a person as a mere means and the notion that people have certain basic rights. Both suggest the existence of limits on what we justifiably can do to people. Both, in that way, seem to be attempts to explicate the notion that persons are independent centers of dignity or value and deserving of respect. In many ways the disputed issues in biomedical ethics reflect the quest to understand precisely what is required of us if we are to respect persons, and perhaps other sentient creatures.[21]

RAWLS'S THEORY OF JUSTICE

The most influential theory of justice developed in this century is that found in John Rawls's *A Theory of Justice*, a work that has altered, in fundamental ways, the thinking and viewpoints of a considerable number of professional moral and political philosophers and whose ideas have generated a fresh dialogue between philosophers and others who work in the fields of economics, jurisprudence, medical ethics, political theory, and public policy. Although Rawls's theory is conceived as a theory of justice, and questions of justice are conceived by Rawls and most philosophers as a subset of ethical questions (i.e., not all questions of right and wrong involve issues of justice), Rawls suggests that it may be possible to extend his basic contractarian procedure for ascertaining principles of justice to all or virtually all questions of right conduct.[22] Initially, one might begin to reflect on the implications of Rawls's principles for questions about the distribution of benefits and burdens in health care. But first let us review the bare essentials of his theory.

Claims about what is a fair or just distribution of goods are often flawed in an obviously suspect way: they exhibit an arbitrary favoritism toward the interests of those making the claims, e.g., defenders of slavery in the southern part of the United States during the nineteenth century often defended existing black-white inequalities on the rather paternalistic grounds that blacks were worse off in Africa and would be worse off if living freely under the difficult industrial conditions prevailing for workers in northern cities). To surmount the barriers of rationalization and arbitrary prejudice, Rawls invites us to conduct a thought-experiment and, imaginatively, to enter into a hypothetical contractual situation in which we are to negotiate what principles or rules will govern our mutual interaction, especially the constraints on basic social institutions (e.g., constitutional ones) that will govern our mutual dealings. Nevertheless, participants in this hypothetical situation, whether ourselves or others, are figuratively placed behind a "veil of ignorance." Such contractors in what he labels the "original position" are construed to be rational choosers of principles designed to protect and promote the good of persons in the society of which they will be members. However, as choosers they are ignorant of certain features about themselves, ones that they might exploit to gain partisan advantage. More fully, such participants are to decide on principles to regulate and determine the basic structure of fundamental social institutions. These in turn will determine the basic forms of social cooperation and interaction among persons in society. The principles impartially chosen would be, in Rawls's view, principles of justice and would identify, at least in part, the sort of just treatment owed to individuals in a just society. The participants, under a veil of ignorance, do not know what their own position in such a society would be, nor their gender, their talents, their particular conception of the good, their race, or even to what generation they would belong. Hence, they would not be able to choose principles that might differentially favor the positions they are to occupy. Their ignorance is to guarantee *impartiality* in the consideration of which principles to adopt. If the rational participants knew they were going to be males, the principles they would choose would be different than those chosen under the Rawlsian veil of ignorance; for example, a "modified Difference Principle" might be chosen: inequalities are permissible only if they maximize the benefits of the least advantaged males.[23] Such a principle would be arbitrary and its implications need no further comment. The original position, then, is designed to prevent a disregarding of the interests of any person or set of persons, or any arbitrary favoring of the interests of some over the interests of others. The choosers, then, are not "self-interested" *or* "altruistic."

What basic principles would be chosen in this hypothetical contractual situation? Rawls's reasoning here is complex, but, in brief, it proceeds as follows. Given that each participant has so much at stake (for personal opportunities and well-being will be greatly affected by which principles are to constrain the basic institutions governing their lives as participants in the society being designed), Rawls claims that they would proceed conservatively by adopting the *maximin rule* of choice: choose that alternative whose *worst* outcome is better than the *worst* outcome of any other available alternative.[24] Hence they would be averse to gambling with their "future" well-being. For example, some initially might argue for a system of slavery. If they should turn out to be masters, after the veil of ignorance is removed and the chosen principles implemented, they would gain immensely. But if they turn out to be slaves, then they would lose immensely. However, since the veil of ignorance prevents them from knowing their actual positions in society, it would not be rational for them to endorse a principle that might condemn them to the worse possible social positions. Without attempting to elaborate fully the reasoning of such participants in the original position, as Rawls projects it, he claims that two principles would be chosen (often labeled [1] the Liberty Principle and [2] the Difference Principle, respectively):

1. Each person is to have an equal right to the most extensive total system of equal basic liberties compatible with a similar system of liberty for all.

2. Social and economic inequalities are to be arranged so that they are both: (a) to the greatest benefit of the least advantaged . . . and (b) attached to offices and positions open to all under conditions of fair equality of opportunity.

Rawls claims that whatever principles are chosen under conditions preventing anyone from arbitrarily pressing for special personal advantage are the *fundamental principles of justice*. Such principles are whichever principles would be selected by concerned, rational choosers under circumstances securing impartiality of choice. In briefest outline, that is the core of Rawls's rich, and more complex, theory.

We note a few of the attractions of Rawls's theory. First, it seems to capture the Kantian and commonsense conviction that principles of morality are in some sense universal, that all persons have certain rights or deserve certain opportunities. In contrast, certain principles favoring certain groups or individuals (e.g., "Aryans should rule," "Only males should own property") seem arbitrary. The veil of ignorance provides a conceptual mechanism that embodies the notion that justice is blind, that it pays no attention to irrelevant differences between persons. The hypothetical choice situation of the original position seems to overcome the arbitrary promotion of self or group interests commonly involved in many actual bargaining situations.

Second, Rawls's theory hardly can be accused of ignoring, or giving peripheral place to, questions of the distribution of benefits and burdens; in Rawls's view, what is right is not to be equated with whatever maximizes the total amount of aggregate net utility. For reasons already mentioned, the contractors would not adopt that as an overriding principle or goal.

Third, Rawls explicitly rejects the assumption that all utility counts morally. Any satisfactions received by the rapist in rape go *no* way toward morally justifying the act of rape. Principles of right action are prior to, and place constraints on, possible efforts to promote the good, or utility.

Fourth, at a theoretical level Rawls's contractarian procedure seems to connect the question of acceptable moral principles to an intelligible notion of rational choice. What is just is determined by principles that rational choosers would adopt under conditions of impartial choice. To invoke considerations of justice is not, then, like banging on a table with a shoe—an incredibly subjectivist view but one actually defended by some. In this respect, Rawls's view is close to the commonsense view that to complain that homicide, rape, or theft involves an injustice is to make a *reasonable* protest.

Rawls's principles have implications in the area of health care ethics. One concerns the distribution of benefits and burdens in the health care system. With regard to those who are sick, one possible basis for distributing health care would be to make it available only to those willing and able to pay for it (rather unadulterated capitalism). Another would be to make it freely available to all those in need. What principles would contractors in the original position adopt regarding such a matter? Given the contingencies of the "natural lottery," some people are born severely handicapped or retarded and are not able to earn money to pay for health care. With a pay-as-you-receive system, they would go without. Knowing this and wishing to avoid this worst possible outcome, the "maximizing" contractors would reject such a system. Given the inordinately high costs of a system of free health care for all who need it and given further questions about whether those who voluntarily make themselves needy (by sloth or risky lifestyle choices) should be aided when the cost is great, it is not obvious that those in the original position would choose, alternatively, a system of free health care for all. Relevant here, of course, is the Difference Principle. If we agree that it is a principle of justice, its implications for the distribution of health care are not straightforward; further investigation is in order. Later essays here will explore questions about justice, efficiency, and individual responsibility for health care (especially the essays by Norman Daniels and Dan Wikler; see chapters XIII and IX).

A second area in which we can profitably examine the implications of Rawls's theory concerns restrictions on liberty (broadly conceived). We may restrict the liberty of others by the use of force, coercive threat, or deception (including the withholding of information). Thus, whether informed consent is necessary in order to proceed justifiably with the risky treatment of patients involves the question of whether we can justifiably restrict liberty. The acceptability of certain forms of experimentation on individuals (both those capable of valid consent and those not capable), therapeutic civil commitment (e.g., to protect the seriously mentally ill from themselves), and the use of randomized clinical trials also call for a principled answer to the question of when we can justifiably restrict liberty. Here it may be important to consider whether there are relevant differences among subjects (e.g., children, competent adults, incompetent adults). Further, it is worth noting that one standard justification for restricting liberty is that it is all right to restrict Smith if Smith is harming or wronging Jones (such as kidnaping him), a principle roughing allowing third parties to intervene coercively to prevent one person (or group) from imposing wrongful harm on others. This principle is fundamental in criminal law. In contrast, considerable restriction of liberty in the context of health care is defended on paternalistic grounds (e.g., A's restriction of S's liberty is defended on the ground that A's doing so is for *S's own good*). Note that, in contrast to the prior case, the aim of the restriction is to prevent harm to, or promote the well-being of, *the subject* of the constraint. Although we find a considerable range of paternalistic intervention with children or incompetents morally unobjectionable, paternalistic intervention with competent persons is a matter of much current controversy.[25] This issue is relevant to deciding whether it is permissible to deceive patients, to prohibit risky activities, to prohibit certain kinds of self-care, to prohibit access to certain drugs, to incarcerate those dangerous only to themselves—"for their own good." In exploring this matter, readers may consider the implications of Rawls's two basic principles or, more generally, whether as a contractor in the original position one would agree to certain principles allowing certain paternalistically oriented restraints on one's behavior.

Finally, we shall note, with little elaboration, that a fuller understanding and assessment of Rawls's theory would require the consideration of various questions.[26] These include: Is the device of the original position adequate to justify the mentioned principles? Would participants in it actually choose the principles that Rawls claims they would choose? Is the veil of ignorance designed to ensure complete neutrality? Are the implications of the two principles independently reasonable? A further point worth contemplating is whether Rawls's theory, commonly described as "contractarian," is contractarian in any important sense. Given the design of the original position, if *any* participants would choose the principles that Rawls proposes, there seems no basis for disagreement, and hence no basis, negotiation or compromise. If no participant could have any basis for disagreement, it is not clear that the notion of contractual agreement has any substance. There would seem to be no distinct individuals with differing preferences or interests who would need to search for mutually satisfactory policies or priciples. There can be no element of "I'll give up this if you give up that." If the original position helps us identify principles of justice or what is a matter of duty, it may not be at all like the case in which duties are generated by mutual contracts or agreements (e.g., that you fix the salad and I'll prepare the pasta). But it is foolish to think that *all* duties arise from voluntary agreements; hence, it may be unimportant whether Rawls's theory is strictly contractarian or not.

Grounds for Restricting Liberty

In our discussion of Rawls's theory, we have briefly sketched the problem of when it is justifiable to restrict liberty. The question is an important one, and it deserves fuller elaboration. If we can sometimes justifiably place limits on the freedom of others to choose or to act, we need to know the grounds for doing so. There are a few leading proposals. As noted, one type of purportedly acceptable ground for interfering in the lives of others is paternalistic; it is thought, roughly, that interfering is justifiable if it promotes the good, welfare, preferences, interests, or, perhaps, rights of the subject of the interference. What counts as an interference or a restriction of liberty is in itself a matter of some dispute. It is worth observing that various modes of influence can be employed to affect another's behavior or, more broadly, his or her destiny. Fair and honest attempts to persuade another person to act or choose in a certain fashion are one such mode. Such attempts, however, seem morally innocuous and, indeed, seem to respect other persons as autonomous choosers and centers of choice. Certain modes of influence are suspect (e.g., the use of brute force, the use of deception, the employment of coercive threats, or certain techniques of brainwashing). It is not clear, however, what counts as deception (do I deceive you if I simply withhold information from you, or only when I have some duty to reveal a truth to you—or what I believe to be true?). Further, even if we were clear about this conceptual issue, whether others consent to deception seems important in contemplating the morality of the deception. Consider, for example, the deception that occurs in poker, bridge, certain sports, or the attitude expressed by a spouse who says, "Do that if you want; just don't tell me about it!" The analysis of 'coercion' also is not entirely clear. A plausible analysis is that A coercively has threatened S if and only if: A has conveyed to S his intent to make S significantly worse off than S is (post-threat) if S fails to comply with A's directive, and if S complies A will not make S worse off than S is (post-threat). The mugger who says, "Your money or your life" thus utters a coercive threat. One may think that, analogously, the prison administrator who (in so many words) says to a prisoner, "If you do not volunteer as a subject for this research project, I will not recommend you for early parole" is employing coercion. In contrast, *seductive offers* seem less suspect. Is it not acceptable to propose to a prospective employee, "If you come to work for us, we'll double your salary." But compare the prison administrator who says, "If you volunteer for the experiment, I will recommend you for early parole." There is, at least, some question about the morality of proposals that seem to constitute "an offer one cannot refuse."

There is, then, a need to identify, sort out, and assess what counts as restrictions on liberty or, at least, morally suspect modes of influencing others. Some forms of influence on patients in health care contexts seem more subtle, such as the use of pressure, promoting guilt, manipulation of information, authoritative intimidation, or what is called "undue influence." Still, we commonly find acceptable the use of suspect modes of influence in certain situations, such as in the prevention of crime, the punishment of criminals, or what is thought to justify self-defense or a just war. A question of enormous importance, in and out of biomedical contexts, concerns identifying legitimate and principled grounds for restricting liberty. We have noted that one proposed type of principle is paternalistic. Various other (allegedly) legitimate grounds are *nonpaternalistic* in nature—that is, they focus on promoting or protecting the good, welfare, preferences, interests, or rights of parties other than those of the subject(s) whose liberty is restricted. There are various ways of classifying nonpaternalistic principles that, purportedly, identify legitimate grounds for restricting liberty. Virtually everyone accepts some formulation of *"The" harm principle.* On one version it simply is this:

It is permissible to restrict the liberty of S to prevent or halt S from harming others.

Note that such a principle appeals to nonpaternalistic grounds to justify a restriction on liberty. The stated principle seems to countenance too much. Unless qualified, it would sanction a rapist's use of violence to subdue his intended victim if she gained the upper hand and was about to harm him. That *his* liberty-limiting efforts are morally justified is hardly obvious. The principle is more plausible if it is amended to read ". . . innocent others." But this leaves us with at least two important questions: (1) what are the criteria for determining innocence, and (2) what counts as harming another?[27] Although there seem to be paradigmatic (perfectly clear) examples of harming, there are also disputed cases. Should we say that S is harmed by A, for example, whenever S is disabled by A or A severs a limb of S? What if S has consented to such acts or requested them? We might conclude then that "no harm was done." Alternatively, we might say that harm did result but that no *wrong* was done; if so, why should we think it right to intervene to prevent harming that does not wrong the one harmed? This type of reflection tempts some to suggest that the connection between an act being wrong and being harmful is not analytic. Perhaps one can wrong another without harming him (e.g., I infringe on your property rights by sitting on your porch while you are gone without your consent). And if you fail to make the team because I win the remaining position, should we conclude that you are harmed but not wronged (assuming the results were generated by fair competition)? For reasons such as these, among others, some conclude that it is more plausible to focus on the infringement of rights as a legitimate nonpaternalistic basis for restricting liberty—as opposed to a "harm principle." These remarks also suggest the considerable importance of determining the moral relevance of voluntary, knowing, consent in determining permissible treatment of others.

If harm is construed somewhat narrowly, one might recognize a distinction between harming another and *offending* another. If so, one might think that there is a further principle identifying another legitimate basis for restricting liberty: namely, some sort of *offense principle*. Although we might think that a policy of coercive prohibition of ordinary insults goes too far, other cases may generate second thoughts. Should Nazis be allowed to parade the swastika in Jewish communities? Should white racists be allowed to excoriate "niggers" on television? Should male chauvinists be allowed to refer to women as "cunts" in the media? Similar worries arise in contemplating analogous acts by black racists or female chauvinists. Should married couples be allowed to copulate in the parking lot of the shopping mall on Saturday afternoon? It is tempting to think that some acts should be prohibited because they are extremely offensive. One worry about such a policy, however, concerns the risks to civil liberties of allowing the state to define "lewd and indecent behavior" or what counts as a "nuisance." A related reservation focuses on the fact that numerous people may be offended seriously by acts that, for other reasons, people seem to have a right to perform (e.g., gay persons expressing affection in public, an interracial couple holding hands, or the use of "guerilla theater" tactics to protest what its users take to be an unjust war).[28] For these reasons a simple offense principle such as

It is permissible to restrict the liberty of S in order to prevent or halt S's engaging in acts seriously offensive to others

seems problematic and in need of emendation or, in the absence of such, not deserving of rational acceptance.

It is worth noting that the principles mentioned here seem to be middle-level principles, principles of moderate scope that purport only to identify legitimate bases for employing presumptively wrongful modes of interference in the lives of others. In general they focus on halting or preventing something—harm, rights infringement, or the occurrence of an offense—as opposed to benefiting others. Further, each seems to focus only on the "direct recipient" of certain kinds of behavior (but this appearance may be only a first impression). Thus, such principles seem to lack the breadth of the principle of utility or a Kantian imperative. One question that arises, then, if we believe that one or more of these liberty-limiting principles is acceptable (or, let us not forget, some sort of paternalistic principle), is: To what more comprehensive ethical outlook does this commit us? Conversely, if we find the principle of utility initially plausible, or we approve of the Kantian proposal to treat each person as an end and never as a mere means, what are the implications of such global normative principles for questions concerning when we can justifiably restrict liberty—especially by one of the suspect means mentioned (e.g., force, coercive threat, or deception)? If these seem to be perplexing and difficult questions, that is because they are. Still, we hardly can afford to ignore them since our answers —explicit, sensitive, and thoughtful or "knee-jerk" and unreflective—substantively affect how we will deal with other persons and how we will be treated, whether as a matter of private conduct, professional practice, or public policy.

Our survey of the standardly mentioned and leading grounds for restricting liberty helps place in a broader context the aforementioned appeal to paternalistic considerations. Although reference to "the principle of paternalism" is not uncommon (or the harm principle or the offense principle), it is clear that various sorts of principles are invoked that purport to identify, and sanction interferences, of more or less invasive sorts, on paternalistic grounds. There are, then, competing "paternalistic principles," and it is worth discussing several of them here. As noted in our discussion of Rawls's theory, it is tempting to think that there is an important difference between paternalistic restrictions placed on individuals who substantially or entirely lack the capacity for autonomous choice (e.g., fetuses, young children, or incompetent adults) and restricting those who possess such a capacity. What counts as having such a capacity is not an unimportant matter, but we will leave that question open. If we restrict our focus to interventions in the lives of competent persons, there is an important sense in which by paternalistically intervening in certain ways, we "substitute our judgment" for theirs with regard to what is "for their own good." The apparently benevolent motive of interveners in such cases need not blind us to the residual question of whether such "well-motivated" but suspect intrusions are a morally permissible way of influencing competent persons.[29]

Defenses of paternalistic intervention can be categorized roughly as appealing to the *consent* of the subject (or recipient) of intervention and others as appealing to *promoting the good* or welfare (or preventing or halting harm to) of the subject. Appeals to consent, further, may take significantly different forms. We will not attempt to assess them fully here, but let us do some sorting. One claim is that intervention with paternalistic aims is all right if the subject previously consented to it. For example, a person may contract with professional therapists and agree to being locked in a room all day for group therapy. The consequent restriction on his liberty may be thought justified because of such prior consent—even if the subject later changes his mind. Another appeal is to *current consent*. For example, suppose that I am wavering about my diet and I agree that you can go ahead and activate the time-lock on the refrigerator. When there is such prior or current consent to a restriction on choice or behavior, some writers will deny that there is any paternalistic interference at all. Although I once agreed, such a view now seems to me to be arbitrarily restrictive. The "cooperative interference" involved may be both a type of interference and paternalistic. Another appeal is to *subsequent consent*. The familiar, possibly parental, claim that "you will be glad we did this" typically expresses the view that paternalistic restrictions are acceptable if (and, perhaps, only if) the subject will later consent to the restriction. It is worth noting that in contrast to the appeal to prior or current consent, there simply is, at the time of intervention, no consent by the subject in the unique cases allegedly sanctioned by this latter principle. Hence, it would sanction a greater range of paternalistic intervention than principles requiring current or prior consent. Another type of appeal to consent also does not require actual overt consent by the subject; rather, it appeals to some form of *hypothetical consent*. In one version, paternalistic interference is permissible with a subject, S, if it is true that a fully rational person would consent to the restriction involved. Even if some competent persons choose to drive on expressways without using seat belts, it may be true that no fully rational person would do so. If so, building automobiles that cannot function, for example, unless seat belts are operative *may* be an instance of permissible paternalism. For similar reasons, attaching criminal penalties to their nonuse may be justifiable in this view. The relevance of these principles to the defense of certain restrictive policies and laws aimed at promoting life or health is not difficult to see. They also have implications for how we ought to think about individual responsibility for risks to life and limb. Another appeal to hypothetical consent maintains that paternalistic interference with a subject, S, is permissible if *S would consent* to the restrictions involved if S were adequately apprised of the consequences of his or her actions. We leave the examination of the differences and implications of these two appeals to hypothetical consent for the reader to consider. With regard to all the liberty-limiting principles noted (paternalistic and nonpaternalistic), we can and should attempt to ascertain whether a principle has any wildly counterintuitive implications, whether it captures part of what we pretheoretically regard as respecting competent persons, and whether it is compatible with, or derivable from, some attractive, more comprehensive, ethical theory (e.g., Kantian, utilitarian, Rawlsian).

Barriers to Inquiry

There was a time when at least some persons (male and female) merited the label "Renaissance man," a person well versed in virtually all the major areas of intellectual inquiry. That time may be past. As we have taken some pains to emphasize, the perplexities of the issues in health care ethics require, for their rational resolution, empirical expertise, sensitivity to conceptual sources of confusion, skill in analyzing slippery arguments, and awareness of the complexities of scientific and ethical theories. As such, inquiry in health care ethics is both important and challenging; it requires patience, persistence, and a surmounting of the myopia engendered by the understandable move toward academic or professional specialization. Progress in resolving the issues requires the skills and information of persons in diverse disciplines and a dialogue among them. If such a dialogue is to proceed unimpeded, we must surrender the crude stereotypes that persist about "all physicians," "all nurses," and the distortions embodied in remarks to the effect that lawyers are casuists, philosophers are logic-choppers or only interested in linguistic matters, scientists are concerned only with empirically testable hypotheses, and so on. A mark of maturity in the practitioners of such disciplines is that they can openly criticize their own disciplines, and are at least minimally aware of, and can readily admit, its limitations, and exhibit a genuine willingness to learn from those with other sorts of expertise. In short, we need to surmount the not uncommon intellectual hubris and pugnaciously clothed insecurity of the dedicated but myopic professional.

In the essays that follow, and generally in the examination of issues in health care ethics, a familiar distinction employed in moral philosophy can help minimize the unnecessary acrimony that is often associated with deep disagreements over certain practices. I shall lead up to it. As this is written, it has been reported that a number of antiabortionists, self-described members of the "Army of God" have abducted a physician and his wife, presumably in order to protest the practice of abortion. *If* abortion is morally wrong and *if* it should be thought of as a wrong as serious as murder, then the abduction is both unsurprising and understandable. Indeed, it is, arguably, an act of justified civil disobedience—as would be a similar rebellion against slavery or the Nazis' extermination of the Jews. A somewhat natural tendency, however, is to think that if murder is an evil, those who murder are evil and blameworthy. In general, if someone does what is wrong, it is tempting to infer that the doer of the wrong deserves blame. In a related manner, health care professionals may be inclined to view attacks on the morality of certain of their professional practices as personal attacks, or attacks of an interprofessional sort (or intra-professional assaults by disloyal members of the profession in question). There are at least two reasons for hesitating before drawing these conclusions. One is the distinction alluded to above but not stated. It is the distinction between (1) the question of the morality of an act or practice, and (2) the question of whether an agent who performs the act is blameworthy (or praiseworthy). Under certain conditions, agents are exonerated from blame otherwise associated with wrongful acts. Most notably, ignorance and compulsion tend to exculpate agents from responsibility for such acts. To argue that a given act or practice is morally impermissible is, then, not necessarily to presuppose that the agent is blameworthy. A second, related, consideration in favor of separating the question of whether certain health care practices are morally permissible (just, and so on) from the issue of whether agents of those practices are to blame derives from the recalcitrant nature of many of the ethical perplexities in question. In the absence of any substantive exculpating conditions,[30] we readily would agree that anyone who poisoned the local water supply is blameworthy; however, that is an act that conscientious, reasonable, "good-hearted" persons would not find morally perplexing. In contrast, many if not all of the disputes in biomedical ethics are perplexing, and there is frequently little or no reason to conclude that practitioners of disputed practices are "moral monsters" even if, when the final word is in, we must conclude that certain practices are intolerable and, hence, must be brought to a halt. I am suggesting, in short, that the genuine difficulty of reaching a reasonable view about the permissibility of certain practices goes some significant way toward exonerating practitioners of the blame that usually attaches to unjustified practices. The burden of identifying those practices is one that all can share. If abortion is wrong, then both physicians who abort and consenting citizens should cease to support the practice. If, alternatively, the practice is permissible and desirable, then dissenting physicians and citizens should cease their attempts to prevent it. Analogously, if attacks on certain forms of paternalism in health care, on examination, turn out to be defensible, citizens should withdraw their cooperation in and support of such practices. Nor should we ignore the fact that such forms of paternalism may have close analogues in the practices of, for example, parents, professors, architects, priests, or others—practices that may deserve equal moral scrutiny or condemnation. Recognition that (1) to question a practice is not necessarily to question the motives or character of the practitioner, and (2) moral scrutiny of health care practices may yield ethical insights for, and a basis for moral criticism of, all agents, whatever their vocation, may facilitate the development of a principled and reasoned health care ethic. It also may help subvert the uncritical defensiveness that is often associated with a sincere commitment to the norms and practices of one's own discipline or vocation.

The serious and lively interest in ethical issues in health care, an interest most manifest in the past decade, is an occasion for optimism. The trend that has begun is likely to increase significantly in the next decade. The current debates are challenging. Coming to grips with the issues can be a personally rewarding, as well as an intellectually demanding, experience. The ensuing essays here— when coupled with an inquisitive, careful, and reflective examination—promise just such an experience.[31]

Notes

1. Note that the expression 'factual claim' is ambiguous between (a) what we mean here by 'empirical claim,' and (b) a true empirical claim.

2. Epistemology is concerned with what counts as knowledge and the justification of claims to know, or to have reasonable beliefs.

3. One begs the question by assuming, in a premise purporting to provide independent support of what one is trying to conclude, the truth of the conclusion. This happens, for example, in the argument that abortion is wrong because abortion is murder—if by murder one means wrongful killing.

4. The essay by Christopher Boorse (see Chapter X) instructively explores these issues.

5. More carefully, this is writing or speaking aimed at establishing what is reasonable or true by argumentation and, hence, excepting most poetry and fiction.

6. Detecting validity or invalidity in more complicated forms of argument and the methods for doing so are matters not elaborated on here; a course in beginning philosophy or logic usually fosters such skills.

7. Suppose a drunken man enters your home with a gun in hand after returning from a hunting trip and, in his stupor, thinks he is entering his own house. You mistakenly think he is your daughter's embittered ex-husband (or, perhaps, the heroin pusher your testimony sent to prison), and shoot him after he, equally mistakenly, takes you to be the person who previously threatened to break into his house and kill him.

8. Or compare the case in which Chico says, "You should not doubt my credibility since Harpo has vouched for me and Groucho has vouched for him; and, of course, I have vouched for Groucho."

9. Another interesting implication, almost always surprising to those who initially contemplate it, is that any argument with inconsistent premises *must be valid*. It often takes some thought to see why. This result also seems troublesome. One step toward relieving any philosophical discomfort is to recall that valid arguments need not "prove" anything—in the

sense of providing a compelling reason to judge that their conclusions are true. This point in turn calls in question certain glib assumptions about what counts as a proof. If all that is required in proving a claim is that it be the conclusion of a valid argument, *any* claim can be proved. This point raises a conceptual question: What counts as proving a claim?

10. A third strategy is possible (constructing a counterdilemma), but we will set it aside here.

11. By 'sentient' is meant: capable of experiencing pain or satisfaction.

12. It is worth observing that 'justify' is often ambiguous between (1) defends, and (2) adequately or successfully defends. One might say that Nixon justified his role in the Watergate episode, but if sense (2) of 'justify' is in question, one may have doubts—to understate the matter. Philosophers usually use 'justify' in sense (2).

13. For example, see R. M. Hare's essay in *Justice and Economic Distribution*, ed. John Arthur and William Shaw (Englewood Cliffs, N.J.: Prentice-Hall, 1978), 116–131.

14. This is not exactly the way Bentham and Mill posed the principle. Also, PU, as formulated here, is equivalent to "act-utilitarianism," a principle distinguished from "rule-utilitarianism"—a version of utilitarianism espoused by some recent advocates. For a more thorough discussion of utilitarianism, see William Frankena, *Ethics* (Englewood Cliffs, N.J.: Prentice-Hall, 1963); Dan Brock, "Utilitarianism," in *And Justice For All*, ed. Tom Regan and Donald VanDeVeer (Totowa, N.J.: Rowman and Littlefield, 1982) pp. 217–40; Fred Feldman, *Introductory Ethics* (Englewood Cliffs, N. J.: Prentice-Hall, 1978) or the admirable critical study by David Lyons, *Forms and Limits of Utilitarianism* (Oxford: Oxford University Press, 1965); a more recent critical treatise is Donald Regan, *Utilitarianism and Cooperation* (Oxford: Oxford University Press, 1980). The discussions by Brock, Feldman, and Frankena are especially good places to start. For an interesting exchange of views see *Utilitarianism: For and Against* by J. J. C. Smart and Bernard Williams (Cambridge: Cambridge University Press, 1973).

15. Unless T is construed to mean the sort failing to yield as much utility as any available alternative.

16. On these points, the reader may wish to explore David Lyons, *Forms and Limits of Utilitarianism* (Oxford: Oxford University Press, 1965) and the writings of Richard Brandt, such as *A Theory of the Good and the Right* (New York: Oxford University Press, 1979). On the last point, see Donald Regan, *Utilitarianism and Cooperation* (New York: Oxford University Press, 1980).

17. See Immanuel Kant, *Groundwork of the Metaphysics of Morals*, trans. H. J. Paton (New York: Harper & Row, 1964). More fully, one might state MP as "treat each person as an end and never as a mere means."

18. This problematic and intriguing type of case is discussed by Joseph Margolis in "Homosexuality," in *And Justice For All*, 42–63.

19. Michael Tooley notes that we could eliminate Smith's identity by,

say, lobotomy or a more radical procedure, without killing Smith's body. See his essay in Joel Feinberg, ed., *The Problem of Abortion* (Belmont, Calif.: Wadsworth, 1984), pp. 120–34.

20. To "infringe a right," as used here, means to deprive a right bearer of that to which he or she has a right. Some writers use "violate a right" to mean the same thing. Others, such as Judith Thomson, use "violate a right" to mean "wrongfully infringe a right." With the latter usage, an infringement of a right may or may not be a violation of a right. Stealing bread to save a starving child might be an example of a justified infringement of the bread owner's right.

21. There is much else that is relevant to understanding and assessing rights theories. The reader may wish to examine Joel Feinberg, *Social Philosophy* (Englewood Cliffs, N.J.: Prentice-Hall 1973), or his *Rights, Justice, and Bounds of Liberty* (Princeton, N.J.: Princeton University Press, 1980), Ronald Dworkin, *Taking Rights Seriously* (Cambridge, Mass.: Harvard University Press, 1978), or, more succinctly, Lawrence Becker, "Individual Rights," in *And Justice For All*, pp. 197–216. An important work that relies heavily on the notion of individual rights is Robert Nozick, *Anarchy, State, and Utopia* (New York: Basic Books, 1974). See also A. I. Melden, *Rights and Persons* (Berkeley: University of California Press, 1977).

22. John Rawls, *A Theory of Justice* (Cambridge, Mass.: Harvard University Press, 1971), 17.

23. Rawls, in contrast, claims that two basic principles would be chosen; one is called the difference principle; loosely stated, it maintains that inequalities in the distribution of primary goods (income, wealth, liberty, opportunity, the bases of self-respect) are permissible only if they redound to the benefit of the least advantaged.

24. This principle is also referred to as the *minimax principle*. It contrasts with other principles such as the less conservative *maximax principle*: choose that alternative whose *best* outcome is better than the *best* outcome of any other available alternative. Both principles are candidates for being the principle or standard of rational choice under *conditions of uncertainty*, i.e., choosing where there is no firm basis for assigning probabilities to different outcomes.

25. See Joel Feinberg, *Harm to Self* (Oxford: Oxford University Press, 1986); John Kleinig, *Paternalism* (Totowa, N.J.: Rowman and Allanheld, 1983); and Donald VanDeVeer, *Paternalistic Intervention* (Princeton: Princeton University Press, 1986).

26. Those interested might consult, in addition to *A Theory of Justice*, Norman Daniels, ed., *Reading Rawls* (New York: Basic Books, 1980), Brian Barry, *The Liberal Theory of Justice* (Oxford: Clarendon Press, 1973), and Robert Paul Wolff, *Understanding Rawls* (Princeton, N.J.: Princeton University Press, 1977).

27. On liberty-limiting principles, see Joel Feinberg's excellent *Social Philosophy* (Englewood Cliffs, N.J.: Prentice-Hall, 1973). More advanced is Joel Feinberg, *Harm to Others* (New York: Oxford University Press, 1984). On

the concept of harm, see the important essays by John Kleinig, "Crime and the Concept of Harm," *American Philosophical Quarterly* 15 (1978): 27–36, and his "Consent as a Defense in Criminal Law," *Archiv für Rechts und Sozialphilosophie* 65 (1979): 329–346. See also Craig Goodrum, "Notes on the Harm Principle," *The Personalist* 57 (1976): 239–250; John D. Harman, "Harm, Consent, and Distress," *Journal of Value Inquiry* 15 (1981): 293–309.

28. On offensive actions, see Joel Feinberg, "Harmless Immoralities and Offensive Nuisances," and Michael Bayles, "Offensive Conduct and the Law," both in *Issues in Law and Morality*, ed. Norman Care and Thomas K. Trelogan (Cleveland: Case Western Reserve University Press, 1973); see also Donald VanDeVeer, "Coercive Restraint of Offensive Actions," *Philosophy & Public Affairs* 8 (Winter 1979). See also (especially) Joel Feinberg's *Offense to Others* (New York: Oxford University Press, 1985).

29. Regarding apparently benevolent motives, it is worth observing that A may restrict the liberty of S because A cares about the well-being of S for its own sake—or because, for example, S is A's slave and A cares about S only in the manner he cares about any other piece of property he owns.

30. Compare, again, ignorance, compulsion—or special conditions, such as the defensibility of "burning your bridges behind you" in a just war.

31. An earlier, pre-natal title of this volume was *Border Crossings*. Prior to actual publication, it is worth noting, some references in the philosophical literature to *Border Crossings* have appeared. Generally, material thus cited will be found in this volume.

CHAPTER I

Euthanasia

Margaret Pabst Battin

Because it arouses questions about the morality of killing, the effectiveness of consent, the duties of physicians, and equity in the distribution of resources, the problem of euthanasia is one of the most acute and uncomfortable contemporary problems in medical ethics. It is not a new problem; euthanasia has been discussed—and practiced—in both Eastern and Western cultures from the earliest historical times to the present. But because of medicine's new technological capacities to extend life, the problem is much more pressing than it has been in the past, and both the discussion and practice of euthanasia are more widespread. Despite this, much of contemporary Western culture remains strongly opposed to euthanasia: doctors ought not kill people, its public voices maintain, and ought not let them die if it is possible to save life.

I believe that this opposition to euthanasia is in serious moral error—on grounds of mercy, autonomy, and justice. I shall argue for the rightness of granting a person a humane, merciful death, if he or she wants it, even when this can be achieved only by a direct and deliberate killing. But I think there are dangers here. Consequently, I shall also suggest that there is a safer way to discharge our moral duties than relying on physician-initiated euthanasia, one that nevertheless will satisfy those moral demands upon which the case for euthanasia rests.

The Case for Euthanasia, Part I: Mercy

The case for euthanasia rests on three fundamental moral principles: mercy, autonomy, and justice.

The principle of mercy asserts that *where possible, one ought to*

58

relieve the pain or suffering of another person, when it does not con-
travene that person's wishes, where one can do so without undue
costs to oneself, where one will not violate other moral obligations,
where the pain or suffering itself is not necessary for the sufferer's
attainment of some overriding good, and where the pain or suffer-
ing can be relieved without precluding the sufferer's attainment of
some overriding good.[1] (This principle might best be called the principle of medical mercy, to distinguish it from principles concerning
mercy in judicial contexts.[2]) Stated in this relatively weak form and
limited by these provisos, the principle of (medical) mercy is not
controversial, though the point I wish to argue here certainly is:
contexts that require mercy sometimes require euthanasia as a way
of granting mercy—both by direct killing and by letting die.

Although philosophers do not agree on whether moral agents have
positive duties of beneficence, including duties to those in pain,
members of the medical world are not reticent about asserting
them. "Relief of pain is the least disputed and most universal of the
moral obligations of the physician," writes one doctor. "Few things
a doctor does are more important than relieving pain," says another.[3] These are not simply assertions that the physician ought "do
no harm," as the Hippocratic oath is traditionally interpreted, but
assertions of positive obligation. It might be argued that the physician's duty of mercy derives from a special contractual or fiduciary
relationship with the patient, but I think that this is in error: rather,
the duty of (medical) mercy is generally binding on all moral
agents,[4] and it is only by virtue of their more frequent exposure to
pain and their specialized training in its treatment that this duty
falls more heavily on physicians and nurses than on others. Hence,
though we may call it the principle of "medical" mercy, it asserts an
obligation that we all have.

This principle of mercy establishes two component duties:

1. the duty not to cause further pain or suffering; and
2. the duty to act to end pain or suffering already occurring.

Under the first of these, for a physician or other caregiver to extend mercy to a suffering patient may mean to refrain from procedures that cause further suffering—provided, of course, that the
treatment offers the patient no overriding benefits. So, for instance,
the physician must refrain from ordering painful tests, therapies, or
surgical procedures when they cannot alleviate suffering or contribute to a patient's improvement or cure. Perhaps the most familiar
contemporary medical example is the treatment of burn victims

when survival is unprecedented; if with the treatments or without them the patient's chance of survival is nil, mercy requires the physician not to impose the debridement treatments, which are excruciatingly painful, when they can provide the patient no benefit at all.

Although the demands of mercy in burn contexts have become fairly well recognized in recent years,[5] other practices that the principles of mercy would rule out remain common. For instance, repeated cardiac resuscitation is sometimes performed even though a patient's survival is highly unlikely; although patients in arrest are unconscious at the time of resuscitation, it can be a brutal procedure, and if the patient regains consciousness, its aftermath can involve considerable pain. (On the contrary, of course, attempts at resuscitation would indeed be permitted under the principle of mercy if there were some chance of survival with good recovery, as in hypothermia or electrocution.) Patients are sometimes subjected to continued unproductive, painful treatment to complete a research protocol, to train student physicians, to protect the physician or hospital from legal action, or to appease the emotional needs of family members; although in some specific cases such practices may be justified on other grounds, in general they are prohibited by the principle of mercy. Of course, whether a painful test or therapy will actually contribute to some overriding good for the patient is not always clear. Nevertheless, the principle of mercy directs that where such procedures can reasonably be expected to impose suffering on the patient without overriding benefits for him or her, they ought not be done.

In many such cases, the patient will die whether or not the treatments are performed. In some cases, however, the principle of mercy may also demand withholding treatment that could extend the patient's life if the treatment is itself painful or discomforting and there is very little or no possibility that it will provide life that is pain-free or offers the possibility of other important goods. For instance, to provide respiratory support for a patient in the final, irreversible stages of a deteriorative disease may extend his life but will mean permanent dependence and incapacitation; though some patients may take continuing existence to make possible other important goods, for some patients continued treatment means the pointless imposition of continuing pain. "Death," whispered Abe Perlmutter, the Florida ALS victim who pursued through the courts his wish to have the tracheotomy tube connecting him to a respirator removed, "can't be any worse than what I'm going through now."[6] In such cases, the principle of mercy demands that the "treatments" no longer be imposed, and that the patient be allowed to die.

But the principle of mercy may also demand "letting die" in a still stronger sense. Under its second component, the principle asserts a duty to act to end suffering that is already occurring. Medicine already honors this duty through its various techniques of pain management, including physiological means like narcotics, nerve blocks, acupuncture, and neurosurgery, and psychotherapeutic means like self-hypnosis, conditioning, and good old-fashioned comforting care. But there are some difficult cases in which pain or suffering is severe but cannot be effectively controlled, at least as long as the patient remains sentient at all. Classical examples include tumors of the throat (where agonizing discomfort is not just a matter of pain but of inability to swallow, "air hunger," or acute shortness of breath), tumors of the brain or bone, and so on. Severe nausea, vomiting, and exhaustion may increase the patient's misery. In these cases, continuing life—or at least continuing consciousness—may mean continuing pain. Consequently, mercy's demand for euthanasia takes hold here: mercy demands that the pain, even if with it the life, be brought to an end.

Ending the pain, though with it the life, may be accomplished through what is usually called "passive euthanasia," withholding or withdrawing treatment that could prolong life. In the most indirect of these cases, the patient is simply not given treatment that might extend his or her life—say, radiation therapy in advanced cancer. In the more direct cases, life-saving treatment is deliberately withheld in the face of an immediate, lethal threat—for instance, antibiotics are withheld from a cancer patient when an overwhelming infection develops, since though either the cancer or the infection will kill the patient, the infection does so sooner and in a much gentler way. In all of the passive euthanasia cases, properly so called, the patient's life could be extended; it is mercy that demands that he or she be "allowed to die."

But the second component of the principle of mercy may also demand the easing of pain by means more direct than mere allowing to die; it may require *killing*. This is usually called "active euthanasia," and despite borderline cases (for instance, the ancient Greek practice of infanticide by exposure), it can in general be conceptually distinguished from passive euthanasia. In passive euthanasia, treatment is withheld that could support failing bodily functions, either in warding off external threats or in performing its own processes;

active euthanasia, in contrast, involves the direct interruption of on-going bodily processes that otherwise would have been adequate to sustain life. However, although it may be possible to draw a conceptual distinction between passive and active euthanasia, this provides no warrant for the ubiquitous view that killing is morally worse than letting die.[7] Nor does it support the view that withdrawing treatment is worse than withholding it. If the patient's condition is so tragic that continuing life brings only pain, and there is no other way to relieve the pain than by death, then the more merciful act is not one that merely removes support for bodily processes and waits for eventual death to ensue; rather, it is one that brings the pain—and the patient's life—to an end *now*. If there are grounds on which it is merciful not to prolong life, then there are also grounds on which it is merciful to terminate it at once. The easy overdose, the lethal injection (successors to the hemlock used for this purpose by non-Hippocratic physicians in ancient Greece[8]), are what mercy demands when no other means will bring relief.

But, it may be objected, the cases we have mentioned to illustrate intolerable pain are classical ones; such cases are controllable now. Pain is a thing of the medical past, and euthanasia is no longer necessary, though it once may have been, to relieve pain. Given modern medical technology and recent remarkable advances in pain management, the sufferings of the mortally wounded and dying can be relieved by less dramatic means. For instance, many once-feared, painful diseases—tetanus, rabies, leprosy, tuberculosis—are now preventable or treatable. Improvements in battlefield first-aid and transport of the wounded have been so great that the military *coup de grâce* is now officially obsolete. We no longer speak of "mortal agony" and "death throes" as the probable last scenes of life. Particularly impressive are the huge advances under the hospice program in the amelioration of both the physical and emotional pain of terminal illness,[9] and our culturewide fears of pain in terminal cancer are no longer justified: cancer pain, when it occurs, can now be controlled in virtually all cases. We can now end the pain without also ending the life.

This is a powerful objection, and one very frequently heard in medical circles. Nevertheless, it does not succeed. It is flatly incorrect to say that all pain, including pain in terminal illness, is or can be controlled. Some people still die in unspeakable agony. With superlative care, many kinds of pain can indeed be reduced in many patients, and adequate control of pain in terminal illness is often quite easy to achieve. Nevertheless, complete, universal, fully reliable pain control is a myth. Pain is not yet a "thing of the past," nor are many associated kinds of physical distress. Some kinds of conditions, such as difficulty in swallowing, are still difficult to relieve without introducing other discomforting limitations. Some kinds of pain are resistant to medication, as in elevated intracranial pressure or bone metastases and fractures. For some patients, narcotic drugs are dysphoric. Pain and distress may be increased by nausea, vomiting, itching, constipation, dry mouth, abscesses and decubitus ulcers that do not heal, weakness, breathing difficulties, and offensive smells. Severe respiratory insufficiency may mean—as Joanne Lynn describes it—"a singularly terrifying and agonizing final few hours."[10] Even a patient receiving the most advanced and sympathetic medical attention may still experience episodes of pain, perhaps alternating with unconsciousness, as his or her condition deteriorates and the physician attempts to adjust schedules and dosages of pain medication. Many dying patients, including half of all terminal cancer patients, have little or no pain,[11] but there are still cases in which pain management is difficult and erratic. Finally, there are cases in which pain control is theoretically possible but for various extraneous reasons does not occur. Some deaths take place in remote locations where there are no pain-relieving resources. Some patients are unable to communicate the nature or extent of their pain. And some institutions and institutional personnel who have the capacity to control pain do not do so, whether from inattention, malevolence, fears of addiction, or divergent priorities in resources.

In all these cases, of course, the patient can be sedated into unconsciousness; this does indeed end the pain. But in respect of the patient's experience, this is tantamount to causing death: the patient has no further conscious experience and thus can achieve no goods, experience no significant communication, satisfy no goals. Furthermore, adequate sedation, by depressing respiratory function, may hasten death. Thus, though it is always technically possible to achieve relief from pain, at least when the appropriate resources are available, the price may be functionally and practically equivalent, at least from the patient's point of view, to death. And this, of course, is just what the issue of euthanasia is about.

Of course, to see what the issue is about is not yet to reach its resolution, or to explain why attitudes about this issue are so starkly divergent. Rather, we must examine the logic of the argument for euthanasia and observe in particular how the principle of mercy functions in the overall case. The canon "One ought to act to end suffering," the second of the abstract duties generated by the principle of mercy, can be traced to the more general principle of beneficence. But its application in a given case also involves a minor premise that is ostensive in character: it points to an alleged case of suffering. This person is suffering, the applied argument from mercy holds, in a way that lays claim on us for help in relieving that pain.

It may be difficult to appreciate the force of this argument if its character is not adequately recognized. By asserting the abstract duty of mercy and pointing to specific occasions of pain, the argument generates the conclusion that we ought not let these cases of pain occur: not only ought we prevent them from occurring if we can, but also we ought to bring them to an end if they do. In practice, most arguments for euthanasia on grounds of mercy are pursued by the graphic evocation of cases: the tortures suffered by victims of awful diseases.

But this argument strategy is problematic. The evocation of cases may be very powerful, but it is also subject to a certain unreliability. After all, pain is, in general, not well remembered by those not currently suffering it, and though bystanders may be capable of very great sympathy, no person can actually feel another's pain. Suffering that does not involve pain may be even harder for the bystander to assess. Conversely, however, bystanders sometimes seem to suffer more than the patient: pain, particularly in those for whom one has strong emotional attachments, is notoriously difficult to watch. Furthermore, sensitivity on the part of others to pain and suffering is very much subject to individual differences in experience with pain, beliefs concerning the purpose of suffering and pain, fears about pain, and physical sensitivity to painful stimuli. Yet here is no objective way to establish how seriously the ostensive premise of the argument from mercy should be taken in any specific case, or how one should respond. Clearly, such a premise can be taken too seriously—so that concern for another's pain or suffering outweighs all other considerations—or one can be far too cavalier about the facts. To break a promise to a patient—say, not to intubate him—because you perceive that he is in pain may be to overreact to his suffering. However, it is morally repugnant to stand by and watch another person suffer when one could prevent it; and it is a moral failing too to be insensitive, when there is no overriding reason for doing so, to the fact that another person is in pain.

The principle of mercy holds that suffering ought to be relieved —unless, among other provisos, the suffering itself will give rise to some overriding benefit or unless the attainment of some benefit would be precluded by relieving the pain. But it might be argued that life itself is a benefit, always an overriding one. Certainly life is usually a benefit, one that we prize. But unless we accept certain metaphysical assumptions, such as "life is a gift from God," we must recognize that life is a benefit because of the experiences and interests associated with it. For the most part, we prize these, but when they are unrelievedly negative, life is not a benefit after all. Philippa Foot treats this as a conceptual point: "Ordinary human lives, even very hard lives, contain a minimum of basic goods, but when these are absent the idea of life is no longer linked to that of good."[12]

Such basic goods, she explains, include not being forced to work far beyond one's capacity; having the support of a family or community; being able to more or less satisfy one's hunger; having hopes for the future; and being able to lie down to rest at night. When these goods are missing, she asserts, the connection between *life* and *good* is broken, and we cannot count it as a benefit to the person whose life it is that his life is preserved.

These basic goods may all be severely compromised or entirely absent in the severely ill or dying patient. He or she may be isolated from family or community, perhaps by virtue of institutionalization or for various other reasons; he or she may be unable to eat, to have hopes for the future, or even to sleep undisturbed at night. Yet even for someone lacking all of what Foot considers to be basic goods, the experiences associated with life may not be unrelievedly negative. We must be very cautious in asserting of someone, even someone in the most abysmal-seeming conditions of the severely ill or dying, that life is no longer a benefit, since the way in which particular experiences, interests, and "basic goods" are valued may vary widely from one person to the next. Whether a given set of experiences constitutes a life that is a benefit to the person whose life it is is not a matter for *objective* determination, though there may be very good external clues to the way in which that person is in fact valuing them; it is, in the end, very much a function of subjective preference and choice. For some persons, life may be of value even in the grimmest conditions, for others, not. The crucial point is this: when a suffering person is conscious enough to have any experience at all, whether that experience counts as a benefit overriding the suffering or not is relative to that person and can be decided ultimately only by him or her.[13]

If this is so, then we can no longer assume that the cases in which euthanasia is indicated on grounds of mercy are infrequent or rare. It is true that contemporary pain management techniques do make possible the control of pain to a considerable degree. But unless pain and discomforting symptoms are eliminated altogether without loss of function, the underlying problem for the principle of mercy remains: how does *this* patient value life, how does he or she weigh death against pain? We are accustomed to assume that only patients suffering extreme, irremediable pain could be candidates for euthanasia at all and do not consider whether some patients might choose death in preference to comparatively moderate chronic pain, even when the condition is not a terminal one. Of course, a patient's perceptions of pain are extremely subject to stress, anxiety, fear, exhaustion, and other factors, but even though these perceptions may vary, the underlying weighing still demands respect. This is not just a matter of differing sensitivities to pain, but of differing values as well: for some patients, severe pain may be accepted with resignation or even pious joy, whereas for others mild or moderate discomfort is simply not worth enduring. Yet, without appeal to religious beliefs about the spiritual value of suffering, we have no objective way to determine how much pain a person *ought* to stand. Consequently, we cannot assume that euthanasia is justified, if at all, in only the most severe cases. Thus, the issue of euthanasia looms larger, rather than smaller, in the contemporary medical world.

That we cannot objectively determine whether life is a benefit to a person or whether pain outweighs its value might seem to undermine all possibility of appeal to the principle of mercy. But I think it does not. Rather, it shows simply that the issue is more complex, and that we must recognize that the principle of mercy itself demands recognition of a second fundamental principle relevant in euthanasia cases: the principle of autonomy. If the sufferer is the best judge of the relative values of that suffering and other benefits to himself, then his own choices in the matter of mercy ought to be respected. To impose "mercy" on someone who insists that despite his suffering life is still valuable to him would hardly be mercy; to withhold mercy from someone who pleads for it, on the basis that his life could still be worthwhile for him, is insensitive and cruel. Thus, the principle of mercy is conceptually tied to that of autonomy, at least insofar as what guarantees the best application of the principle—and hence, what guarantees the proper response to the ostensive premise in the argument from mercy—is respect for the patient's own wishes concerning the relief of his suffering or pain.

To this issue we now turn.

The Case for Euthanasia, Part II: Autonomy

The second principle supporting euthanasia is that of (patient) autonomy: *one ought to respect a competent person's choices, where one can do so without undue costs to oneself, where doing so will not violate other moral obligations, and where these choices do not threaten harm to other persons or parties.* This principle of autonomy, though limited by these provisos, grounds a person's right to have his or her own choices respected in determining the course of medical treatment, including those relevant to euthanasia: whether the patient wishes treatment that will extend life, though perhaps also suffering, or whether he or she wants the suffering relieved, either by being killed or by being allowed to die. It would of course also require respect for the choices of the person whose condition is chronic but not terminal, the person who is disabled though not dying, and the person not yet suffering at all, but facing senility or old age. Indeed, the principle of autonomy would require respect for self-determination in the matter of life and death in any condition at all, provided that the choice is freely and rationally made and does not harm others or violate other moral rules. Thus, the principle of autonomy would protect a much wider range of life-and-death acts than those we call euthanasia, as well as those performed for reasons of mercy.

Support for patient autonomy in matters of life and death is partially reflected in U.S. law, in which a patient's right to passive voluntary euthanasia (though it is not called by this name) is established in a long series of cases. In 1914, in the case *Schloendorff* v. *New York Hospital*,[14] Justice Cardozo asserted that "every human being of adult years and sound mind has a right to determine what shall be done with his own body" and held that the plaintiff, who had been treated against his will, had the right to refuse treatment; more recent cases, including *Yetter*,[15] *Perlmutter*,[16] and *Bartling*,[17] establish that the competent adult has the right to refuse medical treatment, on religious or personal grounds, even if it means he or she will die. (Exceptions include some persons with dependents and persons who suffer from communicable diseases that pose a risk to the public at large.) Furthermore, the patient has the right to refuse a component of a course of treatment, even though he or she consents to others; this is established in the Jehovah's Witnesses cases in which patients refused blood transfusions but accepted surgery and other care. In many states, the law also recognizes passive voluntary

euthanasia of the no longer competent adult who has signed a re-
fusal-of-treatment document while still competent; such documents, called "natural death directives" or "living wills," protect
the physician from legal action for failure to treat if he or she follows
the patient's antecedent request to be allowed to die. (By 1985, 35
states and the District of Columbia had enacted such laws.) Addi-
tionally, the "durable power of attorney" permits a person to designate a relative, friend, or other person to make treatment decisions
on his or her behalf after he or she is no longer competent; these
may include decisions to refuse life sustaining treatment. Many
hospitals have adopted policies permitting the writing of orders not
to resuscitate, or "no code" orders, which stipulate that no attempt
is to be made to revive a patient following a cardiorespiratory arrest.
These policies typically are stated to require that such orders be issued only with the concurrence of the patient, if competent, or the
patient's family or legal guardian. In theory at least, living wills, no-
code orders, durable powers of attorney, and similar devices are designed to protect the patient's voluntary choice to refuse life-prolonging treatment.

These legal mechanisms for refusal of treatment all protect individual autonomy in matters of euthanasia: the right to choose to
live or to die. But it is crucial to see that they all protect only passive
euthanasia, not any more active form. The Natural Death Act of
California, like similar legislation in other states, expressly states
that "nothing in this Act shall be construed to condone, authorize,
or approve mercy killing."[18] Likewise, the living will directs only
the withholding or cessation of treatment, in the absence of which
the patient will die.[19] A durable power of attorney permits the same
choices on behalf of the patient by a designated second party. These
legal mechanisms are sometimes said to protect the "right to die,"
but it is important to see that this is only the right to be *allowed* to
die, not to be helped to die or to have death actively brought about.
However, we have already seen that allowing to die is sometimes
less merciful than direct, humane killing: the principle of mercy demands the right to be killed, as well as to be allowed to die. Thus,
the protections offered by the legal mechanisms now available may
be seen as truncated conclusions from the principle of patient autonomy that supports them; this principle should protect not only
the patient's choice of refusal of treatment but also a choice of a
more active means of death.

It is often objected that autonomy in euthanasia choices should
not be recognized in practice, whether or not it is accepted in princi-

ple, because such choices are often erroneously made. One version of this argument points to physician error. Physicians make mistakes, it holds, and since medicine in any case is not a rigorous science, predictions of oncoming, painful death with no possibility of cure are never wholly reliable. People diagnosed as dying rapidly of inexorable cancers have survived, cancer-free, for dozens of years; people in cardiac failure or long-term irreversible coma have revived and regained full health. Although some of this can be attributed simply to physician error, we must also guard against the more pernicious phenomenon of the "hanging of crepe," in which the physician (usually not intentionally) delivers a prognosis dimmer than is actually warranted by the facts. If the patient succumbs, the physician cannot be blamed, since that is what was predicted; but if the patient survives, the physician is credited with the cure.[20] Other factors interfering with the accuracy of a diagnosis or prognosis include impatience on the part of a physician with a patient who is not doing well, difficulties in accurately estimating future complications, ignorance of a treatment or cure that is about to be discovered or is on the way, and a host of additional factors arising when the physician is emotionally involved, inexperienced, uninformed, or incompetent.[21]

A second argument pointing to the possibility of erroneous choice on the part of the patient asserts the very great likelihood of impairment of the patient's mental processes when seriously ill. Impairing factors include depression, anxiety, pain, fear, intimidation by authoritarian physicians or institutions, and drugs used in medical treatment that affect mental status. Perhaps a person in good health would be capable of calm, objective judgment even in such serious matters as euthanasia, so this view holds, but the person as patient is not. Depression, extremely common in terminal illness, is a particular culprit: it tends to narrow one's view of the possibilities still open; it may make recovery look impossible, it may screen off the possibilities, even without recovery, of significant human relationships and important human experience in the time that is left.[22] A choice of euthanasia in terminal illness, this view holds, probably reflects largely the gloominess of the depression, not the gravity of the underlying disease or any genuine intention to die.

If this is so, ought not the euthanasia request of a patient be ignored for his or her own sake? According to a limited paternalist view (sometimes called "soft" or "weak" paternalism), intervention in a person's choices for his or her own sake is justified if the person's thinking is impaired. Under this principle, not every euthanasia request should be honored; such requests should be construed, rather, as pleas for more sensitive physical and emotional care.

It is no doubt true that many requests to die are pleas for better care or improved conditions of life. But this still does not establish that all euthanasia requests should be ignored, because the principle of paternalism licenses intervention in a person's choices just *for his or her own good*. Sometimes the choice of euthanasia, though made in an impaired, irrational way, may seem to serve the person's own good better than remaining alive. Thus, since the paternalist, in intervening, must act for the sake of the person in whose liberty he or she interferes, the paternalist must take into account not only the costs for the person of failing to interfere with a euthanasia decision when euthanasia was not warranted (the cost is death, when death was not in this person's interests) but also the costs for that person of interfering in a decision that was warranted (the cost is continuing life—and continuing suffering—when death would have been the better choice).[23] The likelihood of these two undesirable outcomes must then be weighed. To claim that "there's always hope" or to insist that "the diagnosis could be wrong" in a morally responsible way, one must weigh not only the cost of unnecessary death to the patient but also the costs to the patient of dying in agony if the diagnosis is right and the cure does not materialize. But cases in which the diagnosis is right and the cure does not materialize are, unfortunately, much more frequent than cases in which the cure arrives or the diagnosis is wrong. The "there's always hope" argument, used to dissuade a person from choosing euthanasia, is morally irresponsible unless there is some quite good reason to think there actually *is* hope. Of course, the "diagnosis could be wrong" argument against euthanasia is a good one in areas or specialties in which diagnoses are frequently inaccurate (the chief of one neurology service admitted that on initial diagnoses "we get it right about 50 percent of the time"), or where there is a systematic bias in favor of unduly grim prognoses—but it is not a good argument against euthanasia in general. Similarly, "a miracle cure may be developed tomorrow" is also almost always irresponsible. The paternalist who attempts to interfere with a patient's choice of euthanasia must weigh the enormous suffering of those to whom unrealistic hopes are held out against the benefits to those very few whose lives are saved in this way.

As with limited paternalism, extended "strong" or "hard" paternalism—permitting intervention not merely to counteract impairment but also to avoid great harm—provides a special case when applied to euthanasia situations. The hard paternalist may be tempted to argue that because death is the greatest of harms, euthanasia choices must always be thwarted. But the initial premise of this argument is precisely what is at issue in the euthanasia dispute itself, as we've seen: is death the worst of harms that can befall a person, or is unrelieved, hopeless suffering a still worse harm? The principle of mercy obliges us to relieve suffering when it does not serve some overriding good; but the principle itself cannot tell us whether sheer existence—life—is an overriding good. In the absence of an objectively valid answer, we must appeal to the individual's own preferences and values. Which is the greater evil—death or pain? Some persons may adopt religious answers to this question, others may devise their own; but the answer always is tied to the person whose life it is, and cannot be supplied in any objective way. Hence, unless he or she can discover what the suffering person's preferences and values are, the hard paternalist cannot determine whether intervening to prolong life or to terminate it will count as acting for that person's sake.

Of course, there are limits to such a claim. When there is no evidence of suffering or pain, mental or physical, and no evidence of factors like depression, psychoactive drugs, or affect-altering disease that might impair cognitive functioning, an external observer usually can accurately determine whether life is a benefit: unless the person has an overriding commitment to a principle or cause that requires sacrifice of that life, life *is* a benefit to him or her. (But such a person, of course, is probably not a patient.) Conversely, when there is every evidence of pain and little or no evidence of factors that might outweigh the pain, such as cognitive capacities that might give rise to other valuable experience, then an external observer generally can also accurately determine the value of this person's life: it is a disbenefit, a burden, to him. (Given pain and complete cognitive incapacity, such a person is almost always a patient.) It is when both pain and cognitive capacities are found that the person-relative character of the value of life becomes most apparent, and most demanding of respect.

Thus, if we view the spectrum of persons from fully healthy through severely ill to decerebrate or brain-dead, we may assert that the principle of autonomy operates most strongly at the middle of this range. The more severe a person's pain and suffering, when his or her condition is not so diminished as to preclude cognitive capacities altogether, the stronger the respect we must accord his or her own view of whether life is a benefit or not. At both ends of the scale, however, paternalistic considerations come into play: if the person is healthy and without pain, we will interfere to keep him or her alive (preventing, for instance, suicide attempts); if his or her life means *only* pain, we act for the person's sake by causing him or her to die (as we should for certain severely defective neonates). But when the patient retains cognitive capacities, the greater is his or her suffering, and the more his or her choices concerning it deserve our respect. When the choice that is faced is death or pain, it is the patient who must choose which is worse.

We saw earlier that in euthanasia issues the principle of mercy is conceptually tied to the principle of autonomy, at least for its exercise; we now see that the principle of autonomy is dependent on the principle of mercy in certain sorts of cases. It is *not* dependent in this way, however, in those cases most likely to generate euthanasia requests. That someone voluntarily and knowingly requests release from what he or she experiences as misery is sufficient, other things being equal, for the request to be honored; although this request is rooted in the patient's desire for mercy, we cannot insist on independent, objective evidence that mercy would in fact be served, or that death is better than pain. We can demand such evidence to protect a perfectly healthy person, and we can summon it to end the sufferings of someone who can no longer choose; but we cannot demand it or use it for the seriously ill person in pain. To claim that an incessantly pain-racked but conscious person cannot make a rational choice in matters of life and death is to misconstrue the point: he or she, better than anyone else, can make such a choice, based on intimate acquaintance with pain and his or her own beliefs and fears about death. If the patient wishes to live, despite such suffering, he or she must be allowed to do so; or the patient must be granted help if he or she wishes to die.

But this introduces a further problem. The principle of autonomy, when there are no countervailing considerations on paternalistic grounds or on grounds of harm to others, supports the practice of voluntary euthanasia and, in fact, any form of rational, voluntary suicide. We already recognize a patient's right to refuse any or all medical treatment and hence correlative duties of noninterference on the part of the physician to refrain from treating the patient against his or her will. But does the patient's right of self-determination also give rise to any positive obligation on the part of the physician or other bystander to actively produce death? Pope John Paul II asserts that "no one may ask to be killed";[24] Peter Williams argues that a person does not have a right to be killed even though to kill him might be humane.[25] But I think that both the Pope and Williams are wrong. Although we usually recognize only that the principle of autonomy generates rights to noninterference, in some circumstances a right of self-determination does generate claims to assistance or to the provision of goods.

We typically acknowledge this in cases of handicap or disability. For instance, the right of a person to seek an education ordinarily generates on the part of others only an obligation not to interfere with his or her attendance at the university, provided the person meets its standards; but the same right on the part of a person with a severe physical handicap may generate an obligation on the part of others to provide transportation, assist in acquiring textbooks, or provide interpretive services. The infant, incapable of earning or acquiring its own nourishment, has a right to be fed. There is a good deal of philosophic dispute about such claims, and public policies vary from one administration and court to the next. But if, in a situation of handicap or disability, a right to self-determination can generate claim rights (rights to be aided) as well as noninterference rights, the consequences for euthanasia practices are far-reaching indeed. Some singularly sympathetic cases—like that of the completely paralyzed cerebral palsy victim Elizabeth Bouvier—have brought this issue to public attention. But notice that in euthanasia situations, most persons are handicapped with respect to producing for themselves an easy, "good," merciful death. The handicaps are occasionally physical, but most often involve lack of knowledge of how to bring this about and lack of access to means for so doing. If a patient chooses to refuse treatment and so die, he or she still may not know what components of the treatment to refuse in order to produce an easy rather than painful death; if the person chooses death by active means, he or she may not know what drugs or other methods would be appropriate, in what dosages, and in any case he or she may be unable to obtain them. Yet full autonomy is not achieved until one can both choose and act upon one's choices. It is here, in these cases of "handicap" that afflict many or most patients, that rights to self-determination may generate obligations on the part of physicians (provided, perhaps, that they do not have principled objections to participation in such activities themselves[26]). The physician's obligation is not only to respect the patient's choices but also to make it possible for the patient to act upon his or her choices. This means supplying the knowledge and equipment to enable the person to stay alive, if he or she so chooses; this is an obligation physicians now recognize. But it may also mean providing the knowledge, equipment, and help to enable the patient to die, if that is his or her choice; this is the other part of the physician's obligation, not yet recognized by the medical profession or the law in the United States.[27]

This is not to say that any doctor should be forced to kill any person who asks that: other contravening considerations—particularly that of ascertaining that the request is autonomous and not the product of coerced or irrational choice, and that of controlling abuses by unscrupulous physicians, relatives, or patients—would quickly override. Nor would the physician have an obligation to assist in "euthanasia" for someone not severely ill. But when the physician is sufficiently familiar with the patient to know the seriousness of the condition and the earnestness of the patient's request, when the patient is sufficiently helpless, and when there are no adequate objections on grounds of personal scruples or social welfare, then the principle of autonomy—like the principle of mercy—imposes on the physician the obligation to help the patient in achieving an easy, painless death.

The Case for Euthanasia, Part III: Justice

Although the term "euthanasia" traditionally was employed in cases in which "good death" meant the avoidance of suffering, in recent years use of the term has been extended to cover cases in which the patient is neither suffering nor capable of choosing to die. Ruth Russell, for instance, includes among cases of euthanasia the ending of "a meaningless existence."[28] For Beauchamp and Davidson, euthanasia can be the termination of an irreversibly comatose state.[29] Termination of the lives of the brain-dead, the permanently comatose, and those who are, as Paul Ramsey puts it, "irretrievably inaccessible to human care"[30] is justified, it is argued, under the principle of justice: euthanasia permits fairer distribution of medical resources in a society that lacks sufficient resources to provide maximum care for all. Once this principle is invoked, however, it may seem that it also applies in cases in which the patient is still competent: to permit earlier, easier dying will be favored not only on grounds of mercy and autonomy but on grounds of justice as well.

Drawing on the principle of mercy advanced earlier, we may assert that each person, by virtue of his or her medical illness, injury, defect, or other medical abnormality that causes pain or suffering, has a claim on whatever medical resources might be effective in the full treatment of his or her condition: since we have an obligation (subject to the provisos mentioned above) to relieve the person's suffering, he or she has a correlative claim (subject to corresponding provisos) to whatever medical treatment can be used. But since there are not enough resources to supply full treatment for every condition for every person, and since the resources typically cannot be subdivided in a way that makes equal apportionment of them possible (half an operation will do you no good), full treatment can be devoted only to some conditions, or only to some persons. In a scarcity situation, not all competing claims can be satisfied, and a principle of distributive justice must be invoked to adjudicate among them.

Various principles can be proposed for allocating medical resources: to those in greatest medical need, to those for whom restoration of function would be most complete; to those who can pay; to those whose societal contributions are or have been greatest; to those who have been most deprived of medical care in the past; to those whose conditions are not self-induced (this might rule out people suffering from smokers' diseases, conditions exacerbated by obesity, suicide attempts, and perhaps venereal diseases and high-risk sports injuries); or to those who are the winners in a coin toss, lottery, or other system of random selection. Alternatively, treatment could be allocated on the basis of the medical condition involved: to end-stage kidney patients, for instance, but not to those with deteriorative heart disease. But, unless we expand the size of the resources pool, treatment will still be denied to some, *whatever* distributive principle is adopted. Hence, whatever the principle (except perhaps one that allocates all available resources simply to staving off death for the last few minutes in every medical condition), some of those denied treatment will die sooner than otherwise would be the case. But this, it can be argued, would be unjust, since it would impose earlier death on some persons on the basis of characteristics that are not legitimate grounds for death—ability to pay, and so on. Rather, it is often argued, if treatment is to be denied to some people with the result that they will die, it is better to deny it just to those people who are (loosely speaking) medically unsalvageable and will die soon anyway: the terminally ill, the extremely aged, and the seriously defective neonate. The practices of euthanasia in accord with this principle—which we shall call the salvageability principle—is justified, this argument then concludes, by the demands of justice in a scarcity situation.

Of course, to deny treatment to a dying patient on grounds of justice cannot properly be called "euthanasia" in the traditional sense, since it is not done for the sake of the patient or to provide a "good death." A congressional decision not to fund artificial heart research or not to provide Medicaid/Medicare payments for heart transplants can hardly be called "euthanasia" for those heart patients who will die. However, as we saw at the outset of this section, policies involving withholding treatment are frequently called "euthanasia" when practiced on the permanently comatose, the brain-dead, the profoundly retarded, or others in non-sapient states. Despite the abuse of the term under the Nazi regime, our linguistic usage is again undergoing rapid change, and it is apparent that we are coming to use the term "euthanasia" not just for pain-sparing deaths but for resource-conserving deaths as well. It is in this newer sense that we can argue that justice requires the practice of euthanasia in certain kinds of scarcity situations.

The argument from justice, though not always put forward in a coherent, comprehensive way, is often initiated with a recitation of facts. The hospital bill for a 500-gram newborn with serious deficits, it is said, may run somewhere between $60,000 and $80,000, or even more than $100,000; this does not by any means guarantee that the infant will survive or live a normal life. The cost of a coronary bypass, a procedure frequently employed even when it does not extend life expectancy (though it greatly increases the quality of life), is somewhere around $30,000. The bill for a series of bone marrow transplants may run to $80,000, even though the transplants may not succeed in staving off death. According to a study published late in 1981, the average intensive care unit bill (total hospital charges, plus ancillary charges) was $7,112—for patients who survived.[31] But for patients who died, the bill was more than double, a staggering $15,874. A vast proportion of medical costs are incurred during the final year of life (this includes unsalvageable neonates as well as adults), most of it in the last few weeks or days. Justice, under the distributive principle articulated above, demands that the dying be allowed to die, and these resources be given instead to other, salvageable competitors for full health care.

This is not to suggest that the dying should be denied palliative and comfort care: indeed, if their claims to therapeutic treatment diminish, the principle of mercy demands that their claims to palliative care increase. Nor is it to suggest that the dying "do not deserve" medical care that could prolong their lives. All parties in the distribution have prima facie claims to care, under the principle of justice, but the claims of the dying are weakest.

This argument from justice is usually employed only to justify the denial of treatment, that is, to justify passive euthanasia; but similar considerations also favor active euthanasia. Passive euthanasia is often practiced upon unsalvageable patients by withholding treatment if a medical crisis occurs: for instance, no-code orders are issued, or pneumonias are not treated, or electrolyte imbalances not corrected if they occur. If justice demands that, despite the prima facie claims of these patients, the resources allocated to their care are better assigned somewhere else, then we must notice that *passive* euthanasia does not provide the most just redistribution of these resources. To "allow" the patient to die may still involve enormous expenditures of money, scarce supplies, or caregiver time. This is most evident in cases of "irretrievably inaccessible" patients, for whom no considerations of mercy or autonomy override the demands of justice in weighing claims. The cost of maintaining a coma patient in a nursing home without heroic treatment is somewhere around $15,000 a year; the cost for a profoundly retarded resident of a state institution is more than $20,000. Whole-brain-dead patients may survive on life supports in hospital settings from several hours to a few days or more; upper-brain-dead patients may live for years. The total cost of maintaining a permanently comatose woman, who was injured in a riding accident in 1956 at age twenty-seven and died eighteen years later, has been estimated at just over $6,000,000; this care provided her with not a single moment of conscious life.[32] The record survival for a coma patient is thirty-seven years and 111 days.[33] The argument from justice demands that these patients, since their claims for care are so weak as to have virtually no force at all, be killed, not simply allowed to die.

Objection to the Argument from Justice: The Slippery Slope

But if justice, under the distributive principle employed here, licenses the killing of permanently comatose patients, will it not also license the killing of still-conscious, still-competent dying patients, perhaps still salvageable, close or not so close to death? What extensions of the scope of this principle might be made, should resources become still more scarce? These concerns introduce the "wedge" or "slippery slope" argument, which holds that although some acts of euthanasia may be morally permissible (say, on grounds of mercy or autonomy), to allow them to occur will set a logical precedent for, or will causally result in, consequences that are morally repugnant.[34] Just as Hitler's 1938 "euthanasia" program for mentally defective, senile, and terminally ill Aryans paved the way for the establishment of the extermination camps several years later, it is argued, so permissive euthanasia policies invite irreversible descent down that slippery slope that leads to mass murder. Indeed, to permit even the most humane euthanasia may do more than set a precedent: by accustoming doctors to ending life, by supplying death technology, by changing the expectations of family members or other guardians of those who become candidates for death, and by changing the expectations of patients themselves, the practice of euthanasia even in humane cases may lead to moral holocaust.

As it is usually posed, the form of the argument that points to the Nazi experience does not succeed: the forces that brought the mass extermination camps into being were not *caused* by the earlier euthanasia program, and, other things being equal, the extermination camps for Jews would no doubt have been established had there been no euthanasia program at all. To argue that permitting euthanasia now will lead to death camps like Hitler's is to overlook the many other political, social, and psychological factors of the Nazi period. Yet the wedge argument cannot be simply discarded; the factors operating to favor the slide from morally warranted euthanasia to murder are probably much stronger than we realize. They are best seen, I think, as misunderstandings or corruptions of the very principles that favor euthanasia: mercy, autonomy, and perhaps most prominently, justice.

A contemporary version of the wedge argument holds that to permit euthanasia at all—including cases justified on grounds of mercy, autonomy, or justice—will in the presence of strong financial incentives lead to circumstances in which people are killed who are not suffering or who do not wish to die. Furthermore, to permit some doctors to allow their patients to die or to kill them would invite cavalier attitudes concerning the lives of the patients and, in addition to financial incentives, ordinary greed, insensitivity, hastiness, and self-interest, would cause some doctors to let their patients die—or kill them—when there was no moral warrant for doing so.[35] Doctors treating difficult or unresponding patients would find an easy way out. Medical blunders could be more easily covered up, and doctors might use euthanasia as a way of avoiding criticism in cases that were medically difficult to treat. Particularly important, perhaps, are societal and political pressures, most evident in cost-containment policies, to which doctors might respond.

After all, to permit earlier, less expensive death would ease the enormous pressures on third-party insurers, public welfare, and the Social Security system: euthanasia is less expensive than continuing medical care. The recently introduced DRG (diagnosis-related group) reimbursement system would particularly favor this since a hospital profits most from the patient who remains hospitalized for the shortest amount of time, but loses money on the one who remains longer than what is average for the DRG. Although passive euthanasia is cheaper than continuing life-prolonging treatment, active euthanasia is cheaper still: killing is the least expensive, most resource-conserving treatment of intractable disease.

Is there any reason to think such practices would actually occur? The reasons are closer to hand than one might imagine. Rather than predicting the future, we need simply look to our present practices for evidence that violations of the moral limits to euthanasia can occur. It is tempting to reply to a wedge argument against any social practice that we will always be able to draw a moral line when the time comes, but the clear evidence in the case of euthanasia is that we are not managing to do so now.

First, contemporary euthanasia practices sometimes involve violations of the principle of mercy. These violations are of two forms, neither conspicuous because neither involves evident physical cruelty. Nevertheless, both are cases of euthanasia that the principle of mercy does not endorse. First, there are cases in which the rhetoric of euthanasia, with its concept of painless, easy death, is used though considerations of mercy cannot possibly apply: these are the cases of the permanently comatose or brain-dead. Since these persons do not suffer, euthanasia as the granting of mercy cannot be practiced upon them, and we mislead ourselves if we claim that they are "better off" dead. Second, there are cases in which the principle of mercy is violated when more than enough relief is given to those who do suffer. The principle of mercy demands euthanasia *only* when no other means of relieving pain will suffice. Yet we fail to acknowledge that the continuous, very heavy use of narcotizing drugs can be functionally equivalent to mercy killing itself: when used in a sustained way, without drug-free, conscious intervals or careful titration against alertness, such therapy effectively ends the patient's sentient life: his or her existence as a person ends when the drugging begins.[36] Of course, it may sometimes be difficult to obtain adequate and effective narcotics; nevertheless, because we do not recognize such drugging as equivalent in some respects to *active* euthanasia, we may be incautious and hasty in its use.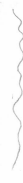

Contemporary euthanasia practices sometimes also involve violations of the principle of autonomy. It is true that much euthanasia, both passive and active, occurs at the request or with the consent of the individual who dies; such practices are provided for in natural death legislation and the use of durable powers of attorney and living wills. But we are also beginning to see the widespread development of hospital policies concerning nonresuscitation, and more frequent, routine physician exercise of this practice. It may even be fair to speak of a widespread consensus that in certain cases, nonresuscitation is the appropriate response. Official policies require that the patient, if competent, or his or her legal guardian be consulted before nonresuscitation orders are written. But such directives are by no means always followed. In Salt Lake City recently (though the story is universal), a physician reminded the granddaughter of an alert, competent eighty-nine-year-old nursing home patient, "You can always have 'do not resuscitate' orders written into her record." ("Why don't you ask her if that's what she wants?" was the granddaughter's reply.) A Stanford University cardiologist says, in contrast, that he would not make such a suggestion to the family—because he "wouldn't want to put them through that"; this physician writes no-code orders on his own, without consulting either patient or family. In some places, no-code orders are written in pencil, so that they can be erased from records if desired; or circumlocutions not intelligible to laypersons ("consult primary physician before initiating treatment") are used.

Most significant among our current euthanasia practices may be the violations of justice. The argument from justice, as discussed so far, favors permitting euthanasia on the grounds that denial of treatment is morally permissible in certain specific cases: those in which the claims of a dying individual to medical resources are overridden by the claims of others in medical need. However, we often see the use of distributive policies that deny treatment to some but do not involve either the weighing of claims between the dying and others or the assurance that resources conserved would in fact be redistributed in accord with justice. The congressional decisions concerning artificial and transplant heart care may be one kind of example; arbitrary age minimums and ceilings for transplants, pacemakers, and dialysis, when they are not medically appropriate, may be another. Yet distributive justice concerns the point at which a dying person's right to medical treatment is outweighed by the claims of others; the distributive principle we considered did not hold that dying deprives one altogether of rights to medical care. In a situation of dire scarcity, like urgent organ transplants, denying a transplant to one person usually means granting a transplant to someone else; if without it each person would die, the distributive principle of salvageability considered here holds that the person more likely to survive and benefit from the procedure has the stronger claim. But many distributive policies do not involve this kind of direct weighing of claims or assurances of reallocation, and much denial of treatment is done simply for thrift. *Thrift,* however, is not the same as *justice in distribution.* To deny treatment to the dying to "conserve resources" or to "save money" is not to show that the claims of the dying are overridden by stronger claims on the part of someone else, or a group of persons, to whom such resources would in fact be redistributed; yet it is this point that is essential in preserving the principle of justice as applied to euthanasia.

In all these areas, then, we see evidence of "euthanasia" practices not justified by moral principle. Given these facts, the wedge argument and its objection to permitting euthanasia may loom larger. We may recall that the wedge argument forecasts a slide down the slippery slope from morally permissible practices to impermissible ones. But if we accept its model at all, there is no reason to assume that we are still at the top of this slope; indeed, the evidence available suggests that we are already slipping. We already engage in "euthanasia" practices not justified on grounds of mercy, autonomy, or justice, and there is no reason to think that such abuses will not become still more widespread.

Nevertheless, I do not agree with the conclusion of the slippery slope argument: that because permissible euthanasia practices would lead (or are leading) to impermissible ones, we ought not allow them at all. We should not cease no-coding; mercy demands it. We should not restrict refusal of treatment or insist that all who can conceivably benefit be given as much treatment as possible; respect for autonomy requires that the patient be permitted to determine what is done to him or her. We should not resist legislative protections for passive euthanasia, like living wills and natural death laws, or oppose legislation permitting voluntary active euthanasia: justice, mercy, and autonomy all demand that euthanasia—both passive and active—be legally protected. Although the wedge argument is a serious one, prohibiting euthanasia is not the appropriate conclusion.

Most advocates of the wedge argument overlook a crucial feature of the structure of the argument itself. The wedge argument is teleological in character: it points to the bad consequence of permitting a morally acceptable type of action (call it A), namely that a morally unacceptable type (B) occurs. But users of the wedge argument err in failing to recognize that B's occurrence is not the sole outcome of A; A and B are *distinct* actions, each with its own set of consequences. Thus, in deciding whether to permit A, one must reckon in the bad consequences of the occurrence of B, but must also reckon in the other, possibly good consequences of A. Or, if one is deciding to prohibit A, the reckoning will include the (good) effects of avoiding B, but must also include the other (bad) effects of not having A occur. The wedge argument against euthanasia usually takes the form of an appeal to the welfare or rights of those who would become victims of later, unjustified practices. Usually, however, when the conclusion is offered that euthanasia therefore ought not be permitted, no account is taken of the welfare or rights of those who are to be denied the benefits of this practice. Hence, even if the causal claims advanced in the wedge argument are true and we are not able to hold the line or avoid the slide, they still do not establish the conclusion. Rather, the argument sets up a conflict. Either we ignore the welfare and abridge the rights of persons for whom euthanasia would clearly be morally permissible in order to protect those who would be the victims of corrupt euthanasia practices, or we ignore the potential victims in order to extend mercy and respect for autonomy to those who are the current victims of euthanasia prohibitions.

Thus, this conflict itself reveals an issue of justice still more fundamental than the distributive problems with which we have begun. The wedge argument assumes, without adequate justification, that the rights of those who may become the victims of abuses of a practice outweigh the rights of those who become victims if a practice is prohibited to whose benefits they are morally entitled and urgently need.

To protect those who might wrongly be killed or allowed to die might seem a stronger obligation than to satisfy the wishes of those who desire release from pain, analogous perhaps to the principle in law that "better ten guilty men go free than one be unjustly convicted."[37] However, the situation is not in fact analogous and does not favor protecting those who might wrongly be killed. To let ten guilty men go free in the interests of protecting one innocent man is not to impose harm on the ten guilty men. But to require the person who chooses to die to stay alive in order to protect those who might unwillingly be killed sometime in the future is to impose an extreme harm—intolerable suffering—on that person, which he or she must bear for the sake of others. Furthermore, since, as we've seen, the question of which is worse, suffering or death, is person-relative, we have no independent, objective basis for protecting the class of persons who might be killed at the expense of those who would suffer intolerable pain; perhaps our protecting ought to be done the other way around. Thus we return to the recurrent problem throughout our discussions: which is the worse of two evils, death or pain? Since there are no prior agreements or claims that are relevant here, justice requires that rights to avoid the worse of the two evils be honored first, before others come into play. This, however, may be an obligation that, because it is person-relative and hence resistant to policy construction, we do not know how to meet.

Justice and Realistic Desire

Is there a workable solution to the problem that euthanasia poses? Certainly we can make some progress by attending to the violations of principle we have discovered. First, we must improve the conditions of dying; mercy will not demand euthanasia, nor the autonomous person choose it, when the conditions of dying are humane. Cicely Saunders, the founder of St. Christopher's Hospice in England and an ardent opponent of euthanasia, is perfectly right when she says of euthanasia, "one should be working to see that it is not needed."[38] Second, we need to improve the quality of the mercy we extend by attending to the element of autonomy in it: we must learn to respond to suffering in a way that takes account of the patient's own wishes and tolerances for pain, so that we give neither too little relief nor too much. Third, we must broaden our respect of autonomy in matters of dying by recognizing that the patient may choose active as well as passive means of coming to die —or none at all. It is crucial that the dying person receive full information about the consequences of accepting treatment or refusing it, so that he or she can rationally choose the way of dying —or staying alive—most in accord with his or her own values.[39] After all, a "good death" must always be a death that counts as good for the patient. For some it is the least painful, for others it is the quickest, for others one that permits final communication with family, and for still others the one that can be delayed the longest possible time. In this most personal of matters, a person's choice deserves the greatest respect.

But attention to mercy and autonomy does not yet seem to solve the problem of justice: the problems of whose rights are to be honored, and who is to be denied care. We saw earlier that all the workable distributive principles we might adopt would have the effect of forcing death on some persons who do not want it—those who cannot pay, those who have made no societal contributions, etc. Even the most plausible of these principles—the salvageability principle—would force earlier death upon the already dying, some of whom may wish to die but some of whom, under their own conception of the relative disvalue of suffering and death, want to continue as long as they possibly can. Thus, I think that the salvageability principle too is in error. Rather, we should favor a distributive principle that would allocate medical resources to whose who want treatment, where "wanting" is interpreted as "realistic desire." This is to say, realistic desire ought to be considered both a necessary and a sufficient condition for providing treatment for those who are seriously ill.

To desire medical treatment in a realistic, reasonable, or rational way, the patient must not only actually have or be about to contract the condition for which treatment is proposed but also must understand the treatment's intended purposes, its possible side effects, the probability of success or failure, and the possible end condition to which the treatment would lead. For, say, an appendectomy, the patient must not only have appendicitis but also must understand at least roughly the nature of the procedure, what could go wrong, the approximate likelihood of success, and the end condition: relief of the acute pain in the abdomen, avoidance of death, and a small scar on the side. In most cases of acute appendicitis, an appendectomy will be the object of realistic desire. In a few cases, however, it is not, such as when the patient believes on religious grounds that the end condition of accepting medical treatment or a blood transfusion includes eventual damnation. Although religious cases are comparatively rare, there are many cases in which the principle of realistic desire would require substantial changes in our current distribution of medical care. Life-prolonging care given to the permanently comatose, decerebrate, profoundly brain-damaged, and others who lack cognitive function is not, even in the case of antecedently executed directives, realistically desire: since such patients cannot want it, they are not entitled to life-prolonging care. Not even supportive care—like feeding or routine hygiene—should be supplied, since this too cannot be realistically desired; patients in these extreme conditions should be allowed—or caused—to die.

Withholding care from permanently comatose patients may not seem morally problematic. But in a serious illness in which a cure cannot be guaranteed yet the patient remains competent, the problem becomes much more complex. Do patients with cancer of the larynx, for instance, *want* surgical treatment that, while providing a better-than-half chance of survival three years later, entails the permanent destruction of the normal voice? Most do, but, according to one study, at least 20 percent do not.[40] In such situations, the new distributive principle articulated here apportions treatment solely on the basis of a patient's desires, not on characteristics like age or social worth. Most patients will receive appendectomies; four-fifths will have surgery on the larynx; permanently comatose patients will receive no care at all.

Would a distributive principle of realistic desire be effective in a scarcity situation? Although one's initial impression may be to the contrary, I believe that it would. It is crucial to remember that medical treatment is not like any ordinary consumer good; getting more of it does not entail that your advantages are increased. (Indeed, in an ideal lifetime, the amount of therapeutic medical treatment a person realistically wants is zero; this is the mark of the perfectly healthy life.) The treatments that are less likely to be realistically desired are, generally speaking, precisely those likely to occur at the end of life—the heroic, last-ditch, odds-against measures, undertaken because nothing else has worked. The chances are that the procedures will be painful, that they will introduce new limitations, and that they will not succeed. And the chance is also that these treatments will be extremely expensive. It is not possible to tell whether the savings in treatment costs under such a distributive policy would make it possible to provide full treatment for all who do want it, but there is no reason to *assume* that such savings would not: we need only recall the huge financial costs for nonsurvivors in an intensive care unit, for severely defective, unsalvageable neonates, or for permanently comatose patients in a nursing home or institution. A vast proportion of medical costs, as stated before, occurs in the last year of life. Most of this can be described as "needed" treatment. No doubt much of this is also "wanted" treatment, but much of it is not.

If use of the "realistic desire" distributive principle should prove inadequate to solve the scarcity problem, then an additional distributive principle would need to be adopted to resolve conflicting claims among competitors who all realistically desired treatment: the salvageability principle, denying treatment to those who will die soon anyway, might then be brought into play. But those who will die soon may nevertheless want every moment of life they can possibly get, and it is unacceptable to adopt a distributive principle that has the effect of depriving some persons of wanted life before there is clear need to do so.

Of course, a distributive principle of realistic desire must have built into it paternalistic proxy procedures for providing medical care for incompetents of a variety of sorts, including infants and children, unconscious accident victims, the mentally ill, and the retarded. But I believe that these procedures should *not* include persons who are capable of realistic desire in the matter of terminal care but who have failed to consider and articulate their desires. Rather, it is becoming apparent that the individual has an obligation, increasingly evident as advances in medical technology both exacerbate the scarcity situation and offer heroic life-prolonging treatment that may not be desired, to stipulate in advance which modes of treatment he or she will accept and which he or she will decline, insofar as the patient's probable future can be foreseen. Only about one death in ten is wholly unexpected,[41] and most result from prolonged, chronic illnesses. Thus, most deaths can be predicted, within a fairly limited range of possibilities, before the event, and the course of the dying in certain general ways anticipated. What, most basically, the patient is obliged to do is indicate, as fully as possible which he or she takes to be worse in situations that can be forseen: pain or death. From this basic choice the treatment alternatives appropriate to the patient's condition can be deduced. By failing to exercise this obligation, the individual may force others—his or her physician, family members, or the courts —to make what are often morally precarious euthanasia decisions for him or her, perhaps on the basis of self-interest, societal pressure, or distributive principles for which there is no moral warrant. Since the patient has rights to medical treatment that he or she realistically desires and since it is the corresponding obligation of others to distribute treatment in accord with these desires, it is in turn the obligation of the patient to make his or her desires known whenever it is possible to do so.

However, it is particularly important to notice that continuous sedation is *not* an option the patient may choose, nor is it a defensible general solution to the problem of euthanasia. The patient's autonomous requests must still conform to the demands of justice, particularly as specified for medical situations by the principle of realistic desire. It is true that continuous sedation may satisfy both the principles of mercy and autonomy, but because there is no ongoing experience or sentient end state to which the treatment leads, the patient cannot realistically desire the treatment that would maintain him. Of course, there may be many cases in which the patient's condition is potentially reversible or the sedation can be interrupted to permit further personal experience, and in these circumstances sedation may indeed be realistically preferred to either pain or death (given the difficulty of accurately predicting circumstances in which continuous sedation will be permanently required without any hope of intervening lucidity, such cases may be the rule rather than the exception); in these cases the patient retains his or her claim to care. There may also be certain special situations in which the needs of, say, family members or transplant recipients outweigh the claims of other patients competing for resources, so that justice will permit maintaining a patient in continuous sedation on the same basis as it might in rare cases permit maintaining a patient who is permanently comatose. But when such conditions do not obtain, even the patient who articulates his or her choices in advance is not entitled to request *permanent* sedation, since the principle of realistic desire prohibits him or her, like the proverbial dog in the manger, from laying claim to resources he or she cannot possibly enjoy. Nor may physicians turn to continuous sedation as a way of avoiding difficult moral dilemmas in terminal care (except, of course, in the frequent situations in which they think that their predictions may be wrong); they are bound to honor the choices of a patient made in accord with the principle of realistic desire, but this principle does not permit such a choice. At least in any scarcity situation, the patient must choose either death or periodically sentient life, though this may involve pain; he or she cannot morally choose to be maintained in a permanently sedated or unconscious state when that means depriving someone else of care.

Conclusion: Euthanasia and Suicide

It may be objected that requiring the patient to choose between death and life, insofar as the patient must antecedently consider treatment decisions that affect the circumstances and timing of his or her own demise, is equivalent to requiring the patient's consideration of suicide. In a sense, it is; but this is also the more general solution to the euthanasia problem. Although euthanasia is indeed warranted on grounds of mercy, autonomy, and justice, these principles can be more effectively and safely honored by permitting suicide, perhaps assisted by the physician who has care of the patient or a family member under the advice of the physicians,[42] and supplemented by nonvoluntary euthanasia *only* when the patient is permanently comatose or otherwise irretrievably inaccessible. Not only do practical reasons like avoiding greed and manipulation on the part of physicians or the institutions controlling them speak for preferring physician-assisted suicide to physician-initiated euthanasia, but there are conceptual reasons as well. The conditions that distinguish morally permissible euthanasia from impermissible murder all involve matters that the patient, not the physician, is in a privileged position to know. To extend mercy, the physician must know how the patient weighs suffering against death, and at what point *for the patient* death becomes the lesser of two evils. To respect the patient's autonomy, the physician must know what his or her preferences are, given the alternatives available, in the matter of dying. And to exercise justice, the physician must know what treatment the patient realistically desires. Perhaps the physician who is painstakingly careful in listening to an articulate and self-aware patient may discover these things, but he or she cannot have the patient's knowledge. Consequently, since the risk of misinterpretation is great and the possibility of manipulation or coercion high, the physician should not be the one to *initiate* the choice. Rather, he or she must be prepared to assist the patient who chooses death, just as he or she is prepared to assist the patient who chooses continuing life. In physician-assisted suicide, it is the person whose death is in question who is responsible for the death; he or she originates and chooses this course of action, rather than having death chosen for him or her. To permit suicide of course increases the risk of encouraging ill-considered suicide among emotionally disturbed or mentally ill persons, but here the physician serves as a check: in the role of assistant to the suicide, the physician will refuse to assist whenever in his or her professional perception the circumstances clearly do not warrant such an act (such as in cases in which there is neither pain nor approaching death, but not in those exhibiting one or both). This is by no means a foolproof policy; the physician will no doubt often influence the patient. But this intrusion is still a far cry from having the physician decide when or why euthanasia is appropriate and initiate the act.

Furthermore, physician-assisted suicide is less subject to the erection of policy requirements than are euthanasia practices. The choices of patients about whether and how to die will vary widely; but then, there is no reason why they should not. These choices are influenced by an enormous range of individual values, past experiences, and moral and religious beliefs. Euthanasia policies developed by physicians or medical institutions may overlook individual differences in patients' wishes by establishing routine, common procedures for dealing with terminal illness, and in this way invite the continuing slide down the slippery slope. We must be prepared to permit and perform mercy killing when the patient desires it and when there is no other way to avoid the sufferings of death. But we do not want doctors to assume the responsibility for such killings, or to appeal to standardized, court-approved procedures, made under economic constraints, for determining when such killings are appropriate. Rather, mercy killing must ideally always be mercy killing of the patient by him- or herself, in which the patient is entitled to the assistance of the physician he or she has chosen. When proxy procedures are required, we must be sure that they approximate as nearly as possible what the person's own decision would have been. It is crucial to exercise mercy; it is essential to respect autonomy, and though we must submit to the demands of justice, we can hope to do so at no one's expense. It is extremely important to avoid any further slide down the involuntary thrift-euthanasia slope. Recognition of physician-assisted suicide, as distinguished from physician-directed euthanasia, comes closest to satisfying all of these moral demands.

After all, we must not forget that we already practice euthanasia on quite a wide scale, but we do not always practice it in a morally defensible way. We practice passive euthanasia by withholding and withdrawing treatment, and we practice active quasi-euthanasia by using sedation sufficient to terminate the personal existence of a human being. Some of this is in accord with the principles of mercy, autonomy, and justice, but much of it is not. What grows dimmer in contemporary practice is the sense that euthanasia, as "good death," must be good *for the person whose death it is;* we are losing any sense that mercy must play a major role or that the patient's choice is crucial in determining whether that death counts as good. Already we are beginning to count resource-conserving deaths under this term. Paul Ramsey remarks that "it is better if you do not know the Greek language or the root meaning of the word"[43];—but, of course, knowing these things permits us to see the shifts in our use of the term, shifts that are perhaps symptomatic of the slide already under way down the slippery slope. Our very language invites us to overlook distinctions that we ought to make. The concept of euthanasia has come to include letting patients die and killings that are not required by mercy, autonomy, or justice, but are simply the product of thrift in medical affairs. Yet at the same time our discomfort with this fact leads us to claim, at least officially, that we reject any practice of euthanasia at all, though of course this is not true. In this way, the increasing distortion of the term itself leads us to overlook a double moral fault: often, we practice "euthanasia" when we should not, and very often, we fail to practice euthanasia when we should.

Notes

Acknowledgments: I'd like to thank Arthur G. Lipman, Pharm. D., and Howard Wilcox, M.D., as well as my colleagues in philosophy, Bruce Landesman and Leslie Francis, for comments on earlier drafts of this paper.

1. Perhaps the principle of (medical) mercy is stronger than this and asserts a duty to relieve the suffering of others even at some substantial cost to oneself, or in violation of others of these provisos. The quite weak form of the principle, as I have stated it here, requires for instance that one ought not stand idly by (all other things being equal) when one could easily help an injured person but does not require feats of physical or financial heroism or self-sacrifice. This is not to say that I think a stronger version of the duty to relieve suffering (as defended, for instance, by Susan James, "The Duty to Relieve Suffering," *Ethics* [October 1982] 93:4–21), could not be supported, but that the stronger version is not necessary for the case I am making here: a duty to participate in both passive and active euthanasia, at least in a more permissive legal climate, is entailed even by the very weak form of the principle of mercy.

Incidentally, although much of the medical literature distinguishes between pain and suffering, I have not chosen to do so here: it would raise difficult mind/body problems, and in any case the two are clearly intertwined. I grant, however, that the principle of (medical) mercy would meet still broader assent if phrased to require the relieving of physical pain alone.

2. It is important not to confuse the principle of (medical) mercy with a principle permitting or requiring judicial mercy. In judicial and political contexts, such as pardons or amnesties, the individual on whom penalties have been or are about to be imposed may have no claim to benevolent treatment, and the issue concerns whether mercy may or should be granted. Many authors treat judicial mercy as a work of individual supererogation, not a requirement or duty, and some suggest that it is morally forbidden: one ought not excuse a person guilty of a crime. However, we are concerned here not with judicial mercy, but rather with mercy as it arises primarily in medical contexts: injuries, illnesses, disabilities, degenerative processes, and genetic defect or disease. Unlike pain or suffering inflicted in judicial contexts, in the medical context these are not warranted by the past actions

of the suffering individual, but are usually of natural or accidental origin and in most cases are beyond the individual's control: pain and suffering are something that happen to him or her, not something the patient has earned. The principle of medical mercy is usually taken to apply even in cases in which a medical condition is caused or exacerbated by the individual's voluntary behavior, as in smokers' diseases or injuries from attempted suicide. It is consistent to hold that mercy is supererogatory (or perhaps morally forbidden) in judicial or political contexts, but also that it is required in medical ones.

3. Edmund D. Pellegrino, M.D., "The Clinical Ethics of Pain Management in the Terminally Ill," *Hospital Formulary* 17 (November 1982): 1,495–1,496; and Marcia Angell, "The Quality of Mercy," *New England Journal of Medicine* 306 (Jan. 1982): 98–99.

4. For instance, I take it to be a moral duty, and not merely a nice thing to do, to help a child remove a painful splinter from a finger, when the child cannot do so alone and when this can be done without undue costs to oneself. (I assume that the splinter case satisfies the other provisos of the principle of medical mercy.) Similarly, I take it to be a moral duty to stop the bleeding of a person who has been wounded or to pull someone from a fire, though in very many of the cases in which such circumstances arise (wars, accidents) this duty is abrogated because we cannot do so without risks to ourselves. The duty of medical mercy is not simply equivalent to either nonmaleficence or beneficence, though perhaps derived from them, since the former is understood as a duty to refrain from causing harm and the latter to do good in a positive sense; the duty of medical mercy requires one to counteract harms one did not cause, though it may not require conferring additional positive benefits.

5. See Sharon H. Imbus and Bruce E. Zawacki, "Autonomy for Burned Patients When Survival Is Unprecedented," *New England Journal of Medicine* 297 (August 11, 1977); 309–311.

6. See Mary Voboril, *Miami Herald,* Saturday, July 1, 1978; see also footnote 17.

7. An extensive discussion of the conceptual and moral distinctions between killing and letting die begins with Jonathan Bennett, "Whatever the Consequences," *Analysis* 26 (1966): 83–97, and, after the American Medical Association's stand prohibiting mercy killing but permitting cessation of treatment, continues in James Rachel's "Active and Passive Euthanasia," *New England Journal of Medicine* 292 (January 9, 1975): 78–80, and many subsequent papers.

8. See Ludwig Edelstein, "The Hippocratic Oath," in *Ancient Medicine: Selected Papers of Ludwig Edelstein,* ed. Owsei Temkin and C. Lilian Temkin (Baltimore: The Johns Hopkins University Press, 1967), esp. 9–15 on the Greek physician's role in euthanasia.

9. Hospice, founded and directed by Cicely Saunders, is a movement devoted to the development of institutions for providing palliative but medically nonaggressive care for terminal patients. In addition to its extraordi-

nary contribution in developing methods of prophylactic pain control, according to which analgesics are administered on a scheduled basis in advance of experienced pain, Hospice has also emphasized attention to the emotional needs of the patient's family. An account of the theory and methodology of Hospice can be found in various publications by Saunders, including "Terminal Care in Medical Oncology," in *Medical Oncology*, ed. K. D. Bagshawe (Oxford: Blackwell, 1975), 563–576.

10. Joanne Lynn, M.D., "Supportive Care for Dying Patients: An Introduction for Health Care Professionals," Appendix B of the President's Commission for the Study of Ethical Problems in Medicine and Biomedical and Behavioral Research, *Deciding to Forgo Life-Sustaining Treatment* (Washington, D.C.: Government Printing Office, 1983), 295.

11. Robert G. Twycross, "Voluntary Euthanasia," in *Suicide and Euthanasia: The Rights of Personhood*, ed. Samuel E. Wallace and Albin Eser (Knoxville: The University of Tennessee Press, 1981), 89.

12. Philippa Foot, "Euthanasia," *Philosophy & Public Affairs* 6 (Winter 1977): 95.

13. To discover what one's own views are, try the following thought-experiment. Imagine that you have been captured by a gang of ruthless and superlatively clever criminals, whom you know with certainty will never be caught or change their minds. They plan either to execute you now, or to torture you unremittingly for the next twenty years and then put you to death. Which would be worse? Does your view change if the length of the torture period is reduced to twenty days or twenty minutes, and if so, why? How severe does the torture need to be?

14. 211 N.Y. 127, 129: 105 N.E. 92, 93 (1914).

15. In re Yetter, 62 Pa. D.&C. 2nd 619 (1973).

16. Satz v. Perlmutter, 362 S. 2d 160 (Fla. App. 1978), affirmed by Florida Supreme Court 379 So. 2d 359 (1980).

17. Bartling v. Superior Court, 2 Civ. No. B007907 (Calif. App. 1984).

18. California A.B. 3060 (1976), Sec. 7195.

19. The living will, recently amended to incorporate a durable power of attorney in states where applicable, is distributed by Concern For Dying and by The Society for the Right to Die, both at 250 West 57 Street, New York, N.Y. 10107; copies are available in many sources.

20. M. Siegler, "Pascal's Wager and the Hanging of Crepe," *The New England Journal of Medicine* 293 (1975): 853–857.

21. See also a study of other factors associated with differences in prognosis and treatment decisions: R. Pearlman, T. Inui, and W. Carter, "Variability in Physician Bioethical Decision-Making," *Annals of Internal Medicine* 97 (September 1982): 420–425.

22. The effects of depression on the choice concerning whether to live or die are described by Richard B. Brandt, "The Morality and Rationality of Suicide," in *A Handbook for the Study of Suicide*, ed. Seymour Perlin (New York: Oxford University Press, 1975), 61–76, and reprinted in part in M.

Pabst Battin and David J. Mayo, eds., *Suicide: The Philosophical Issues* (New York: St. Martin's Press, 1980), 117–132.

23. I've considered elsewhere the symmetrical argument that if death is in some circumstances actually better than life, the paternalist should be prepared to override a patient's choice of life. See my *Ethical Issues in Suicide* (Englewood Cliffs, N.J.: Prentice-Hall, 1982), 160–175.

24. Vatican Congregation for the Doctrine of the Faith, "Declaration on Euthanasia," June 26, 1980; see Section II, "Euthanasia."

25. Peter C. Williams, "Rights and the Alleged Right of Innocents to Be Killed," *Ethics* 87 (1976–77): 383–394.

26. This proviso may appear to resemble similar provisos exempting physicians, nurses, and other caregivers who have principled objections to participating in abortions. But I am much less certain that weight should be given to the scruples of physicians in euthanasia cases, at least at the time of need. As I will suggest in the final section of this chapter, the patient has an obligation to make his or her wishes concerning euthanasia known in advance in a foreseeable decline; if the physician objects, it is his or her duty to excuse himself or herself from the case and from the care of the patient altogether *before* the patient's deteriorating condition prevents or makes it difficult to transfer to another physician; the doctor cannot simply voice his or her objections when the patient finally reaches the point of requesting help in dying. The physician can of course object if, for instance, he or she believes that the patient is acting on faulty information; but the physician cannot introduce a principled objection to participation in euthanasia in general at this late date.

27. To this end, the British and Scottish voluntary euthanasia societies have published booklets of explicit information concerning methods of suicide for distribution to their members; the Dutch voluntary euthanasia society has published a handbook intended specifically for physicians and voluntary physician assisted euthanasia has been legalized in Holland. In the United States, Hemlock, a society advocating legalization of voluntary euthanasia and assisted suicide, also makes available similar information in narrative form.

28. O. Ruth Russell, *Freedom to Die: Moral and Legal Aspects of Euthanasia*, rev. ed. (New York: Human Sciences Press, 1977), 19.

29. Tom L. Beauchamp and Arnold I. Davidson, "The Definition of Euthanasia," *The Journal of Medicine and Philosophy* 4 (September 1979): 301.

30. Paul Ramsey, *The Patient as Person* (New Haven: Yale University Press, 1970), 161.

31. Allan S. Detsky, et al., "Prognosis, Survival, and the Expenditure of Hospital Resources for Patients in an Intensive-Care Unit," *The New England Journal of Medicine* 305 (September 17, 1981): 667–672; figures from Table 1.

32. This case, originally presented in the *Illinois Medical Journal* and reprinted in *Connecticut Medicine* with commentary from medical, ethical,

and legal experts, is summarized in *Concern for Dying* 8 (Summer 1982): 3. This patient did receive treatment for intervening infections, pneumonia, dermatitis, and convulsions, and for the ten days before her death was maintained on oxygen, respiratory therapy, and antibiotics.

33. President's Commission for the Study of Ethical Problems in Medicine and Biomedical and Behavioral Research, *Defining Death: Medical, Legal, and Ethical Issues in the Determination of Death* (Washington, D.C.: Government Printing Office, 1981), 18, citing the *Guinness Book of World Records* regarding the case of Elaine Esposito.

34. See the useful discussion of the form of the wedge argument in Tom L. Beauchamp and James F. Childress, *Principles of Biomedical Ethics* (New York: Oxford University Press, 1979), 109–117. I am concerned primarily with the second, empirical form of the argument here, but disagree with the conclusions Beauchamp and Childress reach.

35. As one physician has pointed out, objecting to the wedge argument's contention that greed would bring doctors to kill their patients, there is "not much financial incentive with a dead patient." In fact, greed may work the other way around: doctors strive to keep their patients alive, whatever the physical or financial costs to the patients, since their income is derived from services provided. As another physician points out, however, not all patients are profitable, and the physician who has enough profitable ones will find that killing off the unprofitable ones further improves the bottom line. Needless to say, greed in any of these varieties will violate the principles of mercy, autonomy, and justice.

36. See the position of Pius XII on the use of painkillers in "The Prolongation of Life," an address to an international congress of anesthesiologists, reprinted in Dennis J. Horan and David Mall, eds., *Death, Dying, and Euthanasia* (Frederick, Md.: University Publications of America, 1980), 281–287. The view of Pius XII is reemphasized by John Paul II (see footnote 24). Although both permit the use of painkillers that shorten life provided they are intended to relieve pain, not intended to produce death, both also warn against the casual use of painkillers that cause unconsciousness, since, in the words of the latter, "a person not only has to be able to satisfy his or her moral duties and family obligations; he or she also has to prepare himself or herself with full consciousness for meeting Christ" (Section III). Advanced pain management techniques may be able to reduce the problem, but in practice the excessive use of painkillers remains common.

37. See the discussion of this analogy in John D. Arras, "The Right to Die on the Slippery Slope," *Social Theory and Practice* 8 (Fall 1982): 301ff.

38. Cicely Saunders, "The Moment of Truth: Care of the Dying Person," in *Confrontations of Death: A Book of Readings and a Suggested Method of Instruction*, ed. Francis G. Scott and Ruth M. Brewer (Corvallis, Ore.: A Continuing Education Book, 1971), 119, quoted in Paul Ramsey, *Ethics at the Edges of Life* (New Haven: Yale University Press, 1978), 152. Dame Saunders is the founder and medical director of St. Christopher's Hospice

near London, which has provided the stimulus and model for the contemporary hospice movement.

39. See my "The Least Worst Death: Selective Refusal of Treatment," *The Hastings Center Report* 13 (April 1983): 13–16.

40. Barbara J. McNeil, Ralph Weichselbaum, and Stephen G. Pauker, "Speech and Survival: Tradeoffs between Quality and Quantity of Life in Laryngeal Cancer," *New England Journal of Medicine* 305 (October 22, 1981): 982–987. The study, however, was performed with healthy volunteers, not actual patients. See Correspondence, *New England Journal of Medicine* (February 25, 1982): 482–483, for other criticisms of this study, including evidence that rehabilitation of speech may be quite satisfactory.

41. John Hinton, *Dying* (Harmondsworth: Penguin Books, 1972) 65–66.

42. It is sometimes argued that physician assistance in a patient's suicide would violate the Hippocratic oath. It is true that the oath, in its original form, does contain an explicit injunction that the physician shall not give a lethal potion to a patient who requests it, nor make a suggestion to that effect (to do so was apparently common Greek medical practice at the time). But the oath in its original form also contains explicit prohibitions of the physician's accepting fees for teaching medicine, and of performing surgery —even on gallstones. These latter prohibitions are not retained in modern reformulations of the oath, and I see no reason why the provision against giving lethal potions to patients who request it should be. What is central to the oath and cannot be deleted without altering its essential character is the requirement that the physician shall come "for the benefit of the sick." Under the argument advanced here, physician assistance in patient suicide may in some cases indeed be for the benefit of the patient. What the oath would continue to prohibit is physician assistance in a suicide for the physician's own gain or to serve other institutional or societal ends.

43. Ramsey, *The Patient as Person,* 145.

Suggestions for Further Reading

Articles anthologized in one or more of the collections listed below are not entered separately.

Battin, M. Pabst. *Ethical Issues in Suicide*. Englewood Cliffs, N.J.: Prentice-Hall, 1982.

Barnard, Christiaan. *Good Life/Good Death: A Doctor's Case for Euthanasia and Suicide.*Englewood Cliffs, N.J.: Prentice-Hall, 1980.

Battin, M. Pabst, and Maris, Ronald W. *Suicide and Ethics*. New York: Human Sciences Press, 1983.

Battin, M. Pabst, and Mayo, David J., eds. *Suicide: The Philosophical Issues.* New York: St. Martin's Press, 1980.

Beauchamp, Tom L., and Childress, James F. *Principles of Biomedical Ethics*. New York: Oxford University Press, 1979.
Beauchamp, Tom L., and Perlin, Seymour. *Ethical Issues in Death and Dying*. Englewood Cliffs, N.J.: Prentice-Hall, 1978.
Behnke, John A., and Bok, Sissela, eds. *The Dilemmas of Euthanasia*. Garden City, New York: Anchor Press/Doubleday, 1975.
Downing, A.B., ed. *Euthanasia and the Right to Death*. London: Peter Owen, 1969.
Fletcher, Joseph. *Humanhood: Essays in Biomedical Ethics*. New York: Prometheus Books, 1979.
———. *Morals and Medicine*. Princeton, N.J.: Princeton University Press, 1954.
Glover, Jonathan. *Causing Death and Saving Lives*. Harmondsworth: Penguin Books, 1977.
Gorovitz, Samuel, et al., eds. *Moral Problems in Medicine*. 2d ed. Englewood Cliffs, N.J.: Prentice-Hall, 1983.
Grisez, Germain, and Boyle, Joseph M., Jr. *Life and Death with Liberty and Justice: A Contribution to the Euthanasia Debate*. Notre Dame and London: University of Notre Dame Press, 1979.
Group for the Advancement of Psychiatry. *The Right to Die: Decisions and Decision Makers*. New York: Jason Aronson, 1974.
Gruman, Gerald J. "An Historical Introduction to Ideas about Voluntary Euthanasia: With a Bibliographic Survey and Guide for Interdisciplinary Studies," *Omega* (Summer 1973): 87–138.
Hinton, John. *Dying*. Harmondsworth: Penguin Books, 1972.
Horan, Dennis J., and Mall, David, eds. *Death, Dying, and Euthanasia*. Frederick, Md.: University Publications of America, 1980.
Humphry, Derek, and Wickett, Ann. *The Right to Die: Understanding Euthanasia*. New York: Harper & Row, 1986.
Kluge, Eike-Henner, W. *The Ethics of Deliberate Death*. Port Washington, N.Y., and London: Kennikat Press, 1981.
———. *The Practice of Death*. New Haven: Yale University Press, 1975.
Kohl, Marvin, ed. *Beneficent Euthanasia*. Buffalo, N.Y.: Prometheus Books, 1975.
———. *The Morality of Killing*. New York: Humanities Press, 1974.
Koop, C. Everett. *The Right to Live: the Right to Die*. Wheaton, Ill.: Tyndale House Publishers; Eastbourne, England: Coverdale House Publishers, 1976.
Ladd, John, ed. *Ethical Issues Relating to Life and Death*. New York: Oxford University Press, 1979.
Larue, Gerald. *Euthanasia and Religion*. Los Angeles: Hemlock Society, 1985.
Maquire, Daniel C. *Death by Choice*. New York: Doubleday, 1973.
McCormick, Richard A., S.J. *How Brave a New World: Dilemmas in Bioethics*. Garden City, N.Y.: Doubleday, 1981.

Oosthuizen, G. C., Shapiro, H. A., and Strauss, S. A. eds. *Euthanasia.* Cape Town: Oxford University Press, 1978.

Portwood, Doris. *Commonsense Suicide: The Final Right.* Los Angeles: Hemlock Society, 1983.

President's Commission for the Study of Ethical Problems in Medicine and Biomedical and Behavioral Research. *Deciding to Forgo Life-Sustaining Treatment.* Washington, D.C.: Government Printing Office, 1983.

Rachels, James. "Euthanasia," in *Matters of Life & Death,* ed. Tom Regan, New York: Random House, 1986.

Ramsey, Paul. *Ethics at the Edges of Life.* New Haven: Yale University Press, 1978.

————. *The Patient as Person.* New Haven: Yale University Press, 1970.

Russell, O. Ruth. *Freedom to Die: Moral and Legal Aspects of Euthanasia.* 2d ed. New York: Human Sciences Press, 1977.

St. John-Stevas, Norman. *Life, Death and the Law.* Bloomington: Indiana University Press, 1961.

Society for the Right to Die. *Handbook of Living Will Laws, 1981–84.* New York: Society for the Right to Die, 1984.

Steinbock, Bonnie, ed. *Killing and Letting Die.* Englewood Cliffs, N.J.: Prentice-Hall, 1980.

Sullivan, Joseph. *Catholic Teaching or the Morality of Euthanasia.* Studies in Sacred Theology No. 22. Washington, D.C.: The Catholic University of America Press, 1949.

Thompson, Ian, ed. *Dilemmas of Dying. A Study in the Ethics of Terminal Care.* Edinburgh: At the University Press, 1979.

Veatch, Robert M. *Death, Dying, and the Biological Revolution.* New Haven: Yale University Press, 1976.

Wallace, Samuel E., and Albin Eser, eds. *Suicide and Euthanasia. The Rights of Personhood.* Knoxville: The University of Tennessee Press, 1981.

Williams, Glanville. *The Sanctity of Life and the Criminal Law.* New York: Alfred A. Knopf, 1957.

CHAPTER II

Informed Consent

Dan W. Brock

The two central aims of the requirement that medical care cannot be given to competent patients without their informed consent are illustrated by the following two cases, in which that requirement is violated.

Case 1. Dr. Smith diagnoses his patient, Mrs. Jones, as having breast cancer. He informs her that a radical mastectomy should be performed as soon as possible, brushes aside her timid attempts to discuss the matter further, and with her silent and grudging acquiescence books her in the hospital for surgery.

Case 2. Mr. Brown is suffering multiple complications and disability, principally from advanced diabetes and renal failure. He has had both legs amputated above the knee and is functionally blind. He is not considered a candidate for a kidney transplant and so faces the necessity of dialysis treatments for the rest of his life. He is mentally alert, has had his medical situation fully explained to him by his attending physicians, and seems to understand his situation well. Two weeks ago, he decided that he wanted no more painful dialysis treatments, knowing that their termination would quickly lead to his death, and he has remained steadfast in that decision since. Despite his decision, his physician refuses to stop the dialysis treatments, believing that to do so would be tantamount to killing his patient.

The importance of informed consent is different in these two cases, and is perhaps most conspicuous in the absence of consent having been obtained. In Case 1, obtaining valid consent would require informing the patient not only of her medical condition but also of the alternatives available for treating it; ascertaining that the patient is sufficiently competent to understand her situation and make a decision; and then permitting the patient freely to decide about treatment. The doctrine of informed consent is an important aspect of the general norms that structure the physician-patient relationship. It has relevance to the great majority of cases in which decisions must be made about treatment, since it requires a mutual process between physician and patient of informing and discussion (whenever the patient is capable of discussion), thereby leading to a mutually acceptable treatment decision. The doctrine ought to shape in important respects the nature of nearly all encounters and decision making between physicians and patients. It is designed to provide the opportunity for the patient to become more actively involved in the ongoing decision-making process than has often been the case in medicine.

The second case illustrates the special importance of informed consent in a much narrower class of cases. In those cases in which patients and their physicians are unable to agree on a course of treatment, the competent patient has the right to refuse any treatment, even if of a life-sustaining nature, no matter how strongly the physician or others believe that the treatment should be undertaken. In the crunch, as it might be put, when disagreement between a physician and a competent patient is irresolvable, it is the patient who has final decision-making authority. The authority of the patient to order a particular treatment, however, is more limited than the authority to refuse one. Although physicians should be flexible in making alternatives available to patients, they cannot be compelled to provide treatments that are outside the bounds of acceptable professional practice or that violate their own deeply held moral beliefs. It is the patient's right to refuse any treatment that is embodied in the informed-consent doctrine and that is violated by the physician's forced treatment in Case 2. Because irreconcilable disagreement between physician and patient is relatively rare, this right seldom will be invoked. Nonetheless, the existence of this right, even when not invoked, helps shape the physician-patient relationship. And the focus of the informed-consent doctrine on the ongoing process of physician-patient communication and decision making is not, of course, unrelated to the right to refuse treatment. The ongoing process of informing and discussion would have less value if the patient's decision could be ignored, and the right to refuse a particular (or any) treatment would be less valuable if there were no means of ensuring the availability of information on which such a refusal reasonably might be based. Together, these requirements aim at ensuring that patients can take an active, full role in the ongoing process of decision making about their medical care, and that no treatment is undertaken that does not first meet their approval.

This is not an uncontroversial view of the proper physician-patient relationship and, more specifically, of the role of patients in decisions about their health care. There is a long and strong authoritarian tradition within medicine that denies patients this role. In its more extreme form, this tradition denies any significant patient participation and leaves the ultimate choice of treatment solely with the physician. In this view, patients should be told what is therapeutically useful for them to know about their condition and treatment, and nothing more. Their role is passively to follow the instructions of their physicians. Because medical knowledge and treatment techniques have expanded dramatically in recent years, this traditional authoritarian relationship might seem even more necessary today. Patients simply will lack the knowledge or ability even to understand the information necessary for sound medical decision-making. Thus, it might seem only sensible that treatment decisions be left to those with the necessary training, experience, and knowledge to make them soundly—physicians. And especially since patients, who at best understand their situation only inadequately, may make decisions positively harmful to themselves, even to the point of resulting in preventable loss of life. In this view, the physician's role is the paternalistic one of directing treatment in the best interests of the patient, and the patient's role is the largely passive one of following the prescribed treatment.

The informed-consent doctrine amounts to a rejection of this traditional authoritarian and paternalistic conception of the physician-patient relationship. But why should that traditional conception be rejected, given its long and important historical role and its seemingly reasonable character? To answer that question, we must examine the values served by the doctrine of informed consent. Only then will we be in a position to understand what is at stake in its acceptance or rejection. Throughout this chapter, our concern will be with the conceptual and moral issues involved in the informed-consent doctrine, and not with the details of its development as a legal doctrine.[1] Our focus will be on the *moral* basis and requirements of informed consent.

The Values Underlying Informed Consent

The informed-consent doctrine serves not only the individual patient in the physician-patient relationship but society as well. Its consequences for the patient are fundamental because the patient is the ultimate recipient of medical treatment. The informed-consent doctrine serves to promote the patient's well-being and to respect his or her self-determination. Both the nature of these values, as well as how the informed-consent doctrine furthers them, must be spelled out.

PATIENT WELL-BEING

Clearly, the fundamental goal of the physician-patient relationship is to protect and promote the patient's health. Medical care treats disease and thereby prevents, eliminates, or ameliorates pain and suffering, disability and premature loss of life. But given the great complexities and sophisticated knowledge involved in such treatment, it is not immediately clear why the patient's health is not best served by vesting ultimate decision-making authority with the physician. Whether a person is healthy or diseased, and what will most effectively treat his or her disease, would seem to be "objective" matters about which well-trained experts such as physicians can best decide. Patients, however, are often confused, anxious, and fearful and as a result sometimes make decisions not in their best interests. They sometimes refuse clearly beneficial treatment, select treatment less efficacious than others available, and fail to complete beneficial treatments. Why then is the patient's well-being best promoted by leaving ultimate decision-making authority with him or her?

The answer lies in three key points: first, and least important, "health" is not a fully "objective" matter, invariant between persons; second, medical criteria alone often do not fully settle which treatment is correct or best for a given medical condition; and third, the relative importance or value of health as compared with other aspects of individual well-being differs for different people.

In perhaps the great majority of cases what constitutes an impairment to health is not controversial—major diseases like cancer or diabetes, fractured limbs, serious infections, and so forth. Because these diseases can have serious adverse effects on an individual's

102 · DAN W. BROCK

normal functioning and even lead to untimely death, it is largely uncontroversial that they are contrary to a patient's well-being. In a few cases, however, it is debatable whether a condition that may lead to a medical intervention represents any impairment to health at all—for example, an unusually large nose or wrinkled skin for which corrective surgery is possible. However, there is general agreement in the great majority of cases about what constitutes impairment to health. If defining health were the only issue, the case for patient participation in decision making in order to promote the patient's health would be weak.

More important, in much of medicine, it takes more than medical facts alone to determine what treatment is "indicated" for a given condition; there usually are several acceptable methods of treatment. A classic example is breast cancer, which can be treated, among other ways, by radical mastectomy, limited mastectomy, and radiation. Many other conditions are similar. Sometimes the choices vary greatly—for example, between surgical and nonsurgical treatment of a slipped disk. In other cases, the differences between alternatives may be small though still significant—for example, the choice between medications having different side effects for the treatment of severe headaches. Moreover, for many conditions, both treatment and nontreatment are considered acceptable alternatives by medical professionals—for example, concerning hemorrhoids. Whenever more than one acceptable alternative exists, the "medical facts" about which the physician is expert will not determine which treatment is best for a particular patient.

What compounds the difficulty of selecting between alternative treatments is that more than health commonly is at issue. The choice is not simply what will maximize a patient's health, but what will best promote his or her overall well-being. Health, for nearly everyone, is only one value among many, albeit an important one. People value their health in part to avoid the evils of pain and unwanted death. But they value it as well for its prevention of disability and its role in making possible the pursuit of the many other goals and activities that they value. People's values and plans of life vary greatly, as does the importance assigned to health, and particular components of health, in comparison with other goals and values. The physician's ultimate responsibility is to use his or her medical skills to serve patients' overall well-being in this broad sense, to facilitate patients' pursuit of their plans of life. The choice of medical treatment now can be seen to be even less objective, since it depends on which alternative best fits a patient's overall goals or life plan. For a given medical condition, appropriate treatments will very greatly because people's goals and values themselves vary greatly. People differ in their tolerance of pain and so, for example, in whether for a slipped disk they prefer surgery with the risks of serious disability or prefer more conservative treatments requiring them to tolerate more pain. An active person may prefer radiation therapy to surgical amputation of a cancerous limb, even if amputation has a higher success rate. Which medical intervention, if any, best will serve a patient's overall well-being must be determined in light of that patient's relevant subjective preferences and overall aims and values. That is what did not happen in Case 1; no attempt was made to determine the importance *to the patient* of minimizing the risk of recurrence of the cancer, of physical disfigurement, and so forth. Following a narrow notion of health in such a case, one that focuses only on minimizing the risk of recurrence of the cancer, may not be in accordance with *the patient's* conception of her well-being and is not the proper sole end of medicine.

It should now be clear why the traditional authoritarian, paternalistic conception of the physician-patient relationship is unacceptable even if the only goal of health care is to promote the patient's well-being. Sound health care decision making involves both objective and subjective components, and both must be taken into account. On the objective side, there are empirical facts about the nature of the expected outcomes for the patient of different treatments (including the alternative of no treatment). These include a determination of the patient's physical status, including his or her prognosis and expected condition under alternative treatments. These are factual or objective matters about which the patient's physician typically will be the best judge. There may often be significant uncertainty concerning these consequences, however, and medical experts will frequently disagree about such factual matters.

The subjective component of decision making involves assessing the relative importance or value to this particular patient of the features and consequences of the alternative treatment outcomes. This evaluation of the outcomes, and of their effects on the patient's well-being, is a subjective component in the sense that it depends on the patient's goals and values. These values and goals may be quite different from the physician's, or from most people's, depending as they do on the patient's preferences, abilities, and opportunities. The authoritarian and paternalistic tradition in medicine fails adequately to recognize the relevance and importance of these subjective components. Because the assessment of the effects on a patient's well-being of treatment alternatives requires a meshing of these objective and subjective components, a process of mutual interaction or shared decision making is called for, with the physician and patient each contributing what each is in the best position to know.

The nature of self-determination

The other principal value promoted by the informed-consent doctrine is patient self-determination. A person's interest in self-determination simply reflects the common desire to make important decisions about one's life oneself, according to one's own aims and values. Self-determination involves the capacities of individuals to form, revise over time, and pursue a plan of life or conception of their good. It is a broad concept applicable at both the levels of decision and of action. Patients' exercise of self-determination in the context of health care involves their deciding which alternative treatment will best promote their own particular goals and values. As we will discuss later, this requires that they become informed about the nature and consequences of alternative treatments. More relevant to the nature of self-determination, it requires as well that patients have formed a minimally stable and consistent conception of their good—that is, a set of goals and values, or plan of life, by which to evaluate those alternatives. Having a conception of one's good is more than merely having a set of desires, instinctual or conditioned. People have a capacity for reflective self-evaluation, for considering what kinds of desires and character they want to have. There are, of course, limits to the extent to which people can change their desires. They can change their particular tastes in food, but not whether they have any desire to eat at all. In broad respects, our natures are fixed and given to us by our biological nature, but within these broad limits we adopt particular values and create a unique self. In these ways, we are capable of shaping our character and of taking responsibility for the kinds of people we are. Self-determination is the name given here to that process.

To say that we are capable of self-determination is neither to deny our interdependence nor that our values are influenced by others. Still, in the evaluation of these influences, one either makes them one's own and incorporates them into one's own conception of what is good, or rejects them. Self-determination does *not* imply that persons create their own character and values free of all causal influence from others. Nor does it require free will in the sense of a will free of causal determination.

The formation of one's values or conceptions of what is good is an ongoing process. In the light of new experience, people revise their values over time. Our interest in taking responsibility for our life by forming a plan of life extends as well to being free to revise and develop our values.

People not only can form and revise a conception of their own good but also can pursue it in action (e.g., in pursuing a particular medical treatment). Thus, interference with self-determination can involve interference with people's deciding for themselves, but also interference with their acting as they have decided they want to act. Respecting self-determination consequently involves avoiding both these interferences, with decision and with action.

Self-determination thus embodies a particular ideal of the person. That ideal is one of a person freely choosing for him or herself, on the basis of personal, reflectively adopted, values, the alternative action to be taken, and then so acting. The spirit of this ideal has been eloquently expressed by Isaiah Berlin:

I wish my life and decision to depend on myself, not on external forces of whatever kind. I wish to be the instrument of my own, not of other men's acts of will. I wish to be a subject, not an object; to be moved by reasons, by conscious purposes, which are my own, not by causes which affect me, as it were, from outside. I wish to be somebody, not anybody; a doer—deciding not being decided for, self-directed and not acted upon by external nature or by other men. . . . I wish, above all, to be conscious of myself as a thinking, willing, active being, bearing responsibility for his choices and able to explain them by reference to his own ideas and purposes.[2]

The value of self-determination

What weight should be given to patient self-determination in health care decision making? This question is particularly pressing in those cases in which a patient has decided on a treatment course seemingly contrary to his or her own well-being. Refusals of life-sustaining therapy are some of the most dramatic examples. In Case 2 above, it may be plausible to suppose that continued treatment would not promote the patient's well-being. But if the patient had not been disabled, were capable of living a rewarding and satisfying life with long-term dialysis treatment, and *then* refused it, respecting his self-determination would appear to require a great sacrifice of his well-being. Evaluating the importance of the impact of medical treatment on a patient's life plan provides a framework for weighing the relative value of medical care for his or her well-being. It is less obvious what the value of self-determination resides in, and so what weight it should be given.

Self-determination typically is valued both for the good consequences that result from respecting it (its instrumental value) and for its own sake, as part of an ideal of the person (its noninstrumental or intrinsic value). Perhaps the most important instrumental value of respecting self-determination lies in its role in promoting a person's good or well-being. This may seem paradoxical, since in discussions both of informed consent and of paternalism it is common to pose individual well-being and self-determination as competing and conflicting values. Indeed, these values sometimes are in conflict, but their relationship is more complex than is suggested by viewing them simply as opposing values. We have argued that a person's well-being or good is subjective in that it is ultimately determined by that person's values and subjective preferences. This is the idea behind the view that the individual is the best judge of his or her own interests. Respecting a person's self-determination leaves a person free to pursue and attain those values and goals. In the exercise of self-determination in purposive, rational action, we pursue our good as we perceive it. An important value of self-determination, and in turn an important reason for respecting it, is then that its exercise commonly results in the promotion of the person's good or well-being. This is not to say that a person can never be mistaken about where his or her good lies. But, when realized, the ideal of self-determination (understood to involve the adoption and pursuit of a plan of life) itself usually contributes to the realization of a person's good or well-being. That this is an important part of the value of self-determination can be seen by the fact that when people's choices bear little relation to their good, for example in cases of severe and wide-ranging psychotic delusion, the extent to which their exercise of self-determination is of any value at all, and certainly of any intrinsic value, is decidedly problematic. Part of the value of respecting people's self-determination then lies in the way in which doing so *normally* contributes to the promotion of their good. This has implications for those instances when persons are confused or ill-informed and so make decisions contrary to their own good. In those cases, not only must protecting their well-being be weighed against respecting their self-determination, but also in that weighing the value of self-determination itself is diminished in comparison with its value in more favorable circumstances.

Although the value of self-determination is then diminished in such cases, it is not lost. That is because respecting self-determination often has other instrumental values such as the avoidance of frustration involved in interfering with a person's liberty of action, the development of individual judgment (especially since people often learn best from their mistakes), the satisfaction people often get from making decisions about their life for themselves, and so forth. The extent to which these instrumental benefits are present in any particular case depends on the facts of that case.

The instrumental consequences of self-determination are not, of course, all good ones. Sometimes persons make choices that are very harmful to themselves or others, experience anxiety from choosing for themselves, and so prefer to have others decide for them, and so forth. The overall instrumental effects of any particular exercise of self-determination must be assessed in context.

The value that many people ascribe to self-determination rests also on a particular noninstrumental ideal of the person—we value being, and being recognized by others as, the kind of person who is capable of determining and taking responsibility for his or her destiny. This is the ideal of the person expressed in the quote from Berlin above. It is a *noninstrumental ideal* in the sense that it offers an attractive vision of what human beings can be, independent of the consequences or satisfactions in realizing that vision. There is a dignity in being self-determining that is lost in even a satisfying subservience. It is this ideal of the person that is expressed in patients' desires to make significant decisions about their lives for themselves, even if others (for example, physicians or computers) might be able to predict how they would decide and so decide for them, or even if others could decide in a way that would more effectively promote their health and well-being.

Waiving self-determination

Patients often do not take an active role in decision making about their own health care. Often they say to their physicians something like, "You do whatever you think is best." This may seem contrary to the account of self-determination as involving people making significant decisions about their lives for themselves. In turn, it might be thought not to satisfy the doctrine of informed consent. *Must* patients ultimately make health care decisions themselves, or may they either waive the exercise of self-determination in particular instances or, perhaps better, exercise it at a different level of decision? The moral doctrine of informed consent as interpreted here *entitles*, but *does not require*, a patient to take an active role in decision making regarding treatment. Patients sometimes have good reasons for avoiding an active role in particular decisions about their health care—for example, they are gravely ill and want to spend what little time remains to them with their families and others, or they know that thinking about the issue at hand makes them distraught and depressed, or they know from past experience that the decisions require technical understanding of which they are incapable and that trying to decide only makes them confused. In any of these circumstances, and especially if a patient has a physician who knows him or her well and who is trusted to act in the patient's best interests, it could be reasonable to let the physician decide. In these cases, the patient waives his or her right to decide and transfers that right to another—his physician or, alternatively, a family member. Doing so is compatible with, and a possible use of, the right to self-determination. What is necessary is that the patient understand that the decision is rightfully his or hers to make, and so also his or hers to transfer to another if the patient so chooses.

By contrast, other patients may leave decisions with their physician because they do not think they have any business interfering in the physician's professional decision about treatment—it never occurs to them that the decision is theirs to make. This would be one plausible rendering of the first case. And this could not possibly be an exercise of self-determination, because a person must first believe that he or she has a right to decide before he or she could intend to transfer it to another. But when a patient does freely and intentionally transfer the right to decide to another, this should be understood as compatible with the right of self-determination and with informed consent. Nevertheless, two qualifications are necessary.

One ideal of self-determination is the self-governing person who makes decisions for him- or herself, after personally weighing alternatives against reflectively adopted values. In turning over a major health care decision to another, a patient does *not* meet that ideal of self-determination. But even that ideal is a matter of degree and not fully realizable—for example, we all rely on much information and accumulated knowledge that we never could evaluate for ourselves. The shortages of time and ability (among other factors) that make such reliance reasonable can also sometimes make turning a health care decision over to another a reasonable and legitimate use of one's right to decide.

The second qualification is that this is one place among others where the moral analysis of informed consent may diverge from the doctrine's optimal legal form. The law and legal policy must be formulated in order to limit well-intentioned misuse and ill-intentioned abuse of its requirements. We want general rules that, when applied by real persons in a variety of circumstances, will produce the best results on balance and over a period of time. The worry here is that permitting true and valid waivings of the right to decide would inevitably bring in its wake other denials of that right, along with failures adequately to inform and involve patients who would want to decide for themselves. It may be that a legal exception to the requirements of informed consent to permit such waivings should be narrowly limited because of the other unavoidable and unjustified denials of patients' rights to decide that it would produce. Whether that is so depends on the particular procedural safeguards that might be devised to permit such waivings while limiting abuses, and empirical investigation of their actual effectiveness.

OTHER VALUES SERVED BY INFORMED CONSENT

In the account of informed consent being developed here, the principal benefits secured by informed consent are benefits for the patient whose consent must be obtained—his or her well-being and self-determination. However, undoubtedly other values are served by informed consent, especially when it is viewed as an institutionalized social practice. It fosters general public trust in the medical enterprise, especially in the context of medical research in which serious concerns would otherwise exist about conflicts of interest between medical researchers and subjects. The requirement that physicians explain and justify treatment recommendations to the patient may also encourage more careful scrutiny and review of those recommendations by the medical profession, thereby resulting in sounder recommendations. There are many other effects of the complex institutional practice of informed consent. Some of those effects are often claimed to be negative; for example, patients may lose some of their trust and faith in the physician's healing powers when all the risks and uncertainties of treatment must be detailed to them. An overall assessment of these institutional benefits and costs is far from clear, and probably too uncertain to serve as the fundamental moral basis of the informed-consent doctrine.

Although the values of patient well-being and self-determination may provide the underlying moral basis for the doctrine, it is helpful to examine the requirements and limitations of the doctrine to see how they do so. As we have already noted, the values of patient well-being and self-determination may be in conflict when a patient's decision is contrary to his or her well-being. (Sometimes, as in the case of a comatose patient, a patient may be unable to make any decision at all.) Only when it is clear how the informed-consent doctrine deals with such conflicts will we know whether, it adequately secures patient well-being and self-determination.

The Conditions for Valid Informed Consent

The requirements of a morally valid consent are commonly considered to be three: that the person giving consent be *competent*; that he or she be *informed* about the proposed intervention; and that his or her consent be *voluntary*. Competence is necessary to ensure that a patient has sufficient decision-making capacities to participate in the decision process and to decide responsibly on a course of treatment. The requirement that the person be informed is to ensure that the patient has received all relevant information concerning available alternative treatments (including no treatment), including the risks and potential benefits of each, in order to be able to judge which alternative is most desirable. The voluntariness condition ensures that the patient's choice not result from coercion, duress, undue influence or manipulation, and thus will serve the patient's own perceived good rather than another's good or another's view of the patient's good. Each of these conditions is complex, both in principle and in practice, and we will examine each in turn. But it is important to emphasize that together these conditions *do* ensure that the patient's consent to treatment is both an exercise of self-determination and a decision reasonably expected to promote his or her well-being.

COMPETENCE

The requirement that a patient be competent in order to give binding consent is more complex than first appearances might suggest. In some cases it is clear whether the patient is competent. Some people are unable to participate in decision making about their health care to any significant extent at all—the comatose, infants and very young children, and some of those who are severely mentally disabled or mentally ill. With these groups, no possibility exists of involving them in decision making about their own health care. Nevertheless, most "normal" adults of average intelligence are usually able to understand their situation and decide about their treatment. In between are the difficult cases—those involving people whose capacities to decide are marginal and whose ultimate competence to decide requires clarity about the nature and function of the determination of competence.

The importance of competence

The importance of the determination of competence can be put simply—it separates those patients whose free and informed decisions must be accepted as binding from those whose decision will be set aside. In other words, the competence determination ultimately establishes when a patient's consent for treatment *must* be secured and honored (i.e., in which cases the requirement of informed consent will be operative). And this suggests that the basic values of patient well-being and self-determination underlying the informed-consent doctrine itself will be at stake in the competence determination, as indeed they are. Consider the issue in personal terms. Suppose you are concerned both for your own well-being and your self-determination. When would you want your own decision about your treatment to be accepted and followed, and when would you want others empowered to decide for you? If your decision-making capacities are sound and are being effectively utilized, your own decision should reflect your view of your well-being—both values will be promoted by your deciding. However, if your decision making is seriously defective, the likelihood increases that your decision will cause you serious harm or the loss of important benefits, and in general not conform to your values. In those circumstances, it is reasonable to want protection against one's choices being honored. A normal concern for our own well-being requires it. The value of self-determination may be diminished in such circumstances; nevertheless, the values of deciding for oneself and protecting one's own well-being are then in conflict. The determination of competence must secure an acceptable balance between allowing persons to decide for themselves while protecting them from the harmful consequences of their own choices when their capacities to decide are seriously limited or defective.

Several points follow from this moral and legal role of competence judgments. First, competence is always relative to a particular task —everyone is competent to do some things and not others. The relevant task here is to make a particular health care treatment decision. It follows that a person may be competent to make a given treatment decision, but incompetent to manage his or her financial affairs or to make other treatment decisions, for example. Second, patient decision-making competence also changes over time, for example, from the effects of medications or in cases of a cyclic mental illness like manic depression. Health care professionals can and should take steps as necessary to enhance patient competence. Third, the capacities contributing to competence are possessed in varying degrees though the determination of a person as either competent or incompetent is an all or nothing judgment. The crucial question will then be *how* defective a person's decision making must be in a particular instance to be deemed incompetent. To understand how to answer that question, we must examine more closely the various elements of decision-making competence.

Elements and standards of decision-making competence

In order to participate in health care decision making and ultimately to give valid consent to treatment, an individual must be able to communicate and understand relevant information, be able to reason and deliberate about alternative treatments, and possess values and goals by which to assess alternatives. The nature of the requirements that a patient be able to understand information and reason about alternatives will be detailed below in discusion of the condition that consent be informed. Understanding and reasoning are together necessary for a patient to be able to acquire and use information to reach an appreciation of the consequences of adopting one or another course of treatment. The patient's values and goals provide the basis for evaluating which course of treatment will best serve his or her ends.

Individuals possess these capacities, and exercise them on particular occasions, in different degrees; or, what amounts to the same thing, the capacities to understand, reason, and value can be imperfect or defective in more or less extensive and important ways. Patients' decision-making competence, as expressed in the making of a particular treatment decision, thus could be measured, at least on a relative scale. While no single, uniform measure of decision-making competence seems possible, this merely reflects the reality that competence involves a complex meshing of a patient's various capacities and skills with the demands of the particular decision situation. The potential situations are too numerous, and the potential arrays of patient abilities and inabilities are too varied to permit a single measure. But from the lack of a formal measure of competence it does not follow, as is often charged, that determinations of competence and incompetence lack any theoretical foundation and are merely "intuitive" in the sense of being inchoate and arbitrary.

This attack on competence determinations as at base intuitive and arbitrary has seemed to some to be reinforced by the widely varying standards or levels of competence actually applied by physicians, courts, and others. However, those differences do not support the "intuitive and arbitrary" charge. Instead they in part reflect confusions and moral disagreements regarding the proper level of competence required and on the issue of paternalism, and in part reflect a quite proper variation in the standard of competence. Standards of competence are divided below into three broad classes, moving from the most minimal to the most stringent standard, in that the alternatives will classify a progressively larger proportion of people as incompetent. We shall argue that the minimal standard is insufficiently paternalistic, the strictest standard overly paternalistic, and that the proper standard lies in the middle category, that evaluates the process of the patient's decision making, though even this standard should vary depending on the decision in question.

Ability to express a preference. This standard of competence considers only whether the patient is able to express a preference for a particular treatment but does not assess the presence or nature of the understanding or reasoning underlying that preference, nor the content of the preference itself. It maximally respects patient self-choice or self-determination, but it provides no protection at all against the consequences of defective decision making. For example, this standard would require accepting an individual's refusal of life-saving therapy when that refusal was caused by psychotic delusions induced by drugs or mental illness. This standard is in fact not a standard of *competent* choice at all, since any choice whatsoever is deemed competent. It fails to provide any protection of patient well-being—one of the two values that the informed-consent doctrine is designed to promote. It fails to balance the values of self-determination and well-being, but instead defers entirely to the former, even under conditions in which the value of self-determination is drastically diminished.

Standards evaluating the content of the patient's decision. While the "mere expression of a preference" standard of competence is insufficiently paternalistic, at the other extreme are standards that determine competence by evaluating the content of the patient's choice and that are excessively and objectionably paternalistic. This is not to deny that it is commonly disagreement with the content of the physician's recommendation that will trigger review of the patient's competence in marginal cases. This is natural and reasonable, given the presumption that the physician's recommendation is in the patient's interests. But it is to say that merely having decided on a course of treatment different from the physician's (or family's) recommendation serves as no basis at all for a determination of incompetence. Basing determinations of incompetence on the content of the patient's decision inevitably requires appeal to some "objective" standard of correct decisions, independent of whether that standard conforms to this patient's values and goals. "Correct" decisions in this view might be those that are rational, or what most would decide, or what the physician would decide, and so forth. But it is highly problematic whether any such objective standard of a patient's good is ultimately defensible. Employing such a standard will seriously compromise the patient's self-determination, without requiring evidence that his capacity for self-determination in the circumstances is deficient. Finding a patient incompetent merely because his treatment choice does not conform to some external, supposedly objective, standard fails to respect the patient's capacity to define his own values. Finally, any such standard in practice risks substantial abuse and unwarranted denial ("for their own good") of patients' rights to decide for themselves.

Standards evaluating the nature of the patient's understanding and reasoning. Any asessment of competence that examines a patient's actual understanding and use of information in reasoning to reach a decision allows protection against serious harms that may result from defective understanding and mistaken reasoning. This standard of competence focuses on the *process* of decision making, rather than either on merely whether the patient has made a choice or on the content of his or her choice. Of course, the first response of health care professionals or others to apparent misunderstandings or mistakes of patients should be further discussion with the patient to seek to remove or remedy the difficulties. Only when such misunderstandings or mistakes prove irremediable is there any warrant for a finding of incompetence. The goal under this standard of competence, as with the informed-consent doctrine generally, is to foster the patient's full participation in decision making that most clearly conforms with his or her own values and goals. This standard seeks a balance between respecting a patient's self-determination and protecting his or her well-being. When information about the nature of available alternatives and their consequences for the patient's values and goals has been understood and appreciated by the patient, then his or her choice must be honored, even if others such as the physician would have chosen differently. But when the patient is clearly unable to understand necessary information and reason to a decision, a standard that focuses on the nature of the patient's decision-making *process* allows a possible finding of incompetence and would justify transferring the decision to a surrogate.

While the general standard of competence should focus on the process of the patient's decision making, this still leaves open two important questions regarding others assessing the patient's competence. What level and degree of understanding and appreciation of the full consequences of alternatives are necessary for competence? How certain must others be that the patient has not achieved the appropriate level before finding him or her incompetent? The answer to both questions is, "It depends." The level of decision-making incapacity that should be required for a finding of incompetence properly varies depending on the decision in question. There is *no* single proper level of decision-making capacity that should be required for all treatment decisions. This is simply a consequence of the fact that what is a reasonable balance between patient self-determination and well-being in setting that level will depend in part on the consequences of the patient's choice for his well-being.

The consequences of acting on a patient's choice can range along a continuum from being substantially better to being substantially worse than other alternatives in their expected effects in achieving the goals of preserving life, preventing injury and disability, and relieving suffering, as against their risks of harm. The relevant comparison should be with other available alternatives, and the degree to which the net benefit/risk balance of the alternative chosen appears better or worse than that for other treatment options. When the net benefit/risk balance appears substantially to favor the patient's choice it is reasonable to require only a low/minimal level of decision-making capacity in the choice; there is no need to compromise his self-determination in order to protect his well-being. At the other extreme, when the expected effects for the patient's life and health appear to be substantially worse than available alternatives, a requirement of a high/maximal level of competence is reasonably required to insure that the patient's well-being is adequately protected and that in exercising his self-determination he has chosen in accordance with his own aims and values. When the expected effects for life and health of the patient's choice are approximately comparable to those of alternatives, a moderate/median level of competence is appropriate to insure that the patient's well-being is adequately protected while respecting his self-determination.

One final and perhaps unexpected consequence of this variability is that the level of competence for consenting to and refusing a treatment need not be the same, because the consequences for the patient's well-being may be dramatically different. It is reasonable to insist that a patient fully understand that he or she is *refusing* a life-saving therapy that has only limited risks, while applying less strict standards to the patient's *acceptance* of that same therapy. While this variability in morally appropriate levels of competence implies the need for discretion on the part of individuals making competence determinations, legal and professional practices must be designed to limit the unjustified use of that discretion wrongly to deny patients' rights ultimately to insist on what they believe will best promote their values and goals. The more reason we have to distrust professional use of such discretion, the more we will reasonably design legal rules and practices to limit it.

Standards evaluating the content of the patient's decision. Although the "mere expression of a preference" standard of competence is insufficiently paternalistic, standards that determine competence by evaluating the content of the patient's choice are excessively and objctionably paternalistic. This not to deny that it is commonly disagreement with the content of the physician's recommendation that will trigger review of the patient's competence in marginal cases. This is natural and reasonable, given the presumption that the physician's recommendation is in the patient's interest. But the mere fact that the patient has decided on a course of treatment different from the physician's (or family's) recommendation serves as no basis at all for a determination of incompetence. Basing determinations of incompetence on the content of the patient's decision inevitably requires appeal to some "objective" standard of correct decisions, independent of whether that standard conforms to this patient's values and goals. "Correct" decisions in this view are rational, or what most people would decide, or what the physician would decide. But it is highly problematic whether any such objective standard of a patient's good is ultimately defensible. Employing such a standard will seriously compromise the patient's self-determination, without evidence that his or her capacity for self-determination in the circumstances is deficient. Finding a patient incompetent merely because his or her treatment choice does not conform to some external, supposedly objective, standard fails to respect the patient's capacity to define his or her own values. Finally, any such standard in practice risks substantial abuse and unwarranted denial ("for their own good") of patients' rights to decide for themselves.

VOLUNTARINESS

For the consent of a competent decision maker to be binding, it must be voluntary or freely given. Consent that is obtained as a result of coercion or duress manipulation or undue influence, is invalid and does not authorize treatment. An involuntary choice will not reflect the aims of the chooser, but the will of the coercer or manipulator instead, and so will violate the chooser's self-determination.

Coercion

A patient's decision is coerced when the patient is threatened, either explicitly or implicitly, with unwanted and avoidable consequences unless the patient makes the desired choice. For example, a gravely ill patient is told that unless he agrees to further treatment, other palliative measures to limit his discomfort will be withdrawn. Outright coercion of patients, at least by health care professionals, is probably relatively rare, though it may be more common in special settings, such as mental hospitals, prisons, and some nursing homes. The great inequalities between involuntarily committed mental patients, prisoners, children, some nursing home populations, and those on whom they are dependent, make these groups especially vulnerable to coercion. Since there is significant potential for conflict of interest between these groups and their caretakers, special scrutiny of the voluntariness of their consent to medical care is warranted. Coercion by family members to force treatment is probably more common than by health care professionals. With relatively few exceptions, such as innoculations for public health purposes or treatment in connection with obtaining evidence in criminal proceedings, coerced or forced treatment of competent patients is not morally justified or legally permitted. Forced treatment without the patient's consent can be distinguished from coerced consent. Forced treatment involves no consent, while coerced consent invalidates the consent; each makes the treatment unauthorized.

It is sometimes said that patients faced with very difficult and unpleasant alternatives, such as whether to undergo painful chemotherapy when it is the only treatment for an otherwise fatal cancer, do not choose the chemotherapy voluntarily because their choice is coerced by the disease itself. Nevertheless, unpleasant and unwanted choices between bad alternatives are not in themselves coercive. When the undesired alternatives are caused, for example, by the patient's illness, rather than by the threat of another person, they represent the unfortunate but inevitable constraints within which the patient must decide about treatment. That all alternatives are "bad" and leave little or no "real choice" provides no sound reason to set aside the patient's choice as involuntary and to transfer the decision to another.

It is also important to distinguish coercion involving threats of unwanted consequences from warnings about the natural history of a disease and the natural consequences of certain decisions. In most cases, the distinction turns on whether the physician acts to bring about the unwanted consequence (threat) or merely informs the patient that it will be a consequence of one of the patient's alternatives (warning). Telling a hypertensive patient of the medical consequences of not taking medication constitutes a warning and does not coerce him or her to take the medication, whereas threatening to withdraw further care unless the patient accepts the physician's preferred treatment generally is coercive. The first is part of a physician's responsibility, while the second is morally wrong.

Manipulation

Although coercion is probably relatively uncommon in health care relationships, manipulation of patient decision making is more widespread. Indeed, it is a common criticism by physicians that the informed-consent process is meaningless because they can get the patient to agree to whatever they want. Manipulation in health care relationships is complex, both in theory and practice, and can take more forms than there is space to discuss here. Many features of the health care setting make it ripe for manipulation. Patients are commonly worried and fearful, uncertain of what is "wrong" with them, and seek reassurance and care. They are explicitly asked to place their trust in physicians who possess special knowledge and capacities to give care. In these circumstances, the disparities in knowledge, status, and authority make manipulation sometimes hard to avoid. Perhaps the most blatant form of manipulation is when information is deliberately withheld from patients in order to affect their choice. For example, they are not told of alternative treatments to the one the physician prefers, or of significant risks or side effects of a recommended treatment. This clearly limits a patient's capacity to make an informed choice that best fits his or her particular needs and values.

Manipulation can, however, be far more subtle than outright deception. For example, a physician's manner and tone of voice can indicate whether a risk is one to worry about, or whether a concern is justified. The way information is presented can affect how the patient responds to it—for example, "This treatment succeeds in two out of every five cases" or "This treatment fails most of the time." In some cases, there may be no fully "objective" or "neutral" form in which necessary information can be conveyed. Nevertheless, it generally is posible to avoid putting information in a form designed to change the patient's decision from what it would have been with a sound understanding of the information. Such manipulation may be conceived as being "for the patient's own good" and producing the "best" decision. Or it may be used merely to avoid the more difficult and time-consuming process of helping the patient clearly understand the situation and how alternative courses of action may or may not serve his aims and needs. But in the former case it both infringes self-determination by denying patients a sound understanding on which to base their choice and fails to respect the extent to which people's own aims and values determine what will best promote their own well-being. In the latter case, although the outcome of patient's decisions may not be different as a result of the manipulation, the manipulation bypasses the patient's own deliberative processes and their self-determination is compromised, making the decision not fully theirs.

None of this is to say that physicians should not make treatment recommendations to patients who want those recommendations, or that such recommendations are inherently manipulative. On the contrary, it is part of physicians' professional responsibility to make such recommendations available, and these recommendations naturally and reasonably influence patients' decisions. If the recommendations are tailored to a particular patient's goals and values and are not manipulative in the ways discussed above, they need not compromise the voluntariness of the patient's decision.

The various forms of involuntariness of treatment decisions occur in different degrees—coercion and manipulation may both be more or less serious, irresistible, and pervasive in undermining self-determination. Ideal physician-patient decision making would involve no kind or degree of involuntariness. The law and other forms of public policy should seek to promote this ideal. Nevertheless, legal remedies in the law for coerced or manipulated consent often require evidence both that (1) the patient's decision was different from what it would otherwise have been as a result of the involuntariness and that (2) the treatment given resulted in harm to the patient. This is only one instance of the general fact that the law is neither a desirable nor effective instrument for preventing or remedying every moral wrong, or every failure to attain a moral ideal.

Informed understanding. The goal of the requirement that consent be informed is for patients to achieve a sufficient understanding of their condition and possible treatments so that they can make a sound assessment of which treatment, if any, will best serve their goals and values. It thereby permits an informed exercise of self-determination and promotes a decision most in accord with the patient's well-being. It is worth adding as an important practical matter that therapeutic benefits can accrue from the patient's being well-informed (for example, increased conformity to a treatment regimen), that the great majority of patients want vital information about their treatment,[3] and that the lack of an adequate explanation of the nature and purpose of a procedure is a major cause of refusals of treatment by patients.[4] Physicians sometimes conceive of informed consent as principally requiring a disclosure of the risks of treatment in order to protect themselves from legal liability should a problem arise. This leads to association of informed consent with the form that the patient signs testifying that such risks have been disclosed. But such forms are neither necessary nor sufficient to protect from legal liability, and although obtaining informed consent can protect against legal liability for negligence or battery (though not from liability for malpractice), that is not its main ethical basis.

The focus on *disclosure* of risks to protect against legal liability also has had the unfortunate result of shifting attention away from the *comprehension* or *understanding* of the information by the patient. A patient's understanding is the result sought by any requirement that a patient be informed. Thus, physicians should tailor the presentation of information to the particular patient so that it is as comprehensible as possible. This usually will involve avoiding technical medical or scientific jargon and helping the patient understand the consequences of various medical procedures. Making information comprehensible to the particular patient also is relevant to meeting the objection often made by physicians that informed consent cannot be achieved because patients only rarely can fully understand the relevant information. In its extreme form, this objection holds that patients would have to be given extensive medical and scientific training if they are to understand fully their medical condition and various treatment alternatives. Such objections, however, largely are misguided. Physicians obviously bring medical knowledge to the treatment decision process that patients nearly always lack, just as patients bring knowledge of their own particular goals and values that physicians lack. It is not necessary for a patient to become a physician in order to give informed consent. In order to make an informed decision about treatment, patients do not require all the medical details and underlying scientific bases of treatment alternatives that their physicians have. Rather, patients need to understand how those treatment alternatives will affect their capacity to pursue their various plans of life. This understanding rarely will require a sophisticated medical or scientific background.

The other aspect of the objection we are now considering concerns the impossibility or unreasonableness of communicating all information possibly relevant to the decision at hand. Even if it all could be communicated, such information would overwhelm the average patient who is unable to integrate it all into his or her decision process. Moreover, telling patients of every risk or possible side effect of treatment, no matter how remote, might so terrify them that they would reject needed treatment. This objection raises questions about both the *kinds* and *amounts* of information that ought to be conveyed to the patient. The broad kinds of information to be conveyed are relatively uncontroversial. They should include: (1) the patient's current medical condition, including a future prognosis if no treatment is pursued; (2) any treatment alternatives that might improve the patient's condition and prognosis, including an explanation of the procedures involved, the significant risks and benefits of the alternatives, with their associated probabilities, and the financial costs of the alternatives; and (3) a recommendation as to the best alternative. We assume for the present that the patient has not expressed a desire *not* to have any of this information. If there is anything not commonly discussed in this list, it is the financial cost of the alternatives. However, when the costs to the patient are significant (and whether they are will vary with a patient's circumstances), they can have a substantial impact on the patient's financial ability to pursue other goals important to him or her—and so on the overall desirability of treatment alternatives, and can affect the likelihood of the patient's actually pursuing a treatment course.

What is controversial is the amount of information that must be conveyed. More specifically, concern has focused on when risks are too remote or inconsequential to require that the patient be told about them. Courts, as well as the state legislatures that have intervened on this matter, have largely been divided between two alternative general standards of disclosure: (1) the standard of professional medical practice for such cases—crudely put, an individual physician must convey particular information, and in particular disclose risks, if most other physicians do or would do so in similar cases; (2) the standard of what a reasonable person would want to know in the case at hand—or, as it is sometimes put, whatever information is "material" to the decision at hand. The first standard probably provides a clearer guide for physicians, as well as greater protection from liability for nondisclosure. However, given the long paternalistic tradition of limited disclosure of information to patients, the "professional practice" standard fails to ensure that patients will have the information necessary for sound decision making. The "reasonable person" standard, though introducing greater uncertainty about just what information must be conveyed, is more likely to result in patients obtaining necessary information. However, as a moral matter, this standard should be amended to require conveying whatever information a reasonable person would want to know, *plus* whatever else the actual person wants to know. For example, a professional athlete may quite reasonably want to know about a risk from treatment that would ruin her career that others would not want disclosed to them. So it is important that physicians consider the particular concerns and values of the actual patient and how these may differ from other persons. Perhaps the simplest way to try to ensure meeting any unusual information needs a particular patient may have is always to invite the patient to ask for any additional information he or she may want after a discussion of information the physician considers material to the decision.

Legal policy. Here, as elsewhere in this chapter, the focus is on the ethically sound basis and nature of informed consent. There may be good reason not to fully individualize the *legal* requirement for disclosure because of the difficulty of establishing in litigation, often taking place long after the event in question, what the particular patient wanted to know. Doing so would create an invitation for self-serving testimony by patients, for whom a remote risk has eventuated in actual harm, that "of course, I would have wanted to know about that." For similar reasons, it may be best for the law not to allow *less* disclosure than a reasonable person would want, even though fully respecting self-determination would seem to support doing so when patients do not want to be told that information. As a matter of public and legal policy, it is probably best not to fully individualize the information requirement, in order to help protect against the abuse of patients being denied information they do or would in fact want.

The requirement that a patient be informed before consenting often is claimed to be limited by a physician's "therapeutic privilege." Specifically, it is claimed that physicians are justified in not informing competent patients of particular risks when doing so would seriously upset the patient. Therapeutic privilege has the potential of seriously undermining the informed-consent doctrine, given that physicians are quite naturally averse to conveying unpleasant information to their patients, and that patients quite naturally become upset at learning it. Consequently, any ethically acceptable exception to the requirement of informed consent based on therapeutic privilege must be carefully and narrowly framed. Rather than merely "upsetting" the patient, it should be the case that disclosing the information would cause serious harm to the patient. And the harm must result from the receipt of the information itself, independent of its causing the patient to make a different treatment decision than he or she would otherwise have made. Moreover, there should be strict evidentiary requirements for the harm, such as clear and convincing evidence of the high probability of imminent and serious harm. Any such standard will require much interpretation in individual cases—when is evidence clear and convincing, what probability is high enough, when is harm imminent and serious? It would permit temporarily withholding from a deeply depressed and suicidal patient devastating information highly likely to trigger a suicide attempt. However, in the interest of limiting its abuse such a standard would rightly set a high burden of proof on physicians who sought to invoke therapeutic privilege. It is probably reasonable as well to require, when therapeutic privilege is invoked and important information is withheld from a competent patient, that the procedures required for incompetent patients involving use of a surrogate decision maker be followed.

Therapeutic privilege is one of the exceptions to the general requirement that treatment cannot be given without the patient's informed consent. We have discussed in detail a second exception —incompetence—and decision-making procedures for incompetent patients are elaborated in another chapter. We have also discussed a third exception—waiver by patients of their right to decide. The final exception to the informed consent requirement is emergency—treatment can be given without a patient's consent when failure to render urgent care would likely result in serious harm or loss of life to the patient, and obtaining the patient's consent is either not possible or would seriously delay the rendering of that care.

The overall argument of this chapter can be summarized in a sentence: giving due weight to the value of personal well-being while respecting individual self-determination morally requires gaining and honoring the informed and voluntary consent of competent patients for their medical treatment. However, such a simple summary should not be allowed to obscure two points. First, even the more detailed analysis of informed consent here is not detailed enough. It leaves many issues unaddressed—for example, what role, if any, should patients' unconscious beliefs and motivations play in determinations of their decision-making competence, voluntariness, and understanding? And it leaves many cases hard cases—for example, in instances in which a patient's well-being and self-determination are in conflict, we lack any precise and uncontroversial basis for assigning a weight to each. But even the best and most detailed analysis leaves genuinely hard cases hard and controversial, though it should help us understand better why they are hard and what conflicting values and arguments make them controversial. Second, the moral ideal of informed consent expressed here is a high ideal, which is often realized imperfectly at best in medical practice. There is not space here to explore the many avenues of change that might help move much medical practice closer to that ideal. But there can be little doubt that realizing the ideal would involve significant transformations of the traditional health care process.

Notes

Acknowledgments: The basic positions, and even some of the language, of this chapter bear a close relation to parts of *Making Health Care Deci-*

sions: The Ethical and Legal Implications of Informed Consent in the Patient-Practitioner Relationship, Volume One: Report, President's Commission for the Study of Ethical Problems in Medicine and Biomedical and
Behavioral Research (Washington, D.C.: U.S. Government Printing Office,
1982). I was a member of the commission staff team that drafted that report,
with special responsibilities for some of the philosophical issues also discussed here. That report's preparation was truly a team effort and my views
on informed consent are deeply indebted to the other principal commission
staff members on that project, Alexander M. Capron, Joanne Lynn, Marian
Osterweis, and Alan J. Weisbard, though none of them is, of course, responsible for any misuse I may have made of their good influences.

    1. Some of the important legal cases bearing on informed consent include
Schloendorff v. Society of New York Hospital, 211 N.Y. 125, 105 N.E. 92, 95
(1914), in which the right to self-determination is asserted; Salgo v. Leland
Stanford Jr. University Board of Trustees, 154 Cal. App. 2d 560, 317 P.2d 170
(1957), in which "informed" was added to the consent requirement to yield
"informed consent"; Natanson v. Kline 186 Kan. 393, 350 P.2d 1093, the
opinion on denial of motion for rehearing, 187 Kan. 186 354 P.2d 670 (1960);
Canterbury v. Spence, 464 F.2d 772 (D.C. Cir.), cert. denied, 409 U.S. 1064
(1972) and Cobbs v. Grant, 8 Cal. 3d 229 104 Cal. Rptr. 505, 502 P.2d 1
(1972), both of which enunciate standards of disclosure of information.
    2. Isaiah Berlin, "Two Concepts of Liberty," in Four Essays on Liberty
(Oxford: Clarendon Press, 1969), 118–138.
    3. See the survey of public and professional attitudes and practices in the
area of informed consent performed for the President's commission by
Louis Harris Associates, in Making Health Care Decisions: The Ethical and
Legal Implications of Informed Consent in the Patient-Practitioner Relationship, Volume Two: appendices, President's Commission for the Study
of Ethical Problems in Medicine and Biomedical and Behavioral Research
(Washington, D.C.: U.S. Government Printing Office, 1982).
    4. See the study of treatment refusal by Paul Applebaum and Loren Roth
in Making Health Care Decisions Volume Two, appendices.

Suggestions for Further Reading

Capron, Alexander. "Informed Consent in Catastrophic Disease Research
    and Treatment." University of Pennyslvania Law Review 123 (December
    1974): 340–438.
Childress, James. F. Who Should Decide? Paternalism in Health Care
    (New York: Oxford University Press, 1983).
Drane, James, "The Many Faces of Competency," Hastings Center Report
    15 (April 1985): 17–21.
Dworkin, Gerald. "Autonomy and Informed Consent. Making Health Care
    Decisions: The Ethical and Legal Implications of Informed Consent in

the Patient-Practitioner Relationship, Volume Three: Appendices, Studies on the Foundations of Informed Consent. President's Commission for the Study of Ethical Problems in Medicine and Biomedical and Behavioral Research. Washington, D.C.: U.S. Government Printing Office, 1982.

Freedman, Benjamin. "A Moral Theory of Informed Consent." Hastings Center Report 5 (August 1975): 32–39.

Kass, Leon. "The End of Medicine and the Pursuit of Health," in Toward a More Natural Science: Biology and Human Affairs (New York: Free Press, 1985).

Katz, Jay. The Silent World of Doctor and Patient (New York: Free Press, 1983).

Lidz, Charles W., et al. Informed Consent: A Study of Decisionmaking in Psychiatry (New York: The Guilford Press, 1984).

Making Health Care Decisions: The Ethical and Legal Implications of Informed Consent in the Patient-Practitioner Relationship, Volumes One through Three. President's Commission for the Study of Ethical Problems in Medicine and Biomedical and Behavioral Research. Washington, D.C.: U.S. Government Printing Office, 1982.

Meisel, Alan; Roth, Loren H.; and Lidz, Charles W. "Toward a Model of the Legal Doctrine of Informed Consent." American Journal of Psychiatry 134 (1977): 285–289.

Roth, Loren; Meisel, Alan; and Lidz, Charles W. "Tests of Competency to Consent to Treatment." American Journal of Psychiatry 134 (1977): 279–284.

Tancredi, Laurence R. "The Right to Refuse Psychiatric Treatment: Some Legal and Ethical Considerations." Journal of Health Politics, Policy and Law 5 (Fall 1980): 514–522.

Veatch, Robert M. "Three Theories of Informed Consent: Philosophical Foundations and Policy Implications." In Appendix B to The Belmont Report: Ethical Principles and Guidelines for the Protection of Human Subjects of Research. DHEW Publication No. (OS) 78-0014. Washington, D.C.: U.S. Government Printing Office, 1978. Vol. II, (26-1)–(26-66).

CHAPTER III

Experimentation on Human Subjects

The Ethics of Random Clinical Trials

Bruce Miller

Sir Patrick: You remember Jane Marsh?
Ridgeon: Jane Marsh? No.
Sir Patrick: You don't?
Ridgeon: No.
Sir Patrick: You mean to tell me that you don't
remember the woman with the tuberculous ulcer
on her arm?
Ridgeon: (enlightened) Oh, your washerwoman's
daughter. Was her name Jane Marsh? I forgot.
Sir Patrick: Perhaps you've forgotten also that you
undertook to cure her with Koch's tuberculin.
Ridgeon: And instead of curing her, it rotted her
arm right off. Yes: I remember. Poor Jane!
However, she makes a good living out of that arm
now by shewing it at medical lectures.
Sir Patrick: Still, that wasn't quite what you
intended, was it?
Ridgeon: I took my chance of it.
Sir Patrick: Jane did, you mean.
Ridgeon: Well, it's always the patient who has to
take the chance when an experiment is necessary.
And we can find out nothing without experiment.
Sir Patrick: What did you find out from Jane's case?
Ridgeon: I found out that the inoculation that
ought to cure sometimes kills.

> Sir Patrick: I could have told you that. I've tried
> these modern inoculations a bit myself. I've
> killed people with them; and I've cured people
> with them; but I gave them up because I never
> could tell which I was going to do.

> —G. B. Shaw, The Doctor's Dilemma

Introduction

Prior to this century, many treatments were thought to be effective on the basis of experiments similar to Ridgeon's experiment on Jane Marsh. Fortunately for patients, most of them were harmless; unfortunately, many were also ineffective. But many treatments widely used in the past were actually harmful, such as bleeding for fever. Before a medical treatment is approved today as effective and safe, a controlled trial of the treatment must be done. This is frequently done in a random clinical trial (RCT), the gold standard of medical research methods. The RCT is a controlled comparison of two treatments whose design uses the techniques of modern statistics. The aim of this chapter is to explore the ethical issues in the use of RCTs.

The Structure of a Random Clinical Trial

The purpose of an RCT is to determine which of two or more treatments is safer or more effective for a given illness. The subjects are selected for admission to a trial on the basis of diagnostic criteria formulated as precisely as possible in order to ensure that they all have the same illness. Next, the subjects are randomly assigned to the treatment alternatives. If an RCT is double-blind, neither the patients nor physicians know which treatment a patient is receiving. Results of the treatments are collected and these data then are analyzed using appropriate statistical techniques. Finally, conclusions are drawn regarding the relative effectiveness of the treatments. The effectiveness of a treatment is measured by relief of symptoms as reported by the subjects or observed by a physician, or by more objective features such as a reduction in the incidence of death, nonrecurrence of the disease, or an alteration in laboratory tests such as blood counts, X-rays, and biopsies. The risks in a treatment are the side effects, which can be anything from death to minor matters like nausea and dizziness. Other items may include whether the two groups of subjects were comparable with respect to influencing factors such as age, sex, prior illness, and severity of illness, whether the results of the research show that one treatment is always to be preferred over the other, or whether one treatment seems best only for a certain class of patients.

ASPECTS OF A RANDOM CLINICAL TRIAL

Five aspects of the RCT need further explanation: (1) the use of a control group; (2) the placebo effect; (3) double-blinding; (4) random assignment; and (5) statistical significance. One of the reasons for a control group is that the knowledge sought is whether the new treatment is better than existing treatments. A trial without a control may show that the new treatment has some effect and that it has certain side effects, but that may not indicate whether it is more effective or safer than an existing treatment. Sometimes there is no existing treatment, or none that has any significant effect; the control group then may be given a placebo. A placebo is something that is believed to have no biological effect on a patient's illness. In drug therapy, a placebo will be a substance like a sugar pill or an injection of sterile water or saline solution.

The reason for using a placebo control group is that there is a placebo effect to every medical treatment. A person who is ill and who believes that a physician can do something that will relieve the illness typically will have some improvement from the belief alone. The physician's belief that he or she is doing something beneficial to the patient may contribute to the patient's improvement. Part of the effect of every treatment is a result of these symbolic aspects of the patient-physician relationship. To determine the effectiveness of a medical treatment in a research trial, the trial must be structured to distinguish the placebo effect of the treatment from the biological effect of the treatment.

Another reason for the use of a control group is to distinguish the effects of the treatment from the effects of other factors. Suppose that a group of patients is diagnosed as having a certain disease to a certain degree; let's call that condition A. Suppose all these patients are given a drug and six weeks later none of them has condition A. One might conclude that the drug caused this, but condition A may have disappeared independent of the drug rather than because of it. Condition A may simply have run its natural course. If the patients were hospitalized, the environmental change may have been the cause. A methodological postulate of science is that if all we know is that one set of events or conditions preceded another event or condition, we cannot conclude that one particular preceding event or condition was the cause of the subsequent event or condition. The RCT attempts to construct two groups that are identical in all respects except that one group receives one treatment and the other group another. If one group shows significantly more improvement than the other, this improvement can be attributed to the treatment, because that is the only relevant difference between the two groups.

Random assignment to alternative treatments randomly distributes the many possible influencing factors so that it can be assumed that the groups of subjects are alike in all respects, and differences in outcome can be attributed to the difference in treatments. Another reason for using random assignments of subjects is to eliminate bias in the selection of treatment. If a decision must be made whether each patient will receive treatment A or treatment B, physicians may assign a greater portion of the less ill patients to one of the treatments without being conscious of doing so.

The reason for using a double-blind is to avoid any bias of subjects or physicians in reporting or recording patients' symptoms. If a patient knows that he or she is receiving a placebo, he or she may not expect to get well and therefore may not. However, if a patient knows that he or she is receiving a newly discovered treatment that is thought by physicians to hold out great promise of a cure, this may influence the patient's beliefs and reports about how the treatment is working. If the physician who examines the patient knows which of the treatments the patient is receiving, this can influence the physician's reports on the patient. A physician need not have a conscious belief that one treatment is better than another to be biased; a mere hunch, or a personal interest in the results of the trial, may be sufficient to cause lack of uniformity in the observation and care of patients in the trial.

The concept of *statistical significance* is of importance in discussions of the ethical issues of RCTs. There are many different methods of determining statistical significance. They will be described briefly and intuitively here. Consider a simple coin-tossing example. Suppose I toss a coin twice and both times it comes up heads. Prior to any toss of this particular coin, the chances of tossing a head and of tossing a tail are equal. This is expressed by saying that the probability of a head is .5 and the probability of a tail is .5. After two successive heads are tossed, suppose someone claims that the coin is rigged so that it always comes up heads. We probably would reply that the conclusion is not warranted because there have only been two tosses; a nonrigged coin might produce two heads in a row. Suppose eight more heads are tossed. Now it is more plausible to say that the coin is rigged, because it is very unlikely that one would toss ten heads in a row. The statistical significance of the claim that the coin is rigged is greater after ten heads in a row than after two heads in a row.

The concept of statistical significance is fairly easy to understand in the coin-tossing example; in other contexts, the notion of statistical significance is more complicated. We now will consider a simple medical example to explain the notion in a more relevant context. Suppose there are two drugs, A and B. Suppose we wish to know whether A or B is more effective in reducing mortality from a given disease. A and B are randomly assigned to patients with the disease, and we determine whether the patients are dead or alive at some particular period of time after receiving the drug. Suppose four patients enter into the trial, and two of them receive drug A and die, while two receive drug B and survive. Prior to the trial, the hypotheses that we might form about drug A and drug B are that there is no difference in their effect on mortality, that there is a 100 percent difference in their effect on mortality, or anything in between. Based on the results in four patients, the no-difference hypothesis seems unsupported, while the alternatives have received some support. We would not have much warrant to conclude that B is 100 percent more effective than A, for there is not much support from the four instances of administering the drugs. Suppose the drugs are administered sixteen more times, with ten patients receiving drug A and ten patients receiving drug B, and, as before, all the patients on A die and all the patients on B survive. Now we could be much more confident of the claim that B is 100 percent more effective than A in preventing death.

This hypothetical example is more more clear-cut than the usual result of medical research; rarely is there a 100 percent difference in mortality for two treatments. This is because of the biological variability of individuals. We are not exactly alike biologically, and thus diseases and treatments affect us differently. A more common result in a trial of the sort we are imagining is that the survival rate for B was 60 percent, and the survival rate for drug A was 40 percent. However, the same point applies regarding the number of subjects in the trial (the sample size). If the 60–40 percent difference were obtained after five patients were put on each drug, that would be less significant statistically than if the same difference were obtained after twenty patients were put on each drug. Statisticians are able to determine the number of patients required in a trial in order to reach a given level of significance. There is a consensus that a certain level of significance is desired. In one version of the test of statistical significance, that level is expressed as $P \leq .05$. This means that there is less than a one in twenty chance (probability of .05) that there is no difference in the medical effects of the two treatments, and that the difference is the result of the chance allocation of more good-prognosis patients to one treatment than another (this assumes that the patients are being randomly assigned to the two treatments). If the significance level is less than .05, then more confidence can be placed in the view that the difference is the result of the treatment, if it is greater than .05, then less confidence is justifiable. Statisticians admit that a significance level of .05 is somewhat arbitrary. Since significance is a matter of degree, no strong arguments can be given that a medical researcher ought to strive for a level of .05 rather than .06 or .07. The importance of this point will be discussed later.

There are many alternatives to the RCT. Some of them are elaborate adaptations of modern techniques of statistical analysis and will not be discussed in this paper. The procedures which will be considered are the RCT and consecutive trials. In a trial of the latter sort, as the name suggests, each subject enrolled, in succession, is given the experimental treatment. Consecutive trials do not have the same kind of controls as the RCTs mentioned above. The next section discusses research on the treatment of a disease, first by a consecutive trial and then by an RCT.

EXAMPLES OF A NONCONTROLLED AND A CONTROLLED TRIAL

A group of researchers were working on the possible beneficial effects of cryogenic therapy (i.e. treating disease by lowering the temperature of all or part of the body). Among the diseases studied was peptic ulcer, a lesion or wound in the stomach wall caused by excess gastric secretion of acid. It is a common disease that can cause death. The technique developed was "gastric freezing." A tube was inserted into the stomach; at the end of the tube was a balloon. The tube was constructed so that a cold liquid could be circulated through the balloon and thereby lower the temperature of the stomach. The procedure initially was tried with dogs, and it was discovered that the freezing reduced the secretion of acids and caused structural changes in the tissue of the stomach wall. The procedure was then tried on patients who had been admitted to the hospital for surgical treatment of peptic ulcer. Thirty-one patients received the gastric freeze. The treatment lasted for about one hour with temperature maintained at − 12 to − 20 degrees centigrade. The investigators stated that all patients reported a marked or complete relief of subjective symptoms (e.g., stomach pain), and thirty of the thirty-one patients showed a significant decrease in the secretion of acid, an objective measure. The researchers concluded that the treatment appeared simple, effective and safe. In an addendum to the article, they reported that 120 patients had now received the treatment without complication.[1]

In the years immediately following this report, the procedure was introduced in many hospitals. Reports began to arise regarding complications, and many physicians raised questions about the long-term effectiveness of the treatment. A prominent medical journal surveyed physicians using the procedure and reported that although there was an initial decrease in acid secretion, there was a return to the previous level of secretion within six weeks to six months. Nonetheless, patients continued to report a significant improvement in symptoms.

At this point, the evidence on the effectiveness of gastric freezing for peptic ulcer was ambiguous. Although the treatment did provide relief of symptoms, the fact that the reduction of acid secretion does not persist raises doubts about the effectiveness. The symptoms of peptic ulcer, abdominal pain and nausea, are the result of excess secretion of acid, but since the treatment did not maintain reduced levels of acid secretion, there were doubts that the symptomatic improvement was a result of the freezing of the stomach. It may be that there was some other physiological mechanism bringing about the improvement in symptoms, or it may have been a placebo effect. To resolve these issues, a controlled trial was needed.

In a controlled trial of gastric freezing, one group of patients would have to receive the treatment and another group would have to receive a treatment that resembles the gastric freezing so closely that neither they nor the physicians examining them could know which they received. It would be easy to keep the examining physicians in ignorance: just don't tell them. The problem was to make the patients in the control group believe that they were receiving a real gastric freeze. The researchers designed a tube and balloon that resembled the equipment for the gastric freeze except that cold liquid did not circulate in the balloon. In the sham procedure, the temperature in the balloon was at 37 degrees Centigrade. Cold liquid did circulate in the tube, so the patients felt the cold in their mouth and throat, and believed their stomachs were being cooled.

One hundred and sixty patients were randomly assigned. Eighty-two received the freeze treatment; seventy-eight received the sham treatment. All patients were followed for thirteen months. Six weeks after the treatment, 47 percent of the freeze patients reported that they were improved or symptom free compared with 39 percent of the sham patients. However, as time passed, most patients in both groups relapsed or became worse: at 12 months, 28 percent in the freeze group and 30 percent in the sham group relapsed. At no time was there a significant difference in the two groups. Measurement of acid secretion was done before and immediately after treatment and at every follow-up visit. There was no significant difference in the levels of gastric secretion before and after treatment. The researchers concluded that "this study demonstrates conclusively that the 'freezing' procedure was no better than the sham in the treatment of duodenal ulcer. . . . It is reasonable to assume that the relief of pain and subjective improvement reported by early investigators was probably due to the psychologic effect of the procedure."[2]

Ethical Issues about Clinical Trials

The ethical issues in the two trials of gastric freezing can be divided into three categories: first, issues about the initiation of a trial; second, issues regarding the termination of a trial; and third, issues regarding informing patients and obtaining their consent to be subjects in the trial of a medical procedure.

ISSUES OF INITIATION

When the uncontrolled trial of gastric freezing was started, was it ethical to treat the patients with a procedure whose effectiveness and safety were not determined? There are standard surgical treatments for patients with ulcers, and the effectiveness and safety of those treatments are known; they are not fully satisfactory, since they do not prevent recurrence and there is a significant risk to any patient who undergoes surgery with general anesthesia. Still, a patient and his or her physician have evidence on which to judge whether or not it is in the interest of the patient to undergo the standard surgical treatments. Though there is some evidence that the gastric freeze will be effective and safe, a patient with an ulcer cannot be assured that the gastric freeze is the best treatment.

Whether the interests of patients were being sacrificed was also a question in the controlled trial of the gastric freeze treatment. After the noncontrolled trial was published, many physicians who adopted the procedure reported that although there was symptomatic relief, there was no evidence that the level of acid secretion was reduced for a significant time. There may have been enough evidence from these reports to determine that gastric freezing was not an effective treatment. The fact that several controlled trials were done shows that medical researchers believed that either (1) there was insufficient evidence to show that the treatment was not effective, or (2) though the evidence was sufficient, a controlled trial had to be done to persuade others. The freeze treatment is more convenient and safer than the usual surgical treatment, and some distinguished medical researchers believed it to be effective; thus, there was some ground for a physician to use the treatment. In order to stop these physicians from using the treatment, a controlled study was done to show conclusively that the treatment is not effective. If it is not, then the patients who were entered into the controlled trial of gastric freezing had their interests sacrificed in the interest of future patients.

A crucial ethical issue in clinical research emerges: *Is it justifiable to sacrifice the interest of current patients by making them subjects in an RCT to determine what is most beneficial for future patients?* If the answer to this question is no, then a significant restraint is placed on progress in medicine. Research on new treatments would not be totally forbidden, but it would be permissible only in those cases in which it could be shown that everything that was done to a patient was in the best interest of *that patient*. Just how much current research would be unjustified is difficult to say. Research on fatal diseases for which there is no effective life-saving treatment would be permissible, as would research on patients whose condition is terminal because they have not responded to conventional treatments. Experimentation with treatments for nonfatal diseases for which there is no effective treatment would be justifiable provided the side effects of the new treatment were known, and known not to be more severe than allowing the disease to run its course.

Another ethical question emerges from consideration of the idea that the justification for medical research is the benefit of future patients. The researchers who did the initial trials of gastric freezing chose to do a noncontrolled trial. Animal trials were done, but all researchers know that such results are not directly transferable to human beings. The researchers also knew, or should have known, that all treatments have a placebo effect; this is especially true for the symptoms of ulcers. Any effectiveness shown in a noncontrolled trial may be the result largely, or entirely, of the placebo effect. To benefit future patients, researchers must show that a treatment has more than a placebo effect and more effect than treatments currently in use. The noncontrolled trial of gastric freezing is not only questionable regarding the interests of patients in the trial, but also questionable regarding the interests of future patients.

Two more ethical issues about the initiation of clinical trials should be mentioned in connection with the gastric freezing research: whether it was justifiable to use a sham treatment for a control, and whether it was justifiable to randomly assign the patients to the sham or real gastric freeze. With regard to the sham control, the physicians had no reason to believe that the procedure could have more than a placebo effect. Since there are treatments that have a real biologic effect on ulcers, it seems clear that the interests of the patients assigned to the sham treatment were being sacrificed. With regard to random assignment, patients usually expect that a physician's decision is based on a judgment of what is best for the patient; when the treatment decision is made by a random method, this expectation of the patient, and obligation of the physician, is not being met.

ISSUES REGARDING TERMINATION

One hundred and sixty patients were studied in the controlled trial of the gastric freeze procedure; at the end of the trial, the researchers concluded that the gastric freeze was an ineffective treatment for peptic ulcer. During the course of the study, data were available on the two treatments. Suppose that after eighty patients there was evidence that the real freeze was no more effective than the sham freeze. In that case, the next 120 patients were receiving a treatment that the researchers had evidence to believe was ineffective. At what point in a controlled trial is there sufficient evidence to reach a conclusion and stop the trial?

When a controlled trial is designed, a determination is made on how many patients will be included in the study. Many factors are used in this determination. An important one is the level of statistical significance. Statisticians can calculate how many patients will be needed in the trial in order to reach an .05 level of significance. Generally, and setting other aspects aside, the larger the number of patients in a trial, the more likely it is that a result significant at the .05 level will be reached.

The researchers in the controlled trial of gastric freezing only reported the results for the total 160 patients. Suppose that after eighty patients were treated, the null hypothesis (that there is no difference in the treatments) is confirmed at the .07 level. This is not the level that statisticians recommend as good enough. The question is, "Good enough for what?" A level of .07 may be enough for a judgment that it is not in the interest of the eighty-first patient to have a gastric freeze rather than one of the standard surgical treatments. The argument for continuing the trial to 160 patients is that the researcher wants to show that the treatment has no more than placebo effect—with as much certainty as is widely accepted in medical research—so that future physicians will have no grounds at all to use the gastric freeze. Again, the conflict is between the interests of patients in the trial and those of future patients.

ISSUES OF INFORMED CONSENT

The topic of informed consent and the ethical and conceptual problems associated with it are all well discussed in Chapter II by Dan Brock. Although Brock's discussion is limited to informed consent to therapy, the basic notion is not any different in the research context. There are several distinct issues regarding informed consent to participation in an RCT. First, must the subjects be informed that they will be assigned to a treatment at random? Second, if a placebo is being used in the trial, must subjects be told of that fact? Third, should the subjects be informed of the preliminary results of a clinical trial and have the option of withdrawing?

The Food and Drug Administration and the Department of Health and Human Services have extensive regulations concerning informed consent to participation in research. Their purpose is recognition of the right of potential subjects to self-determination. The elements of informed consent specified in the regulations include a statement that the study involves research; an explanation of the purposes of the research and the expected duration of the subject's participation; a description of the procedures to be followed; identification of any procedures that are experimental; a description of any reasonably foreseeable risks or discomforts; a description of any benefits to the subject or others; a disclosure of appropriate alternative procedures or courses of treatment; a statement that participation is voluntary, refusal to participate will involve no penalty or loss, and the subject may discontinue participation at any time. None of these clearly requires that subjects be informed of randomization, placebo control, or preliminary results.

The ethical issue that must be answered here is whether the general right of self-determination requires that the doctrine of informed consent be interpreted to mandate that a subject in an RCT be informed of randomization, placebos, and preliminary results. The right of self-determination, like any other right, has a scope that must be determined—that is, it must be determined how far the right goes before other considerations have more weight. A familiar example will help here. The right to speak one's own mind does not have an unlimited scope; a person does not have the right to speak in a manner that is libelous or slanderous, or to speak with the intent to cause a public disturbance. There comes a point at which speaking one's mind can cause harm to others, and the right to free speech does not extend that far.

The following ethical issues about RCTs have been identified in the preceding discussion of the two trials of gastric freezing. Because they are common to many different kinds of clinical research, it will be useful to state them here in a summary manner.

1. Is it justifiable to treat patients with a new and unproven therapy?
2. Is it justifiable to randomize patients to treatments?
3. Should clinical trials be done with an RCT or a consecutive trial?
4. Is uncontrolled research justifiable?
5. Are placebos or sham treatments justifiable in an RCT?
6. Is the random assignment of subjects justifiable?
7. Should a trial be continued when one treatment appears favorable?
8. Should subjects be informed of random assignment, placebo, and preliminary results?

We have also seen that the central issue that underlies all of this is the justifiability of sacrificing the interests of the patients who will be subjects in an RCT for the benefit of future patients.

Two Views of RCTs

THE STRONG DEFENSE OF RCTS

Many commentators have argued strongly for the methodological and ethical superiority of the RCT. There is no one person who has defended a complete position on all the issues of RCTs; rather, various researchers have articulated and defended a view on RCTs that has a certain coherence.[3,4,5,6] The defenders of the RCT take a position on each of the three problems. First, with regard to initiation, they are strongly in favor of starting clinical research with an RCT rather than a consecutive trial. Second, they attempt to circumvent the termination problem by dividing the responsibility for patients in the trial from responsibility for future patients. Finally, they argue that it is not ethically required that patients in a clinical trial be informed of the fact of randomization and of preliminary results. Let us now look at their arguments on these issues:

1. In an RCT, the researcher does not know which of the two or more treatments is better, thus, the interests of the subjects are not compromised. The results of the trial will show which of the treatments is better, if any, and this will benefit future patients.
2. RCTs should be done on the very first patients, rather than beginning with a small number of patients on the new treatment in a preliminary trial and then going to an RCT. The reasons for this are: an initial trial without a control may show unwarranted acceptance or unwarranted rejection of the new treatment, and this is not in the interest of future patients; and the first patients should have a chance to fall into the control group because the new treatment may be ineffective because of inexperience in its use.
3. With many new drugs, especially anticancer drugs, when they are first used, either the risk of toxicity and mortality is greatest or they are used at impotent doses. In this situation, it is more ethical to do an RCT so that one-half of the early patients will receive the better, conventional treatment.
4. If a consecutive trial is done and the results show the treatment to be effective, publication of the results will convince many others of the effectiveness of the treatment, and then those physicians cannot ethically include their patients in an RCT of the new treatment. But an RCT is the

only way to conclude that a new treatment is effective. Therefore, research should not be done without a control.

5. As an RCT progresses, the data may show that one treatment is better: if the physicians attending the patients in the trial knew of this, they could not ethically keep their patients in the trial. It is imperative to discover new, more effective treatments, and this requires continuing an RCT until statistically significant results are reached. To resolve the conflict between the interests of the patients in the trial and the interests of future patients, the patients in the trial and their attending physicians should be kept ignorant of the preliminary results. A steering committee should know the results and make the decision whether to stop or continue the trial from a perspective that includes the interests of future patients.

6. Being informed of the fact that the treatment for a patient is chosen by a random method is not in the interest of the patient for two reasons. First, if patients are told, nine out of ten may refuse to enter the trial and take the conventional treatment; assuming a 50 percent chance that the new treatment will be more effective, then one-half of the patients who are scared off would be mistreated (i.e. they would not receive the best treatment). Second, sick patients should have confidence in the judgment of their physician; if they are informed that their treatment was determined at random, this confidence will be shaken and that may have harmful consequences for the patients.

We will not provide an analysis or evaluation of these arguments at this point. It will be more instructive first to describe a contrasting position.

THE CRITICS OF RCTs

Unlike the previous general position, this view of the ethical issues in the RCT was developed and defended by a single author in a single work: Charles Fried, *Medical Experimentation: Personal Integrity and Social Policy*.[7] Fried's position is as unlike the previous position as one could imagine and still be within the mainstream of current ethical thinking.

Fried's views on RCTs are carefully connected to a view regarding the fundamental ethical obligations and rights in the physician-patient relationship. His view is aptly described as a model of personal care. The components of this view are briefly as follows. First, a physician-patient relationship is a personal relationship of *this* physician and *this* patient; the physician's primary obligation is to serve the interests of *this* patient. The contrast Fried intends is viewing a physician as having an obligation to patients as a class whose collective interest the physician must serve in an optimal way, one that may include sacrificing the interests of some for the interests of others. Second, the physician-patient relationship is characterized by the following rights of the patient and correlative obligations of the physician: lucidity—the patient's right to know all relevant details; fidelity—each acknowledges that his or her conduct creates expectations in the other that are justified and it is a form of deceit knowingly to disappoint them; humanity—the patient's right to have his or her human particularity taken into account, that is, his or her own particular wants, needs, and vulnerabilities; autonomy—the right of the patient to dispose of him- or herself in person and body as he or she wishes in accordance with his or her own plan.

Without more fully exploring Fried's account of and arguments for this particular view of the physician-patient relationship, we will state his views and arguments on the issues of initiation, termination, and informed consent:

1. Initiating an RCT assumes that there is no evidence to prefer one treatment over another, but it is rarely the case that evidence shows two treatments to be equivalent in effectiveness and safety.
2. Even if two treatments are equivalent when considering a large number of patients, for a given patient with particular symptoms, personal history, and set of values and preferences, the two treatments may not be equivalent. Suppose 60 percent of patients on treatment A improved and 60 percent on treatment B improved; if the two groups were simply defined as moderately hypertensive, a particular patient may be moderately hypertensive and sixty-five years old; this additional fact may be a good reason to prefer A over B.
3. Two treatments may be equivalent, or nearly so, with respect to an outcome that physicians regard as most important (e.g., survival), but the treatments may differ in some respect that is highly important to patients. An often-cited example of this is a clinical trial in which women with breast cancer of a certain stage were randomly assigned to radical or simple mastectomy

on the grounds that the evidence did not show that one was more effective than the other with respect to factors like five-year survival and recurrence. The women in the study may well consider that the increased impairment and disfigurement of the radical mastectomy are very good reasons to prefer simple mastectomy.

4. If a physician is involved in an RCT, this may cause him or her to not examine the patient fully and determine his or her particularly condition and what treatment would be best. If the treatment will be determined at random, there is little reason to make difficult treatment decisions.

5. Patients should be informed of all details of an RCT, for even if the physician believes there is no compromise of the patient's interests and no reason to prefer one treatment over another, the patient may have a different set of values and they could provide a good reason for one treatment.

6. Even if two treatments are equivalent in all respects for a given patient, the patient's participation in research as an important social service requires that the patient know that he or she is participating in the research and know the full details of his or her participation.

7. To maintain the integrity of the physician-patient relationship, complete candor is required to respect the autonomy of both parties; thus, the patient must be informed of all details regarding the RCT.

Fried says nothing about termination problems, such as when to stop an RCT and whether patients should be told of preliminary results. This may not be very important for Fried, because he finds hardly any circumstance in which an RCT would be justified. What he says about initiating a trial implies that a trial should be stopped as soon as evidence shows that a patient would be better off on the other treatment; if not, the obligation of personal care is compromised. Also, patients should be informed of preliminary results so that they can make their own decision about continuing. If autonomy requires that the decision to enter a trial demands full information, it would also require that the decision to continue demands full information.

This brief account of Fried's model of personal care and its criticism of RCTs obviously differs radically from the defense of RCTs. Fried emphasizes the rights of individual patients and a physician's obligation of personal care. The defenders of RCTs emphasize the aggregate of benefits for all patients, those in a trial and those in the future. This reiterates the importance of the central issue regarding RCTs: when, if ever, is it justifiable to sacrifice the interests of patients in an RCT to future patients?

Resolving the Conflict

The two views just described take very different positions on the three areas of dispute: initiation, termination, and informed consent. Whenever there are conflicting positions defended with seemingly plausible reasons, a resolution requires an examination of the assumptions that lie behind the reasons. There are two matters on which the strong defenders and critics make very different assumptions. One of these regards the use of evidence gained prior to the RCT about the effectiveness and safety of the treatments, and the other concerns how the interests of subjects in the trial and the interests of future patients should be understood and compared. In order to explain and assess these different assumptions, it will be useful to have two additional examples of RCTs.

THE ARA-A RCT

The Herpes virus is one that has many different manifestations. One of the most severe diseases caused by the herpes virus is herpes simplex viral encephalitis. Encephalitis is an infection of the brain. Herpes encephalitis is characterized by rapid onset (patients become lethargic, then unconscious, and eventually comatose); there is also a high frequency of seizures. There was no treatment or cure for the disease. Since many other diseases have nearly the same symptoms, the only definitive diagnosis is a brain biopsy to determine whether the virus is present in the brain tissue. In studies in which brain biopsies were used, mortality was reported to be 70 percent. Other studies report the mortality rate as lower than this, but it is still reasonable to say the disease is more often fatal than not. Another indication of the severity of the disease is that most survivors have a permanent and severe neurological deficit, so much so that they have to be institutionalized. Very few persons survive the disease to return to a relatively normal life.

Researchers were working on many varieties of herpes infections. One of the drugs they were studying was ara-A (adenine arabinoside). The drug has been shown effective against other herpes infections so it was thought that it might be useful against herpes encephalitis as well. A double-blind RCT with placebo control was designed. Fifty patients were started in the trial. Ara-A and a placebo were administered intravenously. All fifty patients were given brain biopsies. Those patients whose biopsies were positive were continued on ara-A or the placebo for ten days; those patients whose biopsies were negative had ara-A or the placebo stopped after five days. There were twenty-eight brain biopsy positive patients, eighteen of whom received ara-A and ten of whom received the placebo. Mortality in the placebo control group was 70 percent (seven died). Mortality in the ara-A group was 28 percent (five died). Seven of the treated patients (39 percent) are now leading normal lives with minimal deficiencies due to the disease, while only two of the control group (20 percent) are able to do so. These results were statistically significant (P = .03), and when adjustments were made for increased severity of disease in the treated group, the significance was even greater (P = .0018). (The increased severity was attributable to a chance allocation of more severely affected patients to the treatment group than to the control group.) In the research report, the researchers stated, "Since reduction of mortality resulting from adenine arabinoside treatment of herpes simplex proved to be significant, these controlled studies had to be terminated for ethical reasons, even though the number of placebo treated patients was small."[8]

THE FLU-PREVENTION RCT

The next RCT we will examine is a study of the effectiveness and side effects of two drugs for the prevention of influenza type A. Influenza A virus has several subtypes, and some have caused epidemics resulting in some deaths and many more sick people. The two drugs used in the trial were similar; their short names are amantadine and rimantadine. Amantadine was licensed for prevention and treatment of all influenza A subtypes, though it had not been widely used in the United States. Rimantadine was reported to be more active in vitro and in influenza induced in animals. It is widely used in the Soviet Union, and there is evidence that it may be better tolerated than amantadine. The researchers used the two drugs in an RCT in a town that had an outbreak of influenza A. The trial was double-blind and placebo controlled. Rimantadine was given to 147 patients, amantadine to 145 patients, and a placebo to 148 patients. The researchers calculated the efficacy rate of each drug in the following way:

$$\frac{\text{rate of illness in placebo group} - \text{rate of illness in drug group} \times 100}{\text{rate of illness in placebo group}}$$

This yields a percentage figure that is a measure of how much better the drug is than the placebo. Rimantadine was 85 percent more effective than the placebo, and amantadine was 91 percent more effective than the placebo. These results were significant at levels less than 0.001. These are very impressive results on the effectiveness of the two drugs in preventing influenza. The side effects of the two drugs were determined by comparing the withdrawal rates in the two groups on the drugs with the withdrawal rate of the group on the placebo. The only important difference was in regard to withdrawal due to central nervous system side effects, such as insomnia, jitteriness, and inability to concentrate. Only 11 percent and 10 percent withdrew from the placebo or rimantadine respectively, whereas 22 percent withdrew from amantadine. The researchers concluded that rimantadine is the drug of choice for prevention of influenza A. They cautioned that their subjects were healthy young volunteers (the average age was 25.6 years) and that further study was needed to determine whether the same effectiveness and low rate of side effects would be encountered in the elderly and other high-risk persons. This is important because it is these persons who are most at risk of death and serious illness from influenza.[9]

EVIDENCE AND EFFECTIVENESS

The strong defenders of RCTs claim that an RCT does not compromise the interests of the subjects in the trial, that an RCT is preferable to a consecutive trial with regard to the interests of the subjects, and that an RCT is preferable to a consecutive trial with regard to the interests of future patients. The reason given for all these claims is that prior to the RCT it is not known which treatment is better. The critics of RCTs claim that it is rarely the case that the evidence shows that the two treatments in an RCT are equally effective and safe, especially when all relevant factors are taken into account.

This dispute *seems* to be a matter of fact, a dispute that could be resolved only by studying a large representative sample of RCTs. That may be part of the disagreement, but there is more to it. First, the two sides are not just making a factual claim; each is also making a normative claim. They are contending that a condition that justifies initiating research with an RCT is that a physician would have no good reason for choosing one treatment over another when making a clinical judgment about what is most in the interest of the

146 · BRUCE MILLER

patient. A second aspect of the issue concerns what sort of evidence is used to arrive at the view that it is not known which treatment is better. These two points can be elaborated by examining the three examples of RCTs.

Amantadine and rimantadine had both been used clinically to prevent influenza. Data existed regarding the effectiveness and safety of both. These data could be examined to determine whether one appeared more effective and safer than the other. To say that it is not known which drug is better does not require that the data show that the drugs have the same effectiveness and safety; rather, the data need show only that there was not a *large* difference in the two drugs, for any small difference could be the result of the different conditions under which the drugs were used. Notice that it cannot be claimed that the evidence shows that the two drugs are equally effective, which is what the critics say must obtain to justify an RCT. The reason this cannot be claimed is the same reason it cannot be claimed that one is more effective than another; the two drugs had not been used under conditions that were sufficiently similar. A RCT of the two drugs is justified because there is evidence that the two drugs are effective and safe, and there is no evidence that one is significantly more effective or safer than the other.

The problem with the flu RCT is the use of a placebo control group. A physician may have no good grounds for choosing between amantadine and rimantadine when making a judgment in the interest of a patient, but a physician should not consider a placebo injection as one of the options. Amantadine is an approved drug, so the issue is not how much better amantadine and rimantadine are than a placebo, but which of the two drugs is more effective or safer. This could have been done in a RCT that only compared the two active drugs.

In the RCT of the gastric freeze treatment, the situation is very different. The consecutive trial of the gastric freeze led to widespread use of the procedure, but many physicians reported that although there was improvement in patients' subjective symptoms, there was evidence that the level of gastric acid secretion was not reduced. This strongly suggests that the treatment has no more than a placebo effect. One strategy might have been to do an RCT that compared the gastric freeze with the conventional surgical approach. There are two reasons why this would not be useful. First, the trial could not be blind to the patients and physician, and so apparent differences in outcome could have been the result of subjective factors. Second, the gastric freeze was of interest because it was safer, less costly, and more convenient than surgery. Even if it were somewhat less effective than surgery, it would be attractive as a treatment of first choice, with surgery as a treatment for patients whose ulcers persisted. The issue then was whether the gastric freeze had any real biologic effect on ulcers. Taking all the evidence into consideration, the gastric freeze may be no more effective than a treatment that had the same subjective effect on patients and physicians, but had no biologic effect on the ulcer. The sham freeze was cleverly constructed to test this hypothesis.

In the flu-prevention trial, two treatments were in use, amantadine and rimantadine; in the gastric freeze RCT, there were not two treatments in use, real freeze and sham freeze. Rather, the evidence suggested that the real freeze was no different than if a sham freeze were used. It is important to notice that this RCT is not justifiable by evidence from the clinical use of two different treatments. The views of the strong RCT defenders must be modified from the claim that there are two treatments and the evidence on the use of each does not show that one is more effective. The evidence that can be used to justify an RCT will have to include evidence other than that obtained from clinical use of the two treatments; all the evidence that has some bearing on the comparative effectiveness and safety of the two treatments in the trial must be taken into account. In this case, that included knowledge about the placebo effect as well as knowledge about the relationship between certain symptoms and the secretion of gastric acid.

A critic of RCTs would want to know how patients were recruited for the random assignment to gastric freeze or sham freeze. Typically, a physician and patient would have a choice between gastric freeze and surgery. Although available evidence shows that the gastric freeze may have only a placebo effect, a patient and physician may wish to try the freeze because it is safer, less expensive, and more convenient. They could consider surgery as the next treatment. Or they might go directly to a surgical treatment because they are less concerned about safety, cost, and convenience and would rather do the surgery now than later. If the physicians who enrolled their patients in the RCT did not present the option of surgery, then they compromised the interests of the patients.

The RCT of ara-A is unlike the influenza trial and the gastric freeze trial. Neither of the treatments, ara-A and placebo, had any prior clinical use for herpes encephalitis. Was it justifiable to claim that it could not be known which treatment was better and hence that the interests of the subjects were not compromised by random assignment? The researchers who conducted the trial thought so: "When no therapy or even uncertain therapy is available, as was the case when we started our trials, the physician or medical researcher must honestly admit that the answer to the correct therapeutic approach is unknown. Such a conclusion is not an ethical compromise."[10] The matter of concern prior to the start of an RCT is not whether "the correct therapeutic approach" is known; obviously, if it were known, there would be no reason to conduct an RCT. The matter that must be addressed is whether the untried treatment ought to be tested in an RCT or in a consecutive trial. There was no standard treatment of herpes encephalitis to compare with ara-A in an RCT, so the only possible RCT would be ara-A against a placebo. Does the situation justify a trial with a placebo control? There are several factors that support a consecutive trial rather than an RCT: (1) the seriousness of the disease—it is not like a case of the flu, which nearly everyone survives with no lasting disability; (2) there is no placebo effect nor concern for physician bias when the outcome of interest is whether the patient survives or not and the patient is unconscious from an early point in the disease process; (3) there is no reason to believe that a placebo would be effective against herpes encephalitis; (4) there is evidence that ara-A will be effective. This evidence may be overridden by clinical use of ara-A, or ara-A may only be minimally effective, or ara-A may be very effective; this will not be known until the drug is used, but at the time the trial was started, the available evidence was that ara-A was preferable to no treatment or to a placebo treatment.

What could have led the researchers to do the RCT of ara-A? It would be fruitless to speculate on their thoughts and motivation, but there is a view of the design of medical research that could account for their actions. In order to explain this, we will have to digress into some matters of statistics again. Suppose that there are two large urns, each one containing 10,000 marbles. You are told that the marbles are black or white, but not what the proportion is in the two urns. If you draw a black marble from either urn, you will receive five dollars. You are given forty chances to draw, and each draw can be from either urn. Also, you must pay one dollar for each draw. Now, assuming you wish to play the game, you will want to figure out a strategy. A plausible way to reason out a strategy is this: for your first twenty draws, you will alternate between the urns and keep track of how many times you draw a black marble; following that you will draw the next twenty times from the urn that produced the highest proportion of black marbles. Statisticians have mathematical methods of calculating the most effective strategy for such situations. The one just outlined may not be the best but it is not altogether implausible. From examples like this, statisticians have developed designs for clinical research in medicine. When medical researchers consult them, statisticians may give them a methodology that is based on assumptions that are not present. Among them is the assumption in the urn example that, prior to drawing, you have no knowledge of which urn will have the better payoff.

The comparison of ara-A and placebo was approached as if sampling from two urns; rather than drawing marbles of different colors, the two outcomes were death and survival. It was assumed that there was no evidence that one treatment would produce more live patients than the other, just as it was assumed that there was no evidence that one urn would produce more black marbles than the other.

The ara-A and flu trials show that to determine whether an RCT is justified, all the evidence available must be taken into account. It cannot be assumed that there is no evidence about the comparative effectiveness and safety of the treatments. The defenders of RCTs ignore the evidence that leads them to believe that a new treatment may be effective when they uniformly do controlled trials. Controls can be justified, but only when all the evidence is taken into account.

INTERESTS OF SUBJECTS AND FUTURE PATIENTS

In the RCTs of ara-A, gastric freezing, and the flu vaccines, the interests of individuals who were subjects in the trial were compromised. As the arguments of the previous section show, this is not just an after-the-fact judgment. It was contrary to the interests of the subjects to have a 50 percent chance of receiving a placebo rather than the certainty of receiving ara-A or one of the flu vaccines. In the gastric freezing trial, it was contrary to the interests of the subjects not to have the option of the conventional surgical treatment. In the gastric freeze and flu vaccine trials, there was also a compromise of the interests of the subjects if in the course of the trials one of the treatments was turning out to be better than the placebo and the trial was continued in order to reach a desired level of statistical significance.

How do strong defenders of RCTs perceive the relationship between the interests of the subjects and future patients so they can initiate and continue trials of the sort just described without believing that they are doing something wrong? Their approach is to aggregate the interests of the subjects and future patients and to consider them as equal. Here is an example of this type of argument.

If we do the ara-A RCT against a placebo, significant results can be obtained with a specified number of patients, such as fifty. If a consecutive trial is done, the number of subjects required to reach the same level of significance is greater than fifty; assume that it will be seventy-five. (For a given trial, statisticians can tell medical researchers exactly how many subjects will be needed to reach a given level of significance.) Suppose that adding twenty-five subjects in the trial of ara-A will take six months longer and that in this time there are 200 patients in hospitals not involved in the research who will have herpes encephalitis. The defense of the RCT of ara-A is that although twenty-five of fifty patients in the RCT would have their interests compromised, this compares with 200 patients who would not receive ara-A if a consecutive trial were done and it showed ara-A to be effective.

A second example is the RCT of the gastric freeze treatment. If the trial were stopped when the preliminary results were sufficient to show that the subjects in the trial were not being benefited, the level of statistical significance would not reach the level that would persuade all physicians that the treatment has no more than a placebo effect. Thus, some physicians would continue to use the treatment for future patients and thus their interests would be compromised.

Strong defenders of RCTs handle the problem of termination with a steering committee to oversee the trial and be responsible for determining when the trial should be stopped by taking account of the interests of the subjects and the interests of future patients. The committee will balance these interests and make a judgment that will promote the greatest interest of the aggregate of all subjects and all future patients.

In contrast, Fried's model of personal care requires that the physician attending the patient who is a potential subject in an RCT serve the interest of *that* patient first. Only if the RCT would not compromise the interest of that patient could a physician ask the patient to participate in an RCT. The strong defenders of RCTs count the interest of current patients and future patients equally, while Fried puts the interests of current patients ahead of the interests of future patients.

The appeal to equality may seem more commendable then the

preferential treatment Fried seems to support. However, this appearance is not defensible on a fuller examination of widely held views of when a person should, or may, give preference to the interests of some over others. Parents should prefer the interests of their own children over those of their neighbors. Spouses should prefer the interests of each other over friends, and friends should be more concerned with the welfare of one another than of strangers. Contracts of all sorts, including those for the services of a professional, such as a physician, require that the interests of one person, in an area limited by the terms of the contract, be advanced before those who have no professional/client relationship. The physician-patient relationship is a socially defined relationship with prescribed roles for each party. The physician's obligation and the patient's legitimate expectation is that the physician will provide the patient with the medical care most in the interest of the patient. If the treatment a patient receives is determined by the structure of an RCT designed to advance the interests of future patients, then the current patient's interests are being sacrificed, and the implicit contract between physician and patient is violated.

A strong defender of RCTs might reply that although an RCT may sacrifice the interests of the subjects, not doing an RCT will sacrifice the interests of future patients, and since there are many more future patients than subjects in the trial, the least sacrifice is realized by doing an RCT. This argument will not stand up. It fails to appreciate the difference between *sacrificing* someone's interests and *not promoting* someone's interests. The notion of *sacrificing* interests implies that the interests are not promoted, but it also implies that there was some obligation to promote that person's interests. If a father gives a new toy to the neighbor's child rather than his own, he has sacrificed the interests of his child to those of the neighbor's child. If the father gave the toy to his own child, he has not sacrificed the interests of the neighbor's child because he has no obligation to promote that child's interests. A physician has a special obligation to promote the interests of those individuals who are his or her patients and does not have this obligation to future, unidentified patients.

It might be argued that potential subjects have an obligation to participate in research for the benefit of future patients. The source of this obligation could be the obligation that everyone must promote the well-being of other members of the human community (i.e., a principle of beneficence). The obligation could also be a reciprocal obligation. Current patients have benefited from others having served as research subjects; as the beneficiaries of past sacrifice, they have a reciprocal obligation to make their own sacrifice.

There are several reasons why this argument fails. The most obvious is that though there is an obligation to benefit others—such as the obligation to contribute to charitable organizations—each person may determine who will be the objects of his or her beneficence. No one has an obligation to be beneficial or charitable to everyone. Some distinctions make this clearer. Many philosophers make a distinction between perfect obligations and imperfect obligations. A perfect obligation is one that everyone has to everyone else, such as the obligation not to harm another. These obligations may have exceptions, but the presumption is that the obligation will be fulfilled in every case and that the burden of proof is on the one who would not fulfill it. This might be done by showing that there is a conflicting and more important obligation, such as that the obligation not to harm another can be overridden by the obligation to preserve one's own life. An imperfect obligation is one that we all have, but we do not owe it to everyone. Each person may choose when and toward whom to fulfill the obligation. Sacrificing the interests of current patients for the interests of future patients is an imperfect obligation.

The argument for a reciprocal obligation fails because those who are now patients, and whose participation in research is wanted, did not ask prior research subjects to sacrifice their interests. A reciprocal obligation to benefit another is most persuasive when A asks B to do something for A, which B does, and then later B asks for the return of the favor. This shows another disanalogy; the persons who made a sacrifice for current patients are not those who would be benefited, rather, it is future patients who have not provided current patients with a benefit.

The upshot of these arguments is that the obligation to sacrifice one's own interests in medical care to the interests of future patients is not an obligation that can be *imposed* on individuals; rather, it is an obligation that must be *voluntarily* assumed. Hence, the *doctrine of informed consent* is central to questions about the ethics of research. In the next section, attention will be given to whether the doctrine of informed consent can be used to resolve the issues about the initiation and termination of RCTs.

INFORMED CONSENT

The problem of sacrificing the interests of subjects to the interests of future patients might be resolved by obtaining the informed consent of all subjects. Suppose the patients in the gastric freeze RCT were fully informed (i.e., they were told that the treatment might have only a placebo effect and that the purpose of the RCT was to discover if this were so, that subjects would be randomly assigned to a real freeze and a sham freeze, that they could choose not to participate in the RCT and then they would be offered standard treatments, that if they participated the trial would be continued to obtain a given level of statistical significance, that they would not be told of preliminary results because that might effect their results). If this were done, the patients who chose to be in the RCT would be voluntarily making a choice that might sacrifice their interests; this action would be a commendable, altruistic concern for the interests of future patients.

Defenders of RCTs might resist fully informing subjects. They might argue that if the subjects were told all of the above, very few patients would agree to participate, and that those who did may not be a representative sample of patients who are now receiving the treatment. The defenders might argue that the information should be limited so that a sufficiently large and representative sample of patients could be obtained.

The argument is plainly faulty. It simply assumes that it is justifiable to sacrifice the interests of current patients for the interests of future patients and thereby imposes on the current patients the researcher's view of the relationship between the interests of current and future patients. Even if certain information about the RCT is likely to result in refusals, it is relevant and should be given to the subjects.

Suppose the information is given; an important issue is whether it must also be understood and used by the potential subject. Most patients develop trust in physicians and accept their recommendations. When the recommendation is for a treatment that the physician believes is in the best interest of the patient, then the patient's trust may be justified and the patient is not being taken advantage of. But when the physician is also a researcher, or the cooperating agent of a researcher, the ground of the patient's trust has been tainted.

These points demonstrate that the process of obtaining consent for RCTs is very important. How, when, and by whom the consent is obtained will influence the patient's decision. A physician can present the opportunity to participate in such a way that the patient feels the physician wants the patient to do so and would be disappointed if the patient refused; the physician might indicate directly or indirectly to the patient, "Until now I have been doing everything for you and now it's your turn to do something for me." Alternatively, the physician might present the opportunity to participate as entirely up to the patient and indicate that she or he will be fully supportive of the patient whatever decision the latter makes. Clearly, this is the proper course.

Another matter of importance is whether patients can and do understand the information relevant to a decision to participate in an RCT. This is a factual matter that can be researched, but very little research has been done, and what there is provides no clear answers.[11] A primary issue is whether the relevant information is so technical that the average person could not understand it well. For example, can average persons understand the concept of statistical significance well enough to know what they are agreeing to when they agree to continue in an RCT and not be informed of the preliminary results because they may not be statistically significant to the .05 level? Further, a patient's illness may affect his or her ability to make an independent decision to become a subject in an RCT. If a patient is terminally ill, he or she may agree to an RCT because of a belief that it is a chance for a new miracle cure. A sick patient may be so vulnerable and dependent on physicians that he or she may agree to anything recommended by a physician for fear of losing the approval and support of a person who is of great importance to him or her at the time.

Although there are no researched answers to these questions, our common understanding indicates that these matters are serious. Hence, obtaining a patient's consent to an RCT may not involve a deliberate decision to sacrifice one's own interest to that of future patients. The subjects' informed consent to participation in an RCT, therefore, does not eliminate the concern about the sacrifice of interests in the initiation and termination decisions. Discussion of the ethics of research in medicine typically focuses on informed-consent discussion of what information must be included, how the consent should be documented, and who is capable of giving consent. Less attention is given to the ethical issues in the design of RCTs. A major point of this chapter is that the most important ethical decisions are made with the decisions to *initiate* an RCT of a given sort, and that the defenders of RCTs have failed to present adequate arguments for their widespread use.

REVIEW OF RISKS AND BENEFITS

A defender of RCTs may argue that the shortcomings of informed consent as a protection against unjustified sacrifice are overcome by the multiple reviews of risks and benefits. Under current government regulations, every RCT is reviewed at least four times. First, the researcher, with advice from colleagues and supervisors, must decide whether a particular research project is justifiable. The researcher's own beliefs about the risks of the procedure for subjects and the possible benefits to subjects and future patients will be part of this judgment. After the research is designed, it must be submitted to an institutional review board (IRB). In this submission, the researcher must describe the research, its expected risks and benefits, the process by which informed consent will be obtained, and what the subjects will be told. The IRB may approve, disapprove, or require modification of the research. The IRB's principal concern is to protect the rights and welfare of subjects. An IRB must apply the following criteria:

1. Risks to subjects are minimized.
2. Risks to subjects are reasonable in relation to anticipated benefits, if any, to subjects, and the importance of the knowledge that may reasonably be expected to result.
3. The selection of subjects is equitable.
4. Informed consent will be sought from each prospective subject or the subject's legally authorized representative.[12]

The regulations provide great detail about obtaining informed consent, but there is nothing on the matter of sacrifice of the interest of subjects to future patients other than the statement that the risks to subjects should be reasonable in relation to the possible benefits to future patients (concerning the knowledge that may be gained). The next level is a panel of scientists who review the project for its scientific merit. If a proposed project were so lacking in scientific merit that it could not lead to useful knowledge, presumably it would not be approved and subjects would not undergo risks. The final level of review is from prospective subjects; they must decide, perhaps with the advice of others, including their physician, whether they believe the risk-benefit relationship is a sacrifice they are willing to assume.

The fourth level, review by potential subjects, cannot itself resolve the concern about the justification of sacrifice. We must assume that there will be some patients who are recruited whose consent will be based on a less than adequate understanding of the research protocol or on a vulnerability and dependence resulting from illness or misplaced trust. With this in mind, how should an IRB determine that the risk-benefit relationship is justifiable?

One approach might be for IRB members to consider whether they would be willing to enter the RCT if they were in the patients' position. There are two problems with this approach. First, what a person sees as a justifiable sacrifice depends greatly on his or her general set of values and preferences. People vary on such things as risk taking, interest in medical research, avoidance of pain, inconvenience of hospital stays or outpatient clinic appointments, and numerous other relevant particulars. A decision by one person that he or she would find a sacrifice not unreasonable does *not* support the claim that it is justifiable to approve it for others. Second, the IRB members are not in the position of the patients asked to be subjects. Judgments about what one would do if . . . are frequently hedged by statements like, "But of course if I ever really faced the decision, I'm not sure what I would do." Thus, what an IRB member now believes he or she would consent to does not justify a sacrifice for others who will be subjects.

Another defense of the adequacy of an IRB review is that an IRB contains many members; some of them are not researchers and some of them must be persons not associated with the institution at which the research will be done. With a large and diverse membership, an IRB's decision carries the authority of a collective judgment. If the research placed an unjustified risk on some subjects, some members would notice that and the research would be disapproved or returned for modification. The problem with this argument is that it places undue confidence in a committee process, and it ignores the fact that committees of this sort tend to identify with the institution they work for or that appoints them, and that most of the members of an IRB are researchers. They may not be medical researchers, but they will tend to share the values and aspirations of the researchers who designed the RCT.

If neither informed consent or IRB review provides sufficient assurance that the sacrifice of the interests of subjects in RCTs is justifiable, is there any other alternative? Jonas[13] has argued that subjects in medical research should be recruited and selected in a descending order or priority. At the top of the list would be medical researchers themselves, and those who are in related sciences and other fields who can understand the research protocols and who share the researcher's commitment to new knowledge and the interests of future patients. At the bottom of the list would be those who are vulnerable because of illness, ignorance, or economic disadvantage. The priority is not attached to availability, so that if a sufficient number of subjects could not be recruited from the top of the list, it would be legitimate to drop down the list. Rather, the list is tied to the relative urgency of the research. If research is required to find a treatment for an epidemic disease that threatens nearly everyone, then those at the bottom can be recruited. The analogy Jonas gives is with conscription to defend a nation against an unjust aggressor. However, there are no research guidelines that have tried to incorporate ideas like these.

Conclusion

The object of this chapter has been to explore ethical questions about RCTs. The particular emphasis has been on the problem generated by decisions to initiate research with an RCT, to control the research with a placebo or other treatment, and to terminate an RCT. Most discussions of the ethics of medical research pay little attention to these problems and concentrate instead on questions about informed consent and IRB review.

The conclusions of the preceding section come down on the side of critics of RCTs. This should not be taken to imply that it is my view that RCTs are never justified or that medical research in general is unjustified. The three examples of clinical research discussed in this chapter are not meant to be a representative sample. They were chosen largely because they easily demonstrate the difficult ethical problems that can arise in the use of RCTs. It is my view that the strong defenders of RCTs have failed to reply adequately to the objections we have surveyed. Thus, we must conclude that the use of RCTs in which competent subjects do not knowingly and voluntarily risk their own interests are not justifiable. Aggregate benefits to future patients fail to warrant the imposition of serious risks on less than fully informed "consenting" persons.

Notes

1. O. H. Wangensteen, et al., "Achieving 'Physiological Gastrectomy' by Gastric Freezing: Preliminary Report of Experimental and Clinical Study," *Journal of the American Medical Association* 180 (1962): 439–444.
2. J. M. Ruffin, et al., "A Co-operative Double-Blind Evaluation of Gastric 'Freezing' in the Treatment of Duodenal Ulcer," *New England Journal of Medicine* 281 (1969): 16–19.
3. T. C. Chalmers, "The Ethics of Randomization as a Decision-making Technique, and the Problem of Informed Consent," Report of the Fourteenth Conference of Cardiovascular Training Grant Program Directors,

158 · BRUCE MILLER

National Heart Institute, Department of Health, Education and Welfare, June 3–4, 1967, Coronado, Calif.

4. ——— et al., "Controlled Studies in Clinical Cancer Research," *New England Journal of Medicine* 287 (1972): 75–78.

5. D. P. Byar, et al., "Randomized Clinical Trials: Perspectives on Some Recent Ideas," *New England Journal of Medicine* 295 (1976): 74–80.

6. Paul Meier, "Terminating a Trial: The Ethical Problem," *Clinical Pharmacology Therapeutics* 25 (1979): 633–640.

7. Charles Fried, *Medical Experimentation* (New York: American Elsevier, 1974).

8. R. J. Whitley, et al., "Adenine Arabinoside Therapy of Biopsy-Proved Herpes Simplex Encephalitis," *New England Journal of Medicine* 297 (1977): 289–294.

9. Raphael Dolin, et al., "A Controlled Trial of Amantadine and Rimantadine in the Prophylaxis of Influenza A Infection," *New England Journal of Medicine* 307 (1982): 580–584.

10. R. J. Whitley and C. A. Alford, "Encephalitis and Adenine Arabinoside: An Indictment Without Fact," *Hastings Center Report* (1979): 4, 44–46.

11. Alan Meisel and Loren Roth, "What We Do and Do Not Know About Informed Consent," *Journal of the American Medical Association* (1981): 2,473–2,477.

12. Department of Health and Human Services, *Policy for Protection of Human Subjects*, 45 Federal Register 46, 46.111.

13. Hans Jonas, "Philosophical Reflections on Experimentation with Human Subjects," in *Experimentation with Human Subjects*, ed. P. A. Freund (New York: George Braziller, 1970).

Suggestions for Further Reading

Encyclopedia of Bioethics. Entries under human experimentation; informed consent in human research; research: biomedical; and research policy: biomedical. New York: Macmillan, 1978.

Freund, P. A., ed. *Experimentation with Human Subjects.* New York: George Braziller, 1970.

Fried, Charles. *Medical Experimentation: Personal Integrity and Social Policy.* New York: American Elsevier, 1974.

Katz, Jay. *Experimentation with Human Beings.* New York: Russell Sage, 1972.

Levine, Robert J. *Ethics and Regulation of Clinical Research.* Baltimore: Urban and Schwarzenberg, 1981.

The National Commission for the Protection of Human Subjects of Biomedical and Behavioral Research, *Report and Recommendations: Institutional Review Boards.* DHEW Publication No. (OS) 78-0008.

_____. The Belmont Report: Ethical Principles and Guidelines for the Protection of Human Subjects of Research, and appendix. DHEW Publication Nos. (OS) 78-0012, 0013, 0014. Washington, D.C.: U.S. Government Printing Office, 1978.

CHAPTER IV

Abortion and the Abortion Issue

Abortion

L. W. Sumner

Among the assortment of moral problems that have come to be known as biomedical ethics none has received as much attention from philosophers as abortion. Philosophical inquiry into the moral status of abortion is virtually as old as philosophy itself and has a continuous history of more than two millennia in the main religious traditions of the West. The upsurge of interest in the problem among secular philosophers is more recent, coinciding roughly with the public debate of the past fifteen years or so in most of the Western democracies over the shape of an acceptable abortion policy. Despite both the quantity and the quality of this philosophical work, however, abortion remains one of the most intractable moral issues of our time.

Its resistance to a generally agreed settlement stems primarily from its unique combination of two ingredients, each of which is perplexing in its own right. Abortion, in the sense in which it is controversial, is the intentional termination of pregnancy for its own sake—that is, regardless of the consequences for the fetus. Pregnancy, in turn, is a peculiar sort of relationship between a woman and a peculiar sort of being. It is a peculiar sort of relationship because the fetus is temporarily lodged within and physically connected to the body of its mother, on whom it is directly dependent for life support. The closest approximation elsewhere in our experience to this dependency is that of a parasite upon its host. But the host-parasite relationship typically differs in some material respects from pregnancy and is therefore only an imperfect analogue to it.

The fetus is a peculiar sort of being because it is a human individual during the earliest stage in its life history. Although there are some difficult and puzzling questions to be asked about when the life history of such an individual may properly be said to begin, we will assume for convenience that this occurs at conception. It will also be convenient, though somewhat inaccurate, to use the term 'fetus' to refer indiscriminately to all gestational stages from fertilized ovum through blastocyst and embryo to fetus proper. A (human) fetus, then, is a human individual during that period temporally bounded in one direction by conception and in the other (at the latest) by birth. The closest approximations elsewhere in our experience to this sort of being are the gametes (sperm and ovum) that precede it before conception and the infant that succeeds it after birth. But both gametes and infant differ in material respects from a fetus and are also only imperfect analogues to it.

Abortion is morally perplexing because it terminates this peculiar relationship and causes the death of this peculiar being. It thus occupies an ambiguous position between two other practices—contraception and infanticide—of whose moral status we are more certain. Contraception cannot be practiced after conception, while infanticide cannot be practiced before birth. Since an abortion can be performed only between conception and birth, contraception and infanticide are its immediate temporal neighbors. Although both of these practices have occasioned their own controversies, there is a much broader concensus concerning their moral status than there is concerning abortion. Thus, most of us are likely to believe that, barring special circumstances, infanticide is morally serious and requires some special justification while contraception is morally innocuous and requires no such justification. One way of clarifying the moral status of abortion, therefore, is to locate it on this contraception-infanticide continuum, thus telling us whether it is in relevant respects more like the former or the latter.

Of the two ingredients whose combination renders abortion morally perplexing, the peculiar nature of the fetus is the more troublesome. Clarifying the moral status of abortion thus requires above all clarifying the moral status of the fetus. Contraception is less perplexing in virtue of the fact that it operates not on any temporal stage of a human being but only on the materials out of which such a being might be formed. And infanticide is less perplexing in virtue of the fact that it operates on a later temporal stage of a human being, of whose moral status we are more certain. Deciding whether abortion is in relevant respects more like contraception or infanticide therefore requires above all deciding whether a fetus is in relevant respects more like a pair of gametes or an infant. The moral category in which we choose to locate abortion will be largely determined by the moral category in which we choose to locate the fetus. Let us say that a being has *moral standing* if it merits moral consideration in its own right and not just in virtue of its relations with other beings. To have moral standing is to be more than a mere thing or item of property. What, more precisely, moral standing consists in can be given different interpretations; thus, it might be the possession of some set of basic moral rights, or the requirement that one be treated as an end and not merely as a means, or the inclusion of one's interest in a calculus of social welfare. However it is interpreted, whether a being is accorded moral standing must make a great difference in the way in which we take that being into account in our moral thinking. Whether a fetus is accorded moral standing must therefore make a great difference in the way in which we think about abortion. An account of the moral status of abortion must be supported by an account of the moral status of the fetus.

There is also a political question concerning abortion to which we need an answer. Every society must decide how, if at all, it will regulate the practice of abortion. Broadly speaking, three different types of abortion policy are available.[1] A permissive policy allows abortion whenever it has been agreed upon between a woman and a qualified practitioner, while a restrictive policy prohibits it altogether. A moderate policy occupies a middle ground between the other two, imposing either (or both) of two constraints on the practice of abortion: a time limit (which stipulates *when* an abortion may be performed) and recognized grounds (which stipulate *why* an abortion may be performed). A view of abortion should tell us which type of abortion policy a society ought to adopt, and if a moderate policy is favored then it should also tell us where to locate the time limit and/or which grounds to recognize. There will clearly be an intimate relation between the determination of the moral status of abortion and the defense of an abortion policy. If abortion is as morally innocuous as contraception, then that seems a good reason for favoring a permissive policy, while if it is as morally serious as infanticide, then that seems a good reason for favoring a restrictive policy.

A complete view of abortion, one that answers the main moral questions posed by the practice of abortion, is an ordered compound of three elements: an account of the moral status of the fetus, which grounds an account of the moral status of abortion, which in turn grounds a defense of an abortion policy. It is not enough, however, that a view of abortion be complete—it must also be well grounded. If we explore what is required to support an account of the moral status of the fetus, we will discover what it means for a view of abortion to be well grounded. The main requirement at this level is a

criterion of moral standing that will specify the (natural) character-
istic(s) whose possession is both necessary and sufficient for the possession of moral standing. A criterion of moral standing will therefore have the following form: all and only beings with characteristic
C have moral standing. (Charcteristic C may be a single property or
a conjunction or disjunction of such properties.) A criterion of moral
standing thus determines, both exhaustively and exclusively, the
membership of the class of beings with such standing. Such a criterion will define the proper scope of our moral concern, telling us for
all moral contexts which beings must be accorded moral consideration in their own right. Thus it will determine, among other things,
the moral status of inanimate natural objects, artifacts, nonhuman
animals, body parts, superintelligent computers, androids, and extraterrestrials. It will also determine the moral status of (human) fetuses. An account of the moral status of the fetus is well grounded
when it is derivable from an independently plausible criterion of
moral standing. The independent plausibility of such a criterion is
partly established by following out its implications for moral contexts other than abortion. But a criterion of moral standing can also
be given a deeper justification by being grounded in a moral theory.
The function of a moral theory is to identify those features of the
world to which we should be morally sensitive and to guide that
sensitivity. By providing us with a picture of the content and structure of morality, a moral theory will tell us, among other things,
which beings merit moral consideration in their own right and what
form this consideration should take. It will thereby generate and
support a criterion of moral standing, thus serving as the last line of
defense for a view of abortion.

The Established Views

We are seeking a view of abortion that is both com-
plete and well grounded. These requirements are not easily satisfied.
The key elements remain an account of the moral status of the fetus
and a supporting criterion of moral standing. Our search will be fa-
cilitated if we begin by examining the main contenders. The abortion debate in most of the Western democracies has been dominated
by two positions that are so well entrenched that they may be called
the established views. The liberal view supports what is popularly
known as the "pro-choice" position on abortion.[2] At its heart is the
contention that the fetus at every stage of pregnancy has no moral

standing. From this premise it follows that although abortion kills the fetus it does not wrong it, since a being with no moral standing cannot be wronged. Abortion at all stages of pregnancy lacks a victim; circumstantial differences aside, it is the moral equivalent of contraception. The decision to seek an abortion, therefore, can properly be left to a woman's discretion. There is as little justification for legal regulation of abortion as there is for such regulation of contraception. The only defensible abortion policy is a permissive policy. The conservative view, however, supports what is popularly known as the "pro-life" position on abortion. At its heart is the contention that the fetus at every stage of pregnancy has full moral standing —the same status as an adult human being. From this premise it follows that because abortion kills the fetus it also wrongs it. Abortion at all stages of pregnancy has a victim; circumstantial differences aside, it is the moral equivalent of infanticide (and of other forms of homicide as well). The decision to seek an abortion, therefore, cannot properly be left to a woman's discretion. There is as much justification for legal regulation of abortion as there is for such regulation of infanticide. The only defensible abortion policy is a restrictive policy.

Before exploring these views separately, we should note an important feature that they share. On the substantive issue that is at the heart of the matter, liberals and conservatives occupy positions that are logical contraries, the latter holding that all fetuses have standing and the former that none do. Although contrary positions cannot both be true, they can both be false. From a logical point of view, it is open to someone to hold that some fetuses have standing while others do not. Thus while the established views occupy the opposite extremes along the spectrum of possible positions on this issue, there is a logical space between them. This logical space reflects the fact that each of the established views offers a *uniform* account of the moral status of the fetus—each, that is, holds that all fetuses have the same status, regardless of any respects in which they might differ. The most obvious respect in which fetuses can differ is in their gestational age and thus their level of development. During the normal course of pregnancy, a fetus gradually evolves from a tiny one-celled organism into a medium-sized and highly complex organism consisting of some six million differentiated cells. Both of the established views are committed to holding that all of the beings at all stages of this transition have precisely the same moral status. The gestational age of the fetus at the time of abortion is thus morally irrelevant on both views. So also is the reason for the abortion. This is irrelevant on the liberal view because no reason is necessary to justify abortion at any stage of pregnancy and equally irrelevant on the conservative view because no reason is sufficient to do so. The established views, therefore, despite their differences, agree on two very important matters: the moral irrelevance of both when and why an abortion is performed.

This agreement places the established views at odds with both common practice and common opinion in most of the Western democracies. A moderate abortion policy regulates abortion either by imposing a time limit or by stipulating recognized grounds (or both). The abortion policies of virtually all of the Western democracies (and many other countries as well) now contain one or both of these constraints. But neither of the established views can provide any support for a moderate policy. Further, in countries with moderate policies there generally exists a broad public consensus supporting such policies. Opinion polls typically disclose majority agreement on the relevance both of the timing of an abortion and of the grounds for it. On the question of timing there is widepsread agreement that early abortions are less problematic than late ones. Abortion may be induced within the first two weeks following conception by an intrauterine device or a "morning after" pill, both of which will prevent the implantation of a blastocyst. Most people seem to find nothing objectionable in the use of these abortifacients. At the opposite extreme, abortion may be induced during the sixth month of pregnancy (or even later) by saline injection or hysterotomy. Most people seem to have some qualms about the use of these techniques at such an advanced stage of pregnancy. On the question of grounds there is widespread agreement that some grounds are less problematic than others. The grounds commonly cited for abortion may be conveniently divided into four categories: therapeutic (risk to the life or health of the mother), eugenic (risk of fetal deformity), humanitarian (pregnancy resulting from the commission of some crime, such as rape or incest), and socioeconomic (e.g., poverty, desertion, family size). Popular support for abortion on therapeutic grounds tends to be virtually unanimous (especially when the risk is particularly serious), but this unanimity gradually diminishes as we move through the other categories until opinion is about evenly divided concerning socioeconomic grounds. Whatever the detailed breakdown of opinion on these issues, there is a widely shared conviction that it does matter both when and why an abortion is performed. Since these are the very factors whose relevance is denied by both of the established views, there is a serious gap between those views and current public opinion.

The existence of this gap is not in itself a reason for rejecting either of the established views. The majority may simply be mistaken on these issues, and the dominance of moderate policies may reflect nothing more than the fact that they are attractive political compromises when the public debate has been polarized by the established views. Neither political practice nor public opinion can provide a justification for a moderate view of abortion or a moderate abortion policy. But the gap does provide us with a motive for exploring the logical space between the established views a little more carefully.

THE LIBERAL VIEW

Meanwhile, however, it is time for a closer examination of the established views. We have identified the accounts they offer of the moral standing of the fetus. Such an account is well grounded when it is derivable from an independently plausible criterion of moral standing. We will focus attention, therefore, on the criteria that could serve as underpinnings of the established views. The liberal view requires some criterion that will deny moral standing to fetuses at all stages of pregnancy. Obviously no characteristic will serve that is acquired sometime during the normal course of fetal development. One characteristic that would certainly suffice is that of *having been born.* This characteristic cannot (logically) belong to any fetus, and it also serves to distinguish fetuses as a class from all later stages of human beings. Building this characteristic into a criterion of moral standing would thus enable the liberal to distinguish abortion, even late abortion, from infanticide, and thus to condone the former while condemning the latter.

But it is pretty clear that no acceptable criterion of moral standing can be constructed in this fashion; it is simply an ad hoc device designed to yield a liberal view of abortion while avoiding an equally liberal view of infanticide. Nor does it seem to be supportable by some more plausible criterion. Its effect is to mark birth as a crucial moral watershed, separating beings that lack moral standing (gametes, fetuses) from beings that possess it (infants, children, adults). But birth is merely the process where by the fetus ceases to be housed within and physically connected to the body of its mother. It is difficult to see how we could justify denying moral standing to a being simply because it is housed within or physically connected to the body of another. Neither of these characteristics appears to be relevant to the question of whether we must accord the being some degree of moral consideration in its own right. Furthermore, birth is an abrupt discontinuity in the normal course of human reproduction. It seems unlikely on the face of it that moral standing could be acquired so suddenly (i.e., that killing a full-term fetus moments before birth could be morally inconsequential while killing a neonate moments after birth could constitute homicide). But if this is so, then birth cannot be a crucial moral watershed, and being born cannot be a necessary condition of having moral standing.

This way of supporting a liberal view is arbitrary and shallow. Liberals need a more plausible criterion of moral standing that will nonetheless deny standing to all fetuses. It is apparent that any such criterion will need to set a fairly high standard, one that is beyond the reach of any fetus, however highly developed. Liberals who have sought such a standard have tended to favor such capacities as self-consciousness and rationality.[3] Each of these capacities is complex and each is also open to differing interpretations. In order to avoid needless controversy, we will assume that the core of self-consciousness is the capacity to recognize oneself as the "I" who is the unifying subject of all of one's states of consciousness. Such a capacity appears to require, at least in rudimentary form, the ability to distinguish oneself from the contents of one's states of consciousness, and the ability to conceive of oneself as enduring through time. We will further assume that the core of rationality is the capacity to represent to oneself objects or states of affairs that are spatially or temporally distant. Such a capacity appears to require, at least in rudimentary form, the ability to remember the past and to anticipate the future, the ability to manipulate symbols, and the ability to take propositional attitudes toward the world. On these accounts, self-consciousness and rationality are intimately connected and partially overlapping. If some other accounts are preferred, they may be substituted for these without affecting the course of the argument.

The best defense of a liberal view of abortion grounds it in either a self-consciousness or a rationality criterion of moral standing. Such a criterion is not arbitrary or ad hoc, since it could be appealed to in any moral context in order to distinguish between beings that have moral standing and beings that do not. And it will readily yield the result the liberal is seeking for abortion, since even the most highly developed fetus is neither self-conscious nor rational. But such a high standard generates its own difficulties. Some of these will arise in contexts other than abortion. Thus, for instance, some mentally handicapped adults may have difficulty meeting this standard and may therefore be denied moral standing by it. But the problem that is more pertinent to our inquiry concerns newborn infants. If a full-term fetus is neither self-conscious nor rational, so also a newborn infant is neither self-conscious nor rational. But then the liberal view of abortion has become also a liberal view of infanticide.

It certainly appears that liberals will have the greatest difficulty in defending a moral boundary between abortion and infanticide. In all morally relevant respects, a full-term fetus and a newborn infant appear to be identical. A liberal will therefore find it difficult or impossible to support the common conviction of the moral seriousness of infanticide. This may not in itself constitute a decisive reason for rejecting the liberal view. Even if both fetuses and neonates lack moral standing, infanticide may be more difficult to justify than abortion. At least some of the reasons for seeking an abortion cannot apply to infanticide: an infant cannot pose a physical threat to the life or health of its mother and if rearing it would be burdensome, there is the alternative of adoption. Furthermore, when the same reason can apply in both contexts—as in the case of a severe abnormality—it is not obvious that infanticide is morally indefensible. Finally, it is also open to the liberal simply to bite the bullet and challenge the common conviction of the moral seriousness of infanticide as a taboo for which there is no rational justification. Abandoning the taboo would in that case be a small price to pay for an otherwise plausible view of abortion.

However, the liberal's difficulties concerning infanticide are not so easily dealt with. Both self-consciousness and rationality are sophisticated bundles of abilities; they may, for instance, be beyond the reach of all nonhuman animals. They are therefore likely to be lacked not only by newborn infants but also by all infants, and perhaps as well by young children. We would need a much fuller account of these capacities in order to be able to locate the stage in the normal course of human development when they are acquired. But it seems very likely that such a high standard will deny moral standing to all infants and at least some children. This result is more troubling than the denial of moral standing to neonates. It means that killing an infant or a young child cannot be a wrong *to that infant or child*. It may, of course, be a wrong to others who are thereby deprived of an object of affection, but the deprivation—and therefore the wrong—would be the same in principle as if some valued item of property were destroyed. We ordinarily assume that what is wrong with homicide is not primarily the injury that it incidentally does to third parties but the injury that it necessarily does to the victim. There seems no good reason for altering this assessment if the victim is an infant or a young child. If a view of abortion yields the result that the killing of such a victim is really a property offense, then we are entitled to conclude that it has somehow gone seriously wrong.

THE CONSERVATIVE VIEW

When we turn to the conservative view, most of the difficulties that we encounter are counterparts of those that confront the liberal. This discovery should not surprise us, since these difficulties are caused by the adoption of a uniform account of the moral status of the fetus, a feature that is common to both established views. The conservative requires a criterion of moral standing that will confer such standing upon fetuses at all stages of pregnancy. Obviously no characteristic will serve that is acquired sometime during the normal course of fetal development. One characteristic that would certainly suffice is that of *having been conceived*. This characteristic must logically belong to all fetuses, and it also serves to distinguish all temporal stages of human beings from the genetic materials out of which they are formed. Building this characteristic into a criterion of moral standing would thus enable the conservative to distinguish abortion, even early abortion, from contraception, and thus to condemn the former while condoning the latter.

But it is fairly clear that no acceptable criterion of moral standing can be constructed in this fashion; it is simply an ad hoc device designed to yield a conservative view of abortion while avoiding an equally conservative view of contraception. Nor does it seem to be supportable by some more plausible criterion. Its effect is to mark conception as a crucial moral watershed, separating beings that lack moral standing (gametes) from beings that possess it (fetuses, infants, children, adults). But conception is merely the process whereby two haploid cells unit to form a diploid cell. It is difficult to see how we could justify conferring moral standing on a being simply because it possesses a complete set of paired chromosomes. This characteristic does not appear to be relevant to the question of whether we must accord the being some degree of moral consideration in its own right. Furthermore, conception is an abrupt discontinuity in the normal course of human reproduction. It seems unlikely on the face of it that moral standing could be acquired so suddenly (i.e., that killing a pair of gametes moments before conception could be morally inconsequential while killing a fertilized ovum moments after conception could constitute homicide). But if this is so, then conception cannot be a crucial moral watershed, and being conceived cannot be a necessary condition of having moral standing.

This way of supporting a conservative view is also arbitrary and shallow. However, conservatives might have something slightly different in mind. Let us continue to assume that conception marks the beginning of the life history of a human individual. Then conservatives can confer moral standing on all human fetuses (and all infants, children, and adults as well) while denying it to all gametes simply by adopting *being a human individual* or *belonging to the human species* as their criterion of moral standing.[4] Doing so will, by implication, mark conception as a crucial moral watershed. Furthermore, a humanity condition is implicit in both the liberal's birth criterion and the conservative's conception criterion, since liberals mean to confer moral standing upon all (and only) human beings who have been born and conservatives mean to confer such standing upon all (and only) human beings who have been conceived. A birth or a conception criterion that lacked this condition would distribute moral standing in a rather profligate manner. Nevertheless, a humanity criterion of moral standing is also arbitrary and shallow. Whatever our views on the complex issue of the moral status of nonhuman animals, it cannot be true that they lack moral standing simply because they are not human. Membership in some favored species has no more moral relevance than membership in some favored race or nation. If it is true that all and only human beings have moral standing, this must be because of some further, and morally relevant, property that is both common and peculiar to them.

Thus, conservatives need a more plausible criterion of moral standing that will nonetheless confer such standing upon all fetuses. But here we encounter a curiosity, for conservatives have tended to favor a high standard—such as self-consciousness or rationality—since they are not eager to accord moral standing to nonhuman animals.[5] As we have seen, however, a high standard appears to yield the liberal view of abortion, and of infanticide as well. Since both these results are abhorrent to conservatives, there is considerable tension between their favored criterion of moral standing on the one hand and their view of abortion on the other.

At least two strategies are available for resolving this tension. The first of them rests on the notion of a paradigm member of a species (or natural kind).[6] The basic idea is that if the paradigm member of a particular species displays the characteristic—self-consciousness or rationality—that entails possession of moral standing, then all members of that species have such standing whether or not they display that characteristic. Assuming that the paradigm member of our species is an adult of normal faculties, and assuming further that such an adult is both self-conscious and rational, then these facts are sufficient to accord all human beings moral standing—including fetuses, infants, children, the severely handicapped, and so on. This strategy solves the conservative's problem at one blow, but at the cost of apparent inconsistency. The conservative's reason for favoring a high standard is to deny moral standing to those beings (such as nonhuman animals) who fall below that standard. Yet the paradigm-member strategy ends by according moral standing to large numbers of beings, including fetuses, who fall below that standard. Therefore, the strategy seems rather arbitrary. It is, to be sure, less arbitrary than the humanity criterion that it resembles since it will confer moral standing upon all members of any species whose paradigm member is self-conscious or rational. If there are any such species, then some nonhuman beings will have moral standing; if not, then the two criteria will define precisely the same class of beings with moral standing. The difference between them is that the paradigm-member strategy employs as its characteristic the more general *belonging to some species whose paradigm member is rational* in place of the more particular *belonging to the human species.* But it still treats a being's species membership as sufficient for its possession of moral standing.

The second strategy available to the conservative rests on the notion of potentiality.[7] The basic idea is that any being has moral standing who is *either actually or potentially* self-conscious or rational. The added potentiality condition is intended to confer moral standing on fetuses, infants, and children and marks a distinctive break with a liberal criterion of moral standing. The second strategy defines the same class of beings with moral standing as the first— except for one range of cases. Let us assume that a being has the potential for self-consciousness or rationality if that being will in the normal course of its development either come to display these capacities itself or be transformed into a being that displays these capacities. The potentiality strategy will then confer moral standing upon normal but immature members of the species, but not upon sufficiently abnormal ones. It will therefore, like the liberal's criterion, deny moral standing to some handicapped fetuses, infants, children, and adults. This result is an embarrassment for conservatives, who would clearly prefer to distribute moral standing to all members of the species. But the embarrassment appears to be unavoidable if conservatives wish to employ a standard high enough to deny standing to members of other species.

Like the paradigm-member strategy, the potentiality strategy has an air of arbitrariness about it. Recall again that the point of a high standard is to deny moral standing to those beings that fail to meet the standard. A being that is actually self-conscious or rational clearly meets the standard, but a being that is only potentially self-conscious or rational does not yet meet the standard. Conservatives wish to accord these latter beings moral standing in advance of meeting the standard on the ground that they will come to meet it later in the course of their normal development. But there is an obvious, and seemingly more consistent, alternative available: we may say that beings with potential self-consciousness or rationality have potential moral standing. They will come to have moral standing if and when they pass the threshold of self-consciousness or rationality, but they do not have it in advance of passing that threshold. This line of thought, which seems the more straightforward, leads however directly back to the liberal criterion of moral standing and the liberal view of abortion.

If the potentiality strategy is not arbitrary, it is easy to see how it will generate a conservative view of both abortion and infanticide. The conservative therefore has no problem supporting the common conviction of the moral seriousness of infanticide. But a problem does arise at the other temporal boundary of pregnancy. Conception, as we have seen, is the union of two haploid cells to form a diploid cell. If a newly fertilized ovum contains the potential for a self-conscious or rational being, then it appears that the pair of gametes that united to form it must also have contained that potential (otherwise where did it come from?). If every fertilized ovum has moral standing, then it must also be true that every unfertilized ovum and every spermatozoon—or perhaps every pair consisting of one ovum and one sperm—also has moral standing. Artificial means of contraception prevent gametes from realizing their potential, just as abortion prevents a fetus from realizing its potential. But then the conservative view of abortion has become also a conservative view of contraception.

It certainly does appear that conservatives will have the greatest difficulty in defending a moral boundary between abortion and contraception. In all morally relevant respects, a newly fertilized ovum and a pair of gametes appear to be identical. A conservative will

therefore find it difficult or impossible to support the common conviction of the moral innocuousness of contraception. This may not
in itself constitute a decisive reason for rejecting the conservative
view. Conservatives too may choose to bite the bullet—some
clearly choose to do so and reject contraception as well. But this
time there can be no doubt of the practical costs of the awkward result. Such conservatives appear to be committed to the view that
the use of artificial means of contraception is the moral equivalent
of homicide. To be consistent, therefore, they must advocate a restrictive contraception policy as well as a restrictive abortion policy.
But the consequences of such a policy for women's sexuality, as well
as for the problem of overpopulation, are unthinkable.

A MODERATE VIEW

We can now catalogue the defects of the established views. The
common source of these defects lies in their uniform accounts of the
moral status of the fetus. These accounts yield three different sorts
of awkward implications. First, they require that all abortions be accorded the same moral status regardless of the stage of pregnancy at
which they are performed. Thus, liberals must hold that late abortions are as morally innocuous as early ones, and conservtives must
hold that early abortions are as morally serious as late ones. Neither
view is able to support the common conviction that late abortions
are more serious than early ones. Second, these accounts require
that all abortions be accorded the same moral status regardless of
the reason for which they are performed. Thus, liberals must hold
that all abortions are equally innocuous whatever their grounds, and
conservatives must hold that all abortions are equally serious whatever their grounds. Neither view is able to support the common conviction that some grounds justify abortion more readily than others.
Third, these accounts require that contraception, abortion, and infanticide all be accorded the same moral status. Thus, liberals must
hold that all three practices are equally innocuous, while conservatives must hold that they are all equally serious. Neither view is
able to support the common conviction that infanticide is more serious than abortion, which is in turn more serious than contraception.
  Awkward results do not constitute a refutation. The constellation
of moral issues concerning human reproduction and development is
dark and mysterious. It may be that no internally coherent view of
abortion will enable us to retain all of our common moral convic-

tions in this landscape. If so, then perhaps the best we can manage is to embrace one of the established views and bring our attitudes (in whatever turns out to be the troublesome area) into line with it. However, results as awkward as these do provide a strong motive to seek an alternative to the established views and thus to explore the logical space between them.

There are various obstacles in the path of developing a moderate view of abortion. For one thing, any such view will lack the appealing simplicity of the established views. Both liberals and conservatives begin by adopting a simple account of the moral status of the fetus and end by supporting a simple abortion policy. A moderate account of the moral status of the fetus and a moderate abortion policy will inevitably be more complex. Further, a moderate account of the moral status of the fetus, whatever its precise shape, will draw a boundary between those fetuses that have moral standing and those that do not. It will then have to show that the location of this boundary is not arbitrary. Finally, a moderate view may seem nothing more than a compromise between the more extreme positions that lacks any independent rationale of its own.

These obstacles may, however, be less formidable than they appear. Although the complexity of a moderate view may render it harder to sell in the marketplace of ideas, it may otherwise be its greatest asset. It should be obvious by now that the moral issues raised by the peculiar nature of the fetus, and its peculiar relationship with its mother, are not simple. It would be surprising therefore if a simple resolution of them were satisfactory. The richer resources of a complex view may enable it to avoid some of the less palatable implications of its simpler rivals. The problem of locating a nonarbitrary threshold is easier to deal with when we recognize that there can be no sharp breakpoint in the course of human development at which moral standing is suddenly acquired. The attempt to define such a breakpoint was the fatal mistake of the naive versions of the liberal and conservative views. If, as seems likely, an acceptable criterion of moral standing is built around some characteristic that is acquired gradually during the normal course of human development, then moral standing will also be acquired gradually during the normal course of human development. In that case, the boundary between those beings that have moral standing and those that do not will be soft and slow rather than hard and fast. The more sophisticated and credible versions of the established views also pick out stages of development rather than precise breakpoints as their thresholds of moral standing; the only innovation of a moderate view is to locate this stage somewhere during pregnancy. The real challenge to a moderate view, therefore, is to show that it can be well grounded, and thus that it is not simply a way of splitting the difference between two equally unattractive options.

Our critique of the established views has equipped us with specifications for the design of a moderate alternative to them. The fundamental flaw of the established views was their adoption of a uniform account of the moral status of the fetus. A moderate view of abortion must therefore be built on a *differential* account of the moral status of the fetus, awarding moral standing to some fetuses and withholding it from others. The further defects of the established views impose three constraints on the shape of such a differential account. It must explain the moral relevance of the gestational age of the fetus at the time of abortion and thus must correlate moral status with level of fetal development. It must also explain the moral relevance, at least at some stages of pregnancy, of the reason for which an abortion is performed. And finally it must preserve the distinction between the moral innocuousness of contraception and the moral seriousness of infanticide. When we combine these specifications, we obtain the rough outline of a moderate view. Such a view will identify the stage of pregnancy during which the fetus gains moral standing. Before that threshold, abortion will be as morally innocuous as contraception and no grounds will be needed to justify it. After the threshold, abortion will be as morally serious as infanticide and some special grounds will be needed to justify it (if it can be justified at this stage at all).

A moderate view is well grounded when it is derivable from an independently plausible criterion of moral standing. It is not difficult to construct a criterion that will yield a threshold somewhere during pregnancy.[8] Let us say that a being is sentient when it has the capacity to experience pleasure and pain and thus the capacity for enjoyment and suffering. Beings that are self-conscious or rational are generally (though perhaps not necessarily) also sentient, but many sentient beings lack both self-consciousness and rationality. A sentience criterion of moral standing thus sets a lower standard than that shared by the established views. Such a criterion will accord moral standing to the mentally handicapped regardless of impairments of their cognitive capacities. It will also accord moral standing to many, perhaps most, nonhuman animals.

The plausibility of a sentience criterion would be partially established by tracing out its implications for moral contexts other than abortion. But it would be considerably enhanced if such a criterion

could also be given a deeper grounding. Such a grounding can be
supplied by what seems a reasonable conception of the nature of
morality. The moral point of view is just one among many evaluative points of view. It appears to be distinguished from the others in
two respects: its special concern for the interest, welfare, or well-
being of creatures and its requirement of impartiality. Adopting the
moral point of view requires in one way or another according equal
consideration to the interests of all beings. If this is so, then a being's having an interest to be considered is both necessary and sufficient for its having moral standing. While the notion of interest or
welfare is far from transparent, its irreducible core appears to be the
capacity for enjoyment and suffering: all and only beings with this
capacity have an interest or welfare that the moral point of view requires us to respect. But then it follows easily that sentience is both
necessary and sufficient for moral standing.

A criterion of moral standing is well grounded when it is derivable
from some independently plausible moral theory. A sentience criterion can be grounded in any member of a class of theories that share
the foregoing conception of the nature of morality. Because of the
centrality of interest or welfare to that conception, let us call such
theories welfare based. A sentience criterion of moral standing can
be readily grounded in any welfare-based moral theory. The class of
such theories is quite extensive, including everything from varieties
of rights theory on the one hand to varieties of utilitarianism on the
other. Whatever their conceptual and structural differences, a sentience criterion can be derived from any one of them. The diversity of
theoretical resources available to support a sentience criterion is
one of its greatest strengths. In addition, a weaker version of such a
criterion is also derivable from more eclectic theories that treat the
promotion and protection of welfare as one of the basic concerns of
morality. Any such theory will yield the result that sentience is sufficient for moral standing, though it may also be necessary, thus providing partial support for a moderate view of abortion. Such a view
is entirely unsupported only by moral theories that find no room
whatever for the promotion of welfare among the concerns of morality.

When we apply a sentience criterion to the course of human development, it yields the result that the threshold of moral standing
is the stage during which the capacity to experience pleasure and
pain is first required. This capacity is clearly possessed by a newborn
infant (and a full-term fetus) and is clearly not possessed by a pair of
gametes (or a newly fertilized ovum). It is therefore acquired during

the normal course of gestation. But when? A definite answer awaits a better understanding than we now possess of the development of the fetal nervous system and thus of fetal consciousness. We can, however, venture a provisional answer. It is standard practice to divide the normal course of gestation into three trimesters of thirteen weeks each. It is likely that a fetus is unable to feel pleasure or pain at the beginning of the second trimester and likely that it is able to do so at the end of that trimester. If this is so, then the threshold of sentience, and thus also the threshold of moral standing, occurs sometime during the second trimester.

We can now fill in our earlier sketch of a moderate view of abortion. A fetus acquires moral standing when it acquires sentience, that is to say at some stage in the second trimester of pregnancy. Before that threshold, when the fetus lacks moral standing, the decision to seek an abortion is morally equivalent to the decision to employ contraception; the effect in both cases is to prevent the existence of a being with moral standing. Such decisions are morally innocuous and should be left to the discretion of the parties involved. Thus, the liberal view of abortion, and a permissive abortion policy, are appropriate for early (prethreshold) abortions. After the threshold, when the fetus has moral standing, the decision to seek an abortion is morally equivalent to the decision to commit infanticide; the effect in both cases is to terminate the existence of a being with moral standing. Such decisions are morally serious and should not be left to the discretion of the parties involved (the fetus is now one of the parties involved).

It should follow that the conservative view of abortion and a restrictive abortion policy are appropriate for late (post-threshold) abortions. But this does not follow. Conservatives hold that abortion, because it is homicide, is unjustified on any grounds. This absolute position is indefensible even for post-threshold fetuses with moral standing. Of the four categories of grounds for abortion, neither humanitarian nor socioeconomic grounds will apply to post-threshold abortions, since a permissive policy for the period before the threshold will afford women the opportunity to decide freely whether they wish to continue their pregnancies. Therapeutic grounds will however apply, since serious risks to maternal life or health may materialize after the threshold. If they do, there is no justification for refusing an abortion. A pregnant woman is providing life support for another being that is housed within her body. If continuing to provide that life support will place her own life or health at serious risk, then she cannot justifiably be compelled to do so, even though the fetus has moral standing and will die if deprived of that life support. Seeking an abortion in such circumstances is a legitimate act of self-preservation.[9]

A moderate abortion policy must therefore include a therapeutic ground for post-threshold abortions. It must also include a eugenic ground. Given current technology, some tests for fetal abnormalities can be carried out only in the second trimester. In many cases, therefore, serious abnormalities will be detected only after the fetus has passed the threshold. Circumstantial differences aside, the status of a severely deformed post-threshold fetus is the same as the status of a severely deformed newborn infant. The moral issues concerning the treatment of such newborns are themselves complex, but there appears to be a good case for selective infanticide in some cases. If so, then there is an even better case for late abortion on eugenic grounds, since here we must also reckon in the terrible burden of carrying to term a child that a woman knows to be deformed.

A moderate abortion policy will therefore contain the following ingredients: a time limit that separates early from late abortions, a permissive policy for early abortions, and a policy for late abortions that incorporates both therapeutic and eugenic grounds. This blueprint leaves many smaller questions of design to be settled. The grounds for late abortions must be specified more carefully by determining what is to count as a serious risk to maternal life or health and what is to count as a serious fetal abnormality. While no general formulation of a policy can settle these matters in detail, guidelines can and should be supplied. A policy should also specify the procedure that is to be followed in deciding when a particular case has met these guidelines.

But most of all, a moderate policy must impose a defensible time limit. As we saw earlier, from the moral point of view there can be no question of a sharp breakpoint. Fetal development unfolds gradually and cumulatively, and sentience like all other capacities is acquired slowly and by degrees. Thus we have clear cases of presentient fetuses in the first trimester and clear cases of sentient fetuses in the third trimester. But we also have unclear cases, encompassing many (perhaps most) second-trimester fetuses. From the moral point of view, we can say only that in these cases the moral status of the fetus, and thus the moral status of abortion, is indeterminate. This sort of moral indeterminacy occurs also at later stages of human development, for instance when we are attempting to fix the age of consent or of competence to drink or drive. We do not pretend in these latter cases that the capacity in question is acquired overnight on one's sixteenth or eighteenth birthday, and yet for legal purposes we must draw a sharp and determinate line. Any such line will be somewhat arbitrary, but it is enough if it is drawn within the appropriate threshold stage. So also in the case of a time limit for abortion, it is sufficient if the line for legal purposes is located within the appropriate threshold stage. A time limit anywhere in the second trimester is therefore defensible, at least until we acquire the kind of information about fetal development that will enable us to narrow the threshold stage and thus to locate the time limit with more accuracy.

Conclusions

We began by noting the special moral problems that the practice of abortion forces us to confront. A healthy respect for the intricacies of these problems and an equally healthy sense of our own fallibility in thinking through them should inhibit us from embracing any view of abortion unreservedly. Nonetheless, of the available options, we have reason to prefer the one that appears, all things considered, to provide the best account of these difficult matters. While both of the established views have obvious and serious defects, many people seem to feel that there is no coherent third alternative available to them. But a moderate view does appear to provide such an alternative. It does less violence than either of the established views to widely shared convictions about contraception, abortion, and infanticide, and it can be grounded upon a criterion of moral standing that seems to generate acceptable results in other moral contexts and is in turn derivable from a wide range of moral theories sharing a plausible conception of the nature of morality. Those who are dissatisfied with the established views need not therefore fear that in moving to the middle ground they are sacrificing reason for mere expediency.

Notes

1. These categories are adapted from Daniel Callahan, *Abortion: Law, Choice and Morality* (New York: Macmillan, 1970).
2. The terms 'liberal' and 'conservative,' as used in the chapter generally, refer respectively to those who think abortion permissible and those who believe it impermissible. Thus, 'liberal' here is not synonymous with 'political liberal' and 'conservative' is not synonymous with 'political conservative.'

3. A self-consciousness criterion is defended in Michael Tooley, *Abortion and Infanticide* (Oxford: Oxford University Press, 1983). A more complex criterion including both self-consciousness and rationality is defended in Mary Anne Warren, "On the Moral and Legal Status of Abortion," in *Contemporary Issues in Bioethics*, ed. Tom L. Beauchamp and LeRoy Walters. Second ed. (Belmont, Calif.: Wadsworth, 1982).

4. A humanity criterion is defended in John T. Noonan, Jr., "An Almost Absolute Value in History," in *The Morality of Abortion: Legal and Historical Perspectives*, ed. Noonan (Cambridge, Mass.: Harvard University Press, 1970).

5. A rationality criterion is defended in Alan Donegan, *The Theory of Morality* (Chicago: University of Chicago Press, 1977), 82–83, 170–71.

6. Different versions of this strategy may be found in Donegan, *The Theory of Morality*, and Philip E. Devine, *The Ethics of Homicide* (Ithaca, N.Y.: Cornell University Press, 1978), 51–55.

7. This strategy is employed in Devine, *The Ethics of Homicide*, 94–100.

8. The sentience criterion is defended in my *Abortion and Moral Theory* (Princeton, N.J.: Princeton University Press, 1981), 128–46.

9. This position is defended in Judith Jarvis Thomson, "A Defense of Abortion," in *The Rights and Wrongs of Abortion*, ed. Marshall Cohen et al. (Princeton, N.J.: Princeton University Press, 1974); for contrary views, see John Finnis, "The Rights and Wrongs of Abortion," in *The Rights and Wrongs of Abortion*, and Baruch Brody, *Abortion and the Sanctity of Human Life: A Philosophical View* (Cambridge, Mass.: MIT Press, 1975), Chapters 1 and 2.

Suggestions for Further Reading

Brody, Baruch. *Abortion and the Sanctity of Human Life: A Philosophical View*. Cambridge, Mass.: MIT Press, 1975.
Callahan, Daniel. *Abortion: Law, Choice and Morality*. New York: Macmillan, 1970.
Devine, Philip E. *The Ethics of Homicide*. Ithaca: Cornell University Press, 1978.
Donagan, Alan. *The Theory of Morality*. Chicago: University of Chicago Press, 1977.
Feinberg, Joel. "Abortion." In *Matters of Life and Death*, ed. Tom Regan. New York: Random House, 1986.
Finnis, John. "The Rights and Wrongs of Abortion." In *The Rights and Wrongs of Abortion*, ed. Marshall Cohen et al. Princeton, N.J.: Princeton University Press, 1974.
Noonan, John T., Jr. "An Almost Absolute Value in History." In *The Morality of Abortion: Legal and Historical Perspectives*, ed. Noonan. Cambridge, Mass.: Harvard University Press, 1970.

Sumner, L. W. *Abortion and Moral Theory.* Princeton, N.J.: Princeton University Press, 1981.

Thomson, Judith Jarvis. "A Defense of Abortion." In *The Rights and Wrongs of Abortion.*

Tooley, Michael. *Abortion and Infanticide.* Oxford: Oxford University Press, 1983.

Warren, Mary Anne. "On the Moral and Legal Status of Abortion." In *Contemporary Issues in Bioethics,* ed. Tom L. Beauchamp and LeRoy Walters. Second ed. Belmont, Calif.: Wadsworth, 1982.

The Abortion Issue

Mary Anne Warren

Introduction

In recent years, abortion has become one of the most intensely debated social issues in this and many other parts of the world.[1] The issue is whether or not a pregnant woman has the moral right—and hence should have the legal right—to decide to terminate her pregnancy. Few would argue that it would ever be right to force a woman to undergo an abortion against her will; the issue is her freedom of choice. Women's legal right to that freedom has been partially affirmed by the United States Supreme Court, which ruled in the 1973 case of *Roe* v. *Wade* that the Constitutional right to privacy precludes Congress or the states from prohibiting first- or second-trimester abortions.[2] Yet the political struggle over abortion rights has only increased in intensity since this important ruling. At least three Constitutional amendments banning abortion, or permitting states to ban it, have recently been under consideration in the U.S. Senate. Senate and Congressional seats have been won and lost almost entirely on the basis of this single issue.

The abortion issue has become a symbol of the conflict between two vastly different world views. The view that women have the right to terminate unwanted pregnancies finds most support among those whose philosophical orientation is basically liberal, humanist, feminist,[3] tolerant of private sexual activities between consenting adults, and in favor of individual family planning and the voluntary limitation of population growth. The view that abortion should be prohibited tends to be supported by those whose orientation is conservative, rooted in fundamentalist religion, antifeminist, intolerant of nonprocreative sexual activities, and opposed to birth control and population limitation. While there are some liberals who oppose the right to abortion or who would be willing to place some restriction on it, and some conservatives who support it, the general tendencies just noted are pronounced and significant.

But an awareness of political realities of this kind should not prevent us from considering the abortion issue on its own merits. Whatever one's larger philosophical or political perspective, in order to develop a rationally defensible position on abortion it is necessary to grapple with two extremely difficult questions. First, what sort of moral action is abortion, in itself and apart from any social or other consequences that it may have in a particular context? Is it the killing of a human being with the same right to life as you and I or any other human being; and if so is it a form of murder, or can it sometimes or always be justified (e.g., as a form of self-defense)? Or is it not the killing of a human being or a human person at all, and thus not something that requires such special justification? Is it one sort of action if performed early in the pregnancy and another sort of action if performed later? If so, where should the line be drawn, and why?

The second question is: What are the likely *consequences* of the legal toleration or prohibition of abortion, and are those consequences, on the whole, good or bad? The question about the nature of abortion is logically prior to this one, in that it is impossible to evaluate the moral significance of the "consequentialist" arguments for or against the freedom of women to choose abortion without first having a clear understanding of the sort of action abortion is. If abortion could be shown to be a form of murder, then the consequentialist arguments for and against its prohibition would become largely irrelevant, since murder should be prohibited even if the prohibition cannot be shown to have beneficial side effects, and even if tolerating it would arguably have some desirable results.

The question about the nature of abortion depends largely on the moral status of the fetus.[4] Is it a human being with a full-fledged right to life, or not? Does it acquire this status at conception, at birth, or some time in between? (Does it perhaps only acquire full moral status sometime *after* birth?) English common law—and American law, which is modeled upon it—treats the moment of live birth as the point at which a legal person comes into existence. I shall argue that although fetuses are genetically human organisms (i.e., members of the human biological species), there are sound reasons for retaining this traditional outlook and refusing to consider them persons with a full and equal right to life at any time prior to birth.

This does not imply that all legal restrictions on the performance of abortions are unjustified. It is appropriate for the law to require that abortions, like other potentially dangerous medical procedures, be performed only by trained medical practitioners, with the equipment necessary to ensure the patient's safety. There are also good reasons to regard late-term abortions as morally somewhat more problematic than early ones. A third-trimester fetus is very different from a newly fertilized egg; except in size and location, it is hardly distinguishable from a newborn infant, and this cannot help but affect our attitudes toward it. For this and other reasons, late-term abortion may require a stronger justification than does early abortion. In practice, such abortions are rarely performed except when there are serious medical circumstances, such as danger to the woman's life or health, or the risk of severe fetal abnormalities. Yet the distinction is not as sharp as some have argued. Even when abortions are performed for what some would regard as morally dubious reasons—such as that the fetus is the "wrong" sex—late-term abortions are not the moral equivalent of murder. Women, I shall argue, have the right to choose abortion even in the third trimester, and the law should not seek to intervene.

Many people regard debate over the moral status of the fetus as futile and possibly dangerous; they fear that if fetuses are denied full moral status, then none of us will be safe from the same fate. Later in this chapter, we will consider two lines of argument that are designed to make such debate unnecessary, by proving that women have the right to choose abortion even if fetuses are regarded as persons with full moral status. Since neither of these arguments entirely succeeds, we will go on to consider the main argument for assigning full moral status to fetuses from the time of conception, that is, the "argument from genetic humanity." It will be argued that insofar as first-trimester fetuses are presentient—not yet capable of having sensations or experiences—they are not the sort of beings to which it makes sense to ascribe moral rights. We will examine the moral significance of the fetus's *potential* for developing into a human person, and argue that the "argument from potentiality" is not an adequate basis for the ascription of moral rights.

We will also approach the much more difficult problem of the moral status of the late-term and probably sentient fetus. It will be argued that although late-term fetuses are genetically human beings with some moral status, they should not be viewed as persons with full moral rights; for to view them in this way inevitably jeopardizes women's rights in ways that are unacceptable. (This is a type of consequentialist argument.) We will also examine other consequentialist arguments for and against restrictive abortion policies and argue that the social effects of maintaining legal access to abortion are far more desirable than those of further restricting or eliminating it. Finally, we will briefly examine the issue of the father's rights in the abortion situation, arguing that these depend entirely on the prior agreements (if any) existing between the woman and the genetic or social father; genetic fatherhood in itself confers no right either to demand or to veto an abortion.

Does the Moral Status of the Fetus Matter?

Opponents of abortion usually argue that fetuses are human beings with a full and equal right to life, and that abortion is therefore murder, or some other form of culpable homicide. Defenders of abortion rights may attack either the premise of this argument, or the inference from the premise to the conclusion. Those who prefer to attack the inference rightly point out that the general wrongness of abortion cannot be made to follow in any simple way from the alleged humanity or personhood of the fetus. For it is generally recognized that killing other human beings is sometimes justifiable (e.g., when there is no other way to defend oneself or others against an unjust attack). Furthermore, one person may sometimes *allow* another to die by failing to do what might have preserved their life, without being held to have *killed* them. Perhaps abortion can be shown to be analogous to one of these classes of justifiable killing or letting die.

Such a strategy might seem attractive for several reasons. The question of whether or not fetuses, at any given stage of development, should be regarded as persons with a full and equal right to life is an extremely difficult and obscure one, about which there is no social consensus. Furthermore, there is something vaguely disturbing about any discussion of whether or not certain members of the human species are persons with full moral rights. Whenever any such question is raised—whether about fetuses, brain-dead persons, anencephalic neonates (severely brain-damaged newborn infants), or persons in cryogenic suspension—there will be those who raise the specter of Nazi concentration camps, and who see no difference between this and the most atrocious forms of genocide. It would be a great advantage to be able to discuss the ethics of abortion without stirring up this particular hornets' nest. Yet, as we shall see, it is extremely difficult to reconcile the claim that fetuses are full-fledged persons with the claim that abortion is morally justifiable.

188 · MARY ANNE WARREN

It seems easy enough to argue that abortion is (at least sometimes) a morally justified form of self-defense. Both the law and common-sense morality permit individuals to use lethal force to defend themselves against unwarranted physical assault when there is no other way of escaping that assault. An unwanted pregnancy can be just as physically and psychologically traumatic as an assault by an external aggressor; so why shouldn't the right to self-defense apply?

One obvious difference between abortion and the more standard cases of self-defense—such as against a mugger or a rapist—is that in the standard case the attacker may be presumed to be deliberately acting in a way that he knows, or ought to know, is wrong, and hence to "deserve" whatever harm they may come to should the intended victim prove capable of effective self-defense. Fetuses, on the contrary, are innocent of deliberately trying to harm anyone. Another apparent difference is that any assault severe enough to warrant lethal means of self-defense exposes the victim to a serious danger of death—or at least it is rational for the victim to assume that it does. Given modern medical technology, however, pregnancy and childbirth are usually survivable.

Jane English presented an analogy designed to answer these objections to the self-defense argument.[5] Suppose that a mad scientist were to hypnotize or otherwise "program" innocent persons to attack other innocent persons with knives. In such a case, the absence of moral guilt on the part of the attacker, even if known to the victim, would not preclude the latter from using lethal means of self-defense if there were no other way to escape serious harm. Furthermore, even if the victim knew that the attacker was not programmed to kill, but only to inflict some lesser (but still serious) physical or psychological damage, the right to self-defense would still obtain.[6]

Another prominent philosopher, Judith Thomson, has used an equally imaginative analogy to argue that abortion is not essentially an act of killing at all, but rather a (sometimes) justifiable refusal to act as an "extremely good Samaritan."[7] Imagine that you have been kidnaped and hooked up to an ailing violinist, who needs the use of your kidneys for nine months in order to survive. (No one else can save the violinist because no one else has the right blood type.) Thomson points out that while it would be extremely generous of you to agree to spend nine months in bed with the violinist, if you were to refuse to do so you would not be guilty of murder or any other form of homicide, even if the violinist died as a result. For even though there may be a general moral duty to help those in distress, it would be intolerable for the law to require that individuals be prepared to make so extreme a sacrifice in order to aid a needy stranger. Seen in this light, abortion is a less than saintly act, but it is not morally wrong, and certainly not murder.

As different as they are, these two arguments suffer from the same weakness. Neither the kidnap victim nor the victim of the hypnotized knife-wielder is in any way morally responsible for her predicament. The victim of an unwanted pregnancy, however, unless she was raped, coerced or deceived, bears at least some of the responsibility for her situation. If it is because of her own deliberate risk-taking that there is now an innocent person whose survival depends on her, then it is not obvious that she retains the right to refuse to be a good Samaritan toward that person, or to kill it in defense of her own bodily integrity. This is part of what opponents of abortion rights mean when they say that women who wish to terminate unwanted pregnancies are refusing to accept responsibility for their own actions. If fetuses are assumed to be persons with full moral rights, and if women's heterosexual activities are assumed to be generally more or less voluntary, then this comment makes a good deal of sense.

One response to this objection is to deny that heterosexuality is a fully voluntary and socially optional choice, which a woman can reasonably be expected to avoid if she does not want to bear a child. Even though the majority of *individual* acts of heterosexual intercourse may be more or less voluntary,[8] women of reproductive age are subjected to enormous social pressure to engage in heterosexual activity *of some sort*. Psychology and popular wisdom insist that virtually all adults need some regular sexual outlet for mental health and happiness; and all of the alternatives to "normal" heterosexual copulation—sodomy, masturbation, or homosexuality—are considered by most people to be at best inferior substitutes for "the real thing," and at worst perversions, sins, or symptoms of mental illness. Sterilization is not a viable option for most women, since they may want to have children later; and contraceptives tend to be either unreliable or medically dangerous—or both. Besides, it is difficult for some women, particularly those who are underage, to obtain and use contraceptives without potentially disastrous social repercussions. For all of these reasons, it is highly unrealistic to tell women that if they do not want to have babies then they should simply not choose to do things that are apt to result in pregnancy.

In my view, these considerations of social pressure and need provide an entirely appropriate response to those who maintain that voluntary indulgence in heterosexual intercourse obligates a woman to complete any resulting pregnancy. Yet it is a response that can be fully persuasive only for those who do not assume that fetuses are persons with a full right to life. To assume that they are forces us to view the issue in a very different light. If fetuses are persons from the time of conception, then a policy of legal abortion amounts to a deliberate decision to condemn hundreds of thousands of innocent persons to death every year, in order to permit persons who do not want to become parents (again) to enjoy the fleeting pleasures of heterosexual copulation. Perhaps it would be unreasonable to condemn individuals who are caught up in such a social policy; but an ongoing "national tragedy"[9] of such dimensions would certainly call for some kind of remedial social action. To simply condone abortion as the result of individual exercises of the right to self-defense, or individual refusals to act as an extremely good Samaritan, would be inadequate.

These are just some of the reasons why it is impossible to deal adequately with the moral issues surrounding abortion without first addressing the moral status of the fetus. Further reasons will emerge as the argument proceeds.

Are Fertilized Human Eggs Persons?

The cornerstone of the argument against the moral permissibility of abortion is the claim that a human person, a being with a full and equal right to life, begins to exist at the moment that a human ovum is fertilized by a human spermatozoon.[10] Why at that particular moment? The tiny one-celled ovum, along with hundreds of others, has existed for years within one of the woman's ovaries. At maturity, it is thousands of times larger than a single sperm and has a far greater chance of developing into a mature human being—though the odds are still strongly against it. Yet no one is tempted to call it a human being, since it contains only about half of the genetic material, or DNA, necessary for further development. The zygote (the fertilized egg[11]), however, though only marginally different in size and appearance, contains a complete genetic "blueprint," all of the "information" necessary to guide its transformation into a human organism composed of billions of cells, performing millions of biological functions. It is no more (and no less) *alive* than an egg or sperm, but its greater genetic completeness gives it a better claim to membership in the human species. But is it a human *person* with full moral rights?

Before we can answer this question, we need to ask what it means. How do we decide, in other contexts, what sorts of entities are to count as persons? The concept of a person has both a moral and an empirical dimension. A person, in what we may call the *moral* sense of the term, is any entity to which moral rights and (sometimes) moral responsibilities may be ascribed. It does not necessarily follow that all rights-bearers are persons; nonhuman animals may be said to have rights, without thereby being said to be persons. Moral *person*hood is defined by the fundamental moral postulate that all persons have full and equal basic moral rights, such as the right to life. Nonbasic moral or legal rights, such as the right to vote or to drive an automobile, are sometimes justly accorded to some persons and not to others; and even basic rights can sometimes be waived or overridden by the rights of other persons. Yet no person has stronger basic rights than any other; this is a truth so central to moral reasoning that to reject it is tantamount to rejecting morality itself.

The empirical elements of the concept—the criteria for who or what is to count as a person—are much more controversial. The principle implicit in the antiabortion stance is that all and only those entities that are biologically human count as persons. This principle works reasonably well in most ordinary contexts: it does justice to the conviction that human beings of all races, religions, and nationalities count as persons; whereas rocks, trees, and nonhuman animals (of the sorts with which most of us are familiar) do not. But there are other actual or conceivable contexts in which the principle does not work well at all. It implies that no nonhuman being could ever count as a person, regardless of how sensitive, intelligent, kindly, or cooperative he, she, or it might be. Language-using dolphins or chimpanzees, sapient extraterrestrials, self-aware robots or androids, and even our own descendants, should they evolve into a biologically distinct species, are all ruled out. Indeed, should some subgroup of us be unexpectedly discovered to be biologically nonhuman (perhaps as a result of their parents' exposure to some environmental contaminant), these individuals would automatically become nonpersons, ineligible to hold full and equal moral rights. But surely this is absurd. Our moral rights do not depend on our membership in some particular biological species. It is only an accident of evolutionary history that we all belong to a single species. If we knew nothing about the properties whereby particular organisms may be classified as belonging to the same or to distinct biological species, we could still know that we and other postnatal humans, whatever their color, sex, nationality, or religion, are persons.

The reason we could know this is that the empirical aspect of the concept of a person is not essentially biological. The empirical concept of a person is that of a being who has certain sorts of mental and behavioral capacities.[12] People obviously vary widely in their mental capacities, as well as in their ability to demonstrate those capacities at a given time. However, a typical or paradigm person has all or most of the following capabilities:[13]

1. *Consciousness or sentience*—the capacity to have feelings or sensations, and thereby to be aware of one's environment and one's own inner states.
2. *Rationality*—the capacity to respond in appropriate ways to new and relatively difficult situations (e.g., problems, threats or opportunities).
3. *Self-awareness or self-concept*—the capacity to understand the sort of being one is (e.g., a sentient being persisting in time[14]).
4. *Self-motivated behavior*—the capacity to determine one's own goals and the means of achieving them; and to act in ways that are neither entirely instinctive nor entirely the result of the action of outside forces.
5. *Linguistic capacity*—the capacity to use a conventional symbol system to convey messages of indefinitely many types and contents.

These capacities, together with the right kinds of social learning, make possible another capacity that is central to the concept of a person: the capacity for moral autonomy.[15] Not all of us have this capacity, and none of us has it at all stages of our lives; but the fact that some of us have it is crucial to our understanding of ourselves as persons. It is because we are persons in the empirical sense that we must learn to accept one another as persons in the moral sense. Animals that are not persons are generally able to act in a fashion conducive to their species survival without any explicitly formulated moral code. But beings who are rational, self-aware, self-motivated, and capable of using language require such a moral code in order to make social existence possible (or at least *human* beings do); and in the long run, the only workable moral codes are those based on the postulate of the basic moral equality of all persons.

It is clear that newly fertilized human eggs and very small embryos do not yet have any of these mental or behavioral capacities. We know this because we know that they do not yet have functioning sense organs, brains, or nervous systems, which are in every known case necessary conditions for mental functioning in a biological organism. It follows from this that they are not persons in the empirical sense. Empirically, a zygote is far more similar to a single cell taken from a more mature human being than to a postnatal human being or a late-term fetus; and even late-term fetuses have fewer of the capacities that are distinctive of persons than do many nonhuman animals that are not considered persons. Yet it does not follow immediately from the fact that fetuses are not persons in the empirical sense that it is improper to consider them persons in the moral sense. For there is general agreement that all (or virtually all) *postnatal* human beings are persons in the moral sense, even though some of them—infants, and severely retarded, insane or senile persons—appear to lack most of the mental capacities listed above. The question is: Why should fetuses not be placed in the same moral category as (other) mentally undeveloped or handicapped persons?

This question is most easily answered in the case of first-trimester fetuses, which are not yet sentient. Nonsentient organisms, such as trees, microbes, and the like, are not centers of conscious experience; they are not capable of pain or pleasure, frustration or satisfaction. They are teleological or goal-oriented systems, and as such they may be harmed or benefited; but because they have no desires, hopes, or fears, because they can neither suffer nor enjoy their own condition, they cannot be harmed or benefited *in a way that matters to them.* We may value such organisms and consider them worthy of protection. We may even value them for what they are, and not just for the uses we hope to put them to. But it makes no sense to speak of them as having moral *rights*, because moral rights are protections designed to safeguard the interests of the rights-bearer, and nonsentient entities do not have interests of their own. This is why, when a protected plant or other nonsentient object is illegally damaged, we do not say that its rights have been violated. The law may have been violated, or the property rights of the owner; but the plant itself is not thought of as having either legal or moral rights.[16]

These considerations suggest that the capacity for sentience is a necessary condition for having moral rights. This is true even in the case of postnatal human beings. Sleeping persons and persons who are unconscious or in temporary comas are still persons with full moral rights, because they still have the neurological equipment necessary for sentience and the capacity to use it again, sooner or later. Eike-Henner Kluge refers to this neurophysiologically based capacity for sentience as a "constitutive potential," in order to highlight the fact that it is the way that an organism's nervous system is constituted that determines its capacity for sentience.[17] People who have irreparably lost this constitutive potential for sentience through the permanent destruction of the relevant parts of the brain are legally defined as dead in many states. The moral plausibility of this legal definition arises from the fact that such "brain dead" individuals are forever beyond the reach of any harms or benefits that can matter to them. Although it may be morally right to respect certain of their former wishes, this is not because they are still living persons with full moral rights, but because it is right to respect certain of the wishes of *any* recently deceased person.

If this argument is correct, then the biologically human structure of zygotes and presentient fetuses is not a valid basis for regarding them as persons with full moral rights. This conclusion accords with Western legal tradition and commonsense morality. Although abortion has often been prohibited by legal and religious codes, early abortions or miscarriages have never been viewed by either the law or the social mores as the deaths of human persons: death certificates are not issued, names and "conception dates" are not recorded, funerals are not held, nor funerary memorials erected. Nor are the parents of a spontaneously aborted fetus regarded as having suffered the same tragic loss as if a child of theirs had died. A loss it may be, but a different and generally a much lesser one, for them. For the fetus itself it is no loss at all. *It* has not suffered pain, frustration, or disappointment of any sort.

Fetuses as Potential Persons

I have argued that early abortion is not a form of homicide, because presentient fetuses are not yet the sort of entity to which it makes sense to ascribe moral rights, just as permanently brain-dead persons are no longer such entities. But there is a significant difference between presentient fetuses and brain-dead persons: fetuses have the potential to *become* sentient human beings.[18] They have what might be called the *developmental* potential for sentience, as opposed to the *constitutive* potential that sleeping or temporarily unconscious persons have. Spermatozoa and ova, in mixed pairs, also have this developmental potential, even though the probability that it will be realized is much smaller. Does this developmental potential imply a right to life? If so, then doubt is cast not only on the morality of abortion, but also on the use of contraceptives, voluntary sterilization, coitus interruptus, and even (in a weaker sense) celibacy; for all of these practices prevent potential persons from developing into actual persons.

The moral status of human gametes (spermatozoa or unfertilized ova) is indeed somewhat different from that of other nonsentient entities, which are not potential persons. But this difference arises solely from the fact that the former may later *become* beings with full moral rights. That they may later come to have certain rights in no way implies that they have those rights now. Joel Feinberg points out that

> to infer actual possession of rights from future qualification is a mistake that seems peculiar to the abortion controversy; we are rarely tempted to make it in other contexts. A twelve year old American child, for example, is a potential voter in American elections in the sense that he will have an actual right to vote six years from now if all goes well in the natural course of his adolescence. But we are not tempted to admit him to the voting booths now simply on the grounds that he is a "potential voter" who will be qualified later.[19]

Why are some people tempted to think of potential persons as already having the rights that they may later come to have, when they are not similarly tempted in the case of potential voters, potential presidents, potential property owners, and the like? One reason is that certain sorts of damage done to potential persons can result in violations of the rights of the people they later become. There are, for instance, certain chemicals (teratogens) that can cause birth defects, either by damaging the genetic material in the gametes of prospective parents, or by interfering with the normal course of fetal development. To carelessly expose people of reproductive age to dangerous levels of such chemicals can be a violation not only of their rights, but also those of their future children, who may be born physically or mentally handicapped as a result of such negligence.

But to say this is not to ascribe moral rights to presentient fetuses, let alone to ova or spermatozoa. It is the future children (and their families) who may suffer in such cases, and it is *their* rights that may be violated. It may sound odd at first to say that people can be wronged by actions performed before they even begin to exist; but a little reflection shows that this is so. For instance, if a person were to recklessly squander money left her in trust for her younger sister's future children (should any be born), then she would arguably have wronged any children her sister might have ten, twenty, or

thirty years later. Whether or not these children already existed—
even as gleams in their parents' eyes—at the time the money was
squandered would be irrelevant to whether or not their rights had
been violated; for the rights in question would not be those of presently existing gametes or fetuses, but rather those of future people.

A second reason why it may be tempting to think of potential people as having a right to life is that some people may value them
highly—particularly people who want to have or to adopt children.
It seems self-evidently wrong, in all but the most extraordinary circumstances, either to sterilize a person against his or her will or to
force a woman to have an abortion when she wants to carry the pregnancy to term. But the value that potential persons may have for
others is not a sufficient reason for asserting that they have moral
rights. The wrongness of involuntary sterilization or abortion is better explained by an appeal to the rights of the actual persons affected, such as the right to decide for oneself whether and when to
have children,[20] and the right to security against unwarranted physical assault. The first of these rights is also violated when people are
deliberately denied access to voluntary sterilization, contraception,
or abortion.

Another way in which some people may come to believe that potential persons have a right to life is through reflecting on the fact
that they themselves developed from tiny fetuses, which in turn developed from still tinier gametes. If I enjoy my life and am glad that I
was born, then it may seem to me that it would have been wrong,
and a violation of my rights as a (potential) person, for anyone to
have prevented me from being conceived and born.[21]

This argument is easier to deal with if we divide it into two separate lines of argument. The first says that the existence of happy
people—whoever they are—is a morally good thing, and that therefore it is wrong to fail to bring into existence people who will probably be happy, if and when one has it in one's power to do so. The fallacy in this argument is that even if having children who predictably
turn out to be glad that they exist is a morally good thing to do, it
does not follow that it is a moral obligation. There are innumerable
ways of contributing to the welfare of society, and no compelling
reasons to insist that everyone ought to contribute in *this* way. On
the contrary, there are compelling reasons *not* to insist on a universal obligation to reproduce (provided that one's children would probably be happy), such as the threat of global and national overpopulation, and the fact that some people are happier, healthier, and more
socially productive if they do not have children—or more than one
or two children.

The second line of argument here is that for anyone to have prevented *me*—a particular person—from existing would have been a wrong *against me*, since it would have deprived me of the chance to lead a happy life. The fallacy here is that of supposing that it is possible to wrong a potential person, or the actual person it might have become, by failing to allow it to become an actual person. This supposition appears to be a coherent one only if one wrongly imagines that potential persons are real persons of a special ghostly sort, waiting in some limbo for someone to confer upon them the benefit of existence. In Greek mythology, the souls of unborn persons were conceived in exactly this way, which probably shows that it is a fairly natural way of thinking. But there is absolutely no reason to believe that anything of the sort is true. In reality, potential persons are simply possibilities that are as yet unrealized. If they never develop into actual persons—or at least actual sentient beings—then there is no way in which they can be harmed or victimized, hence no way in which they can be morally wronged.

If this response to the second line of argument fails to dispel the conviction that it would have been a very bad thing *for me* had I never existed, it is probably because we tend to have great difficulty in imagining a state of affairs that consists in our own complete nonexistence. When I try to imagine the situation in which my parents never had me, I tend instead to imagine the quite different situation in which I, an actual and reasonably happy person, am suddenly deprived of my entire life—my past as well as my future. If it were possible for someone to do such a thing to me, then it would certainly be a very bad thing to do; very bad, that is, for me. But had I never existed at all, then no one could have done this or anything else to me. Persons who do not and never will exist cannot be harmed by anything that we do or fail to do, any more than trees that never exist can be cut into firewood.

There are, in short, no valid reasons for concluding that nonsentient potential persons already have the rights that actual persons have. As nonsentient entities, they do not yet have any moral rights at all, although those that *will* develop into persons *will* have rights, some of which can be violated by things that we do now. Like other nonsentient entities, potential persons may have value *for us*; but their potential existence does not as yet have value *for them*. Hence the failure to have children is never a wrong committed against the children one might have had. Contraception, voluntary sterilization, sexual abstinence, and early abortion are all legitimate exercises of the right to reproductive autonomy; they essentially involve no one's rights other than those of the potential parents.

Are Sentient Fetuses Persons?

The later in the pregnancy an abortion is performed, the more dangerous and painful for the woman it is apt to be— though generally less so than giving birth to a full-term infant. This is one important reason for making early abortion fully legal and readily available to all women; for where it is illegal or available only on a restricted basis, many women are forced to wait weeks or months for abortions that could otherwise have been performed early in the first trimester, when the risk of medical trauma is minimal.

But it is not just concern for women's welfare that makes late abortions harder to justify than early ones. Also important is the fact that late-term fetuses are very different sorts of entities from zygotes or tiny embryos. They are not only larger, but also much more similar to infants in their appearance and degree of development. One of the most powerful weapons of the antiabortion factions has been the display of corpses or photographs of aborted third-trimester fetuses. Of course, appearance alone is not a sufficient reason for ascribing moral rights; no one would say that a greatly magnified and vividly colored *photograph* of a tiny fetus has rights, even though it may be a great deal more emotionally evocative than was the fetus itself. More important than their appearance is the fact that late-term fetuses are probably sentient to some degree. They have brains in which the major physiological structures are not only formed but already beginning to function as well. There is evidence that they can react to environmental stimuli such as sound, motion, and light. They are probably capable of experiencing pain or discomfort. While there is probably no *precise* point in its development when a fetus begins to have such sensory capacities, it is thought that at least some rudimentary elements of sentience probably begin to appear at some point in the second trimester.

This fact has evident moral significance. Sentient beings are capable of suffering, and there is (or should be) general agreement that the deliberate infliction of unnecessary suffering is morally wrong. Thus, it is reasonable to suggest that all sentient beings have some moral status, and perhaps some moral rights. But not all sentient beings are persons with *full and equal* moral rights. Nonhuman beings (animals) that are not persons in the empirical sense, but that clearly possess a rather high degree of sentience, are nevertheless not regarded—even by animal liberationists—as moral persons with rights identical to those of human persons.

It is always wrong to treat persons in the empirical sense as if they were not persons in the moral sense. It is the essence of what is morally wrong with slavery, racism, sexism, and other radical negations of the moral equality of all persons. But the very fact that morality requires that all persons be treated as moral equals, with the same basic moral rights, means that we must be careful about how we go about admitting *other* entities to the class of moral equals, entities that—unlike women, children, members of minority races, and other victims of social oppression—are clearly not persons in the empirical sense. The expansion of the class of moral persons beyond the class of empirical persons is not intrinsically illegitimate; it is something that we have a right and even a duty to do, where there are sufficiently compelling reasons. It must, however, be done in a way that is consistent with the basic moral rights and responsibilities of those who are persons in the empirical sense.

The alternative to this view is the view that morality requires us to treat all sentient beings as our moral equals, recognizing them as having not just *some* moral status, but essentially the *same* moral status as we ourselves have.[22] This suggestion is appealing for its theoretical simplicity and its avoidance of human chauvinism. But a little reflection shows that it is impossible to put into practice. We cannot treat all sentient beings as our moral equals without entirely negating our own rights. Insects are sentient beings, though they probably enjoy a lesser *degree* of sentience than do, say, birds or mammals.[23] Some moral or religious idealists do try to live without ever harming any sentient being; but most of us would be unable to carry out many of the daily activities on which our lives ultimately depend given such a restriction. (I cannot even sit quietly at my desk without occasionally causing a loss of insect life, such as by moving my foot and accidentally crushing a passing ant.) Such idealists can survive only because other people are doing things that do sometimes result in harm to sentient beings, such as cultivating crops and protecting food supplies from insects and rodents. If *everyone* refused to do anything that might harm a sentient being—except under circumstances that would justify doing the same thing to a fellow human person—we would all die of starvation or sheer physical inactivity.[24]

We are, therefore, necessarily selective in the ascription of *full* moral status to beings that are sentient, but that are not persons in the empirical sense. There is no single and universally valid principle that will enable us to decide just how much and what sorts of protection should be accorded to any given class of such beings. To reach a morally satisfactory conclusion in any particular case, we must consider a variety of factors, such as the creature's level or degree of sentience, its numerosity and ecological importance, and the probable effects of protecting (or not protecting) it on human interests. Some sentient beings, those whose existence is radically inconsistent with human well-being (e.g., malaria-carrying mosquitoes) are rightly given *no* moral or legal protection other than the general injunction against needless cruelty—and rightly so. At the opposite extreme, our society regards all mentally incompetent postnatal human beings (who are still capable of sentience) as persons in the moral sense, even though some of them may not be persons in the moral sense. There are many good reasons for this, reasons that are somewhat different with respect to each of the various categories of the mentally incompetent—that is, those who are not yet, are no longer, or who never will be capable of rationality, self-awareness, and the use of language. In the case of infants, for example, the reasons include:

1. The affection that most people feel for helpless newborn babies, which makes the thought of their being harmed a painful one.
2. The realistic concern that maltreated infants may become asocial or antisocial children or adults.
3. The fact that there are many more potentially good parents who wish to adopt infants than there are infants available for adoption.
4. The relative wealth of our society, which makes it possible to provide reasonably good care for orphaned or abandoned infants who are not adoptable.
5. The willingness of a majority of people to pay taxes to provide such care, rather than allowing unwanted infants to be neglected.

Some of these reasons (with the necessary changes in wording) are also relevant to the moral status of older human beings who are so severely retarded, deranged, or brain-damaged that their empirical personhood may be doubted. But in these cases, there are additional reasons for retaining the presumption of moral personhood, such as:

6. Respect for the wishes of persons who have established (as it were) personal relationships with the afflicted individual, such as family members and friends.
7. The concern that we or others we care about may someday lose the mental capacities that are distinctive of persons (without

at the same time losing the capacity for sentience), and the
desire to protect our or their interests should this occur.

8. The natural and morally desirable empathy and compassion
that most of us feel for *any* sentient human being, even one
less cute and lovable than a newborn infant.

9. The danger that some human beings who are in fact persons in
the empirical sense would be treated as if they were not
persons in the moral sense, were we to attempt to decide
this sometimes obscure empirical question in each individual
case—or in the case of other races, sexes, nationalities, and
the like.

Considerations of this sort compel us to recognize the moral personhood of all human beings who have been born and who remain
capable of some degree of sentience. The question is whether there
are equally compelling reasons for regarding unborn fetuses as persons with full and equal moral rights. Several philosophers have recently argued for such a sentience criterion of fetal personhood.[25] It
is true, and significant, that some of the above considerations (e.g.,
1, 3, 4, and 8) have some application to the case of sentient fetuses.
Furthermore, insofar as the capacity for sentience seems to be an appropriate criterion for the moral personhood of *postnatal* human beings, the suggestion that we simply extend this criterion to cover
unborn human beings has the virtue of simplicity. Since a human
being's spatial location (e.g., inside or outside a woman's body) does
not appear—at least at first glance—to be a relevant factor in determining its moral status, the fetal sentience criterion might seem to
represent a gain in consistency as well as simplicity.

But there is one crucial factor that has been left out of the argument thus far: the rights of the pregnant woman. The above considerations are compelling in the case of human beings *who have already been born*, because there is no inescapable inconsistency
between the moral personhood of mentally incompetent postnatal
human beings and that of any class of empirical persons—at least
not in a society as wealthy as ours still is. Whether or not we actually do so, we can afford to treat all human beings who are born with
a capacity for sentience as moral persons, without in the process
depriving any set of persons of their most basic moral and legal
rights. There is, however, an unavoidable inconsistency between ascribing full moral rights to unborn fetuses and respecting the full
moral rights of women who are pregnant. Birth is a morally significant event, and a reasonable point from which to date the emergence of a new, separate, and distinct person, primarily because it

constitutes the point at which it becomes possible to treat *both* the woman and her progeny as moral persons.

It is true that the ascription of full moral personhood to sentient fetuses would not necessarily preclude late-term abortion in every case.[26] Some fetuses are so severely abnormal that they do not have and will never have any capacity for sentience; presumably these would not be considered persons and thus could justifiably be aborted or allowed to die after birth. Women's right to self-defense would probably justify at least a few other late-term abortions.

Consider, however, some of the other likely consequences of ascribing full moral status to sentient fetuses, and building this premise into our legal system. First, this would have the result that every spontaneous or induced miscarriage that took place after some specific point in the pregnancy would be liable to be investigated by law enforcement agencies as a possible criminal homicide. Women who abort late for what they (but not the local prosecutor) consider sufficiently compelling reasons could be charged with first-degree murder. Women who miscarry could be indicted for manslaughter on the basis of their having done any of an indefinite number of things that they typically would have every right to do—such as walking, running, drinking, smoking, having sexual intercourse, not taking some prescribed or prescribable medication, or not getting enough sleep—if someone suspected that these activities might have caused the miscarriage and that they constituted negligence. Physicians who perform late-term abortions, for whatever reasons, would also face the threat of criminal prosecution.

Furthermore, if such abortions had to be justified on the grounds of self-defense, physicians would probably be forced to wait much too long before terminating a pregnancy that endangered a woman's health (i.e., until the danger were both immediate and severe). Such a policy would cost some women their lives, and others would sustain needless suffering and injury because late-term abortions could not be performed before the predicted medical crisis actually occurred. For the right to self-defense has never been legally construed to include the right to kill innocent persons who are merely likely to endanger one's life or health in the nonimmediate future; in any context other than abortion, such "preventive strikes" count as murder, not self-defense.

The view that sentient fetuses are moral persons would also seem to preclude the abortion of even very severely abnormal late-term fetuses, unless the abnormality would prevent the emergence of any capacity for sentience. Such "genetic" abortions often cannot be performed early in the pregnancy, because amniocentesis, currently the only way to diagnose many severe fetal anomalies, cannot be performed safely in the first trimester. The fetal sentience view implies that late-term "genetic" abortions are morally equivalent to the killing of physically or mentally handicapped persons at some point *after* their birth (i.e., they are equivalent to active or direct euthanasia). *Voluntary* euthanasia—that is, deliberately causing the death of a person who has made an informed and uncoerced decision to die at such a time and in such a way—is arguably a form of assisted suicide, and something that ought to be permitted, although at present its legal status is at best uncertain. But *nonvoluntary* euthanasia, the killing of a person who has not made and perhaps cannot make such a decision, is considerably more difficult to justify. Nonvoluntary euthanasia may be justifiable in some cases, as in cases in which the person's quality of life is so dismal that continued survival is manifestly contrary to his or her own best interests. But it is extremely difficult to specify the class of cases in which this is true, and for this reason it will be a long time before the legalization of nonvoluntary euthanasia becomes feasible, if it ever does. Hence the extension of the sentience criterion to fetuses would probably result in the prohibition of most "genetic" abortions, at least until the early diagnosis of fetal abnormalities becomes possible in a much wider range of cases than it is at present.

The consequences of such a prohibition would be extremely unfortunate. Inevitably, more infants would be born with medical problems that doom them to an early death, or that preclude their ever leading a decent human life. Family members, and society as a whole, incur extremely heavy burdens in providing care for such individuals. Without the option of selective abortion, would-be parents who are at risk of having a severely abnormal child would have no way to avoid that outcome except by remaining childless, which often would be a great loss for them.

Another risk inherent in the classification of sentient fetuses as moral persons is that pregnant women will be denied the right to refuse surgical operations and other medical treatments that are thought by others to be necessary for the health or survival of the fetus. There have already been several reported cases in which American courts have ordered women to submit to Cesarean sections, against their will, in order to protect the fetus from the supposed risks of vaginal delivery.[27] Other court cases have established that parents do not have the legal right to refuse life-saving medical treatment for their children.[28] Thus the danger exists that if sentient fetuses are given the same legal status as infants and children, pregnant women may be involuntarily subjected to more and more invasive, painful, dangerous, and expensive medical interventions, as the medical treatment of fetuses in utero becomes more feasible and more common. Such a situation would be intolerable and would probably lead increasing numbers of women to avoid professional prenatal medical care altogether, out of an understandable fear of being victimized in this way.

It is necessary to stress that none of these dangers would in any way count against the claim that sentient fetuses should be treated as full-fledged moral persons *if they were persons in the empirical sense.* If they were highly sentient, rational, self-motivated, self-aware, language-using beings—say, just like two-year-olds, only smaller—then none of these probable violations of women's rights could possibly justify refusing to treat them as persons with full and equal moral rights. As long as infants are born of women, and not gestated in artificial wombs, it will be impossible to treat *both* fetuses and women as persons; and since women are persons in the empirical sense and fetuses are not, it is women's rights that should prevail.

This conclusion in no way precludes us from recognizing that sentient fetuses have some moral status. The applicability of some of the conditions listed above is enough to justify regarding them as having a somewhat more significant moral status than do most sentient nonhuman animals. But this moral status, while it is sufficient to preclude the cruel treatment or casual destruction of fetuses, cannot override a woman's right to choose abortion. The basic moral rights of persons outweigh those of sentient beings that are not persons, whenever there is a severe and irreconcilable conflict between them. Reasonable people may disagree about whether it is morally optimal for a woman to choose abortion in the absence of what they consider to be compelling reasons; but it is nevertheless something that the woman has the right to do, and that no one else has the right to coercively prevent her from doing. If some medical practitioners refuse to perform abortions because of their own moral convictions, they too are arguably within their rights; but they overstep those rights when they attempt to force others to refrain from performing abortions as well.

It is important to realize that even where they are legally tolerated, late-term abortions constitute a very small proportion of the total number of abortions performed. Neither women nor physicians are likely to make such decisions lightly. Furthermore, it is reasonable to hope that continued improvements in prenatal care and the early diagnosis and treatment of fetal ailments will make possible a continual reduction in the number of late-term abortions that must be performed. A concern not just for the lives of fetuses but also for the well-being of women, their families, and those involved in providing medical care makes this a necessary goal.

Consequences of the Freedom to Choose

If the arguments presented thus far are correct, then abortion is never a form of homicide. But it might still be thought to be something that has harmful personal or social consequences. If the predictable consequences of a permissive abortion policy were extremely harmful, then it might be possible to argue that women's freedom of choice with regard to their own medical care must be limited, either for their own good or for that of others. Thus, we need to consider the major consequentialist arguments against the freedom to choose abortion, and weigh them against the consequentialist arguments in favor of such freedom.

Historically, one of the most important arguments for the prohibition of abortion has been that it will promote population growth. One reply to this argument is that in this era of shrinking resources and chronic severe poverty throughout much of the world, rapid population increase is no longer a desirable goal. Those nations that have smaller populations than their resources could readily support ought to count their blessings; or, if they really need a larger population, they should open their doors to immigrants from the overpopulated parts of the world, rather than attempting to increase their own birth rate. Besides, even if an increased birth rate were desirable, placing legal restrictions on abortion would be an unjust and inefficient way of bringing it about: unjust because it abridges women's most basic rights for the sake of an optional social goal, one that does not involve the basic rights of others, and inefficient because people who do not want to have (more) children tend to find ways of avoiding it, (e.g., through dangerous illegal abortions).[29]

A second consequentialist argument against abortion is that it is physically or psychologically harmful to the woman who undergoes it. This argument was influential in bringing about the passage of antiabortion laws in the nineteenth century, when abortion typically was attempted through the administration of substances that were more apt to harm the woman than to safely terminate the pregnancy.[30] But the argument is irrelevant under current conditions, when it has been amply demonstrated that a freely chosen abortion, properly performed, is much less apt to prove either physically or psychologically harmful than is carrying an unwanted pregnancy to term.

A third argument is that legal abortion encourages women to be "promiscuous." Those who argue in this way are, in effect, advocating the use of pregnancy and childbirth as a way of punishing women—whether married or unmarried—for having sexual intercourse with (fertile) men. (No comparable penalty is suggested for the male party to the act.) If such a strange and discriminatory use of the punitive power of the state is to be justified, it must be shown not only that it is socially harmful (and harmful to an extreme degree) for women to enjoy nonprocreatively motivated sex, but also that it is *not* socially harmful for men to do so. This is an unlikely prospect. Short of appealing to empirically unprovable religious premises, there is no way to show that private sexual activities between consenting adults have any social consequences dire enough to justify their legal prohibition, let alone the imposition of so severe a penalty as involuntary motherhood.

A fourth argument is that sex is more meaningful, or more valuable as an expression of love and commitment, if it is liable to have unavoidable reproductive consequences. Whereas some religions view nonprocreative sex as sinful, this argument maintains only that it yields a subjectively inferior experience, or one that is a less significant part of a person's life. While this is probably true for some people, it is certainly false for many others. If one does not *want* to have a child, then the fear of accidental pregnancy can only detract from the experience of lovemaking. More to the point, even if all of us did find procreative sex subjectively superior to any other sort, it would hardly follow that all other sorts ought to be legally penalized; the argument confuses what is personally preferable with what is socially necessary.

But of all the consequentialist arguments against abortion, the one that is probably the most influential today is what has been called the slippery slope argument. The argument is that to legally condone the taking of "human life" through abortion will erode our society's respect for the lives of all persons. The result, it is feared, will be an increase in the frequency of wrongful homicides, in particular the killing of persons who are thought to be socially or economically unproductive. Although this fear is real enough, it is not realistic. Abortion has been legally available in the United States for about a decade, but there is no evidence that our alarmingly high rate of homicide has been even slightly increased by this fact. Other countries, which have permitted abortion for considerably longer than the United States (e.g., Japan and the Soviet Union), have a far lower incidence of homicide; furthermore, they provide—relative to their resources—*more* support for those members of society who are not economically self-sufficient.

Empirically, then, the claim that abortion will lead to an increase in the homicide rate is unfounded. On logical grounds, the slipperiness of the slope that is supposed to run from abortion to homicide could be expected to depend on whether or not most people perceive a morally significant difference between the two cases. That most people throughout Western history have perceived such a difference is strongly suggested by the fact that no legal system has ever equated abortion with murder. While abortion has often been treated as a serious crime, it has always been treated as a different crime from murder. It is also suggested by the fact that in our culture—as in most others—birth, and not some earlier point, is treated as the beginning of a person's life and legal existence. Though few people could give a coherent account of *why* birth is morally so significant, few doubt that it is indeed significant. This being the case, we have little reason to fear that many people will interpret the legal toleration of abortion as an endorsement of murder, genocide, or other forms of wrongful killing.

We have seen that none of the consequentialist arguments for banning abortion is at all plausible. What about the consequentialist arguments *against* banning abortion? If fetuses are not persons in the empirical sense, and if there are no compelling arguments for treating them as persons in the moral sense, then there is no need to rely on further consequentialist arguments to establish women's right to choose abortion; women's basic rights to life, liberty, and the pursuit of happiness are sufficient to carry the weight of the argument even in the absence of any further social benefits. Nevertheless, the "pro-choice" position can be further strengthened by a consideration of the social benefits of freedom and the social costs of a return to prohibition.

In the first place, there are all of the dangers to women that are inherent in the substitution of illegal for legal abortion. The prohibition of abortion does not prevent abortions from occurring, often with about the same frequency. It only forces women to procure the procedure illegally, and too often from persons who lack the proper training and equipment. Or women may seek to induce abortions themselves, invariably by unsafe means. Before abortion was legalized in the United States, hundreds of women annually died from botched abortions, and thousands more were left infertile or otherwise severely injured; since legalization, such casualties have become extremely rare.

Second, there are all of the harms to individuals and to society of depriving ourselves—men as well as women—of the right to decide whether and when to have children. If we care about the welfare of parents and children, then we must respect the right of individuals to enter into parenthood only under circumstances which *they* judge to be appropriate.

Third, there are the consequences of further aggravating the problem of overpopulation—consequences that are too well known to require extensive comment here. Some people still doubt that the population problem is a real one, since it seems that a more optimal exploitation of the earth's food-producing resources, plus a more egalitarian distribution system, would permit the planet to support an even larger human population than at present. But this argument ignores various harsh realities, such as that there is no realistic prospect for an even remotely egalitarian worldwide distribution system in the near future, and that soil deterioration and climatic changes threaten to erode the earth's capacity to support even current population levels. The argument also ignores the environmental deterioration that more or less inevitably accompanies human population growth: the destruction of natural ecosystems, of nonhuman species and populations. Even those who see no value in nonhuman life must recognize that in the long run we cannot hope to prosper on a biologically devastated planet. If totally reliable contraceptives were universally available, or if most people were prepared to be sterilized after their first or second child is born, or to abandon heterosexuality in favor of some other lifestyle, then we would not need abortion as a means of limiting population increase; as it is, we do.

Fourth, the prohibition of abortion greatly reduces the enjoyment that many people could otherwise find in heterosexual intercourse. Where abortion is illegal, some people (relatively few) avoid heterosexual intercourse entirely, because of the risk of unwanted pregnancy; but most women live a large portion of their lives in persistent fear, knowing that even the most conscientious use of contraceptives cannot ensure that an "accident" will not occur.

Fifth, the criminalization of abortion creates an enormous class of pseudocriminals, generally law-abiding persons who are forced to violate an unjust law and incur the consequent anxiety and risk. Even where restrictive laws are rarely enforced, this is never a trivial consideration; like other unjust and pragmatically unenforceable laws, it creates a contemptuous attitude toward law in general, along with the risk that selective enforcement will be used to persecute persons whose political views or activities the state wishes to suppress.

Last but not least, the denial of legal access to abortion contributes significantly to nearly every aspect of sexual inequality, from the notorious double standard about sexual activity to the prejudice of employers against women. The lack of a reliable means of controlling her own reproductive life makes a woman's fertility a perpetual liability, a sword of Damocles continually poised to strike down whatever life plans she may have made and whatever economic security she may have managed to win for herself and her family. Sexual equality is impossible without reproductive freedom; and reproductive freedom, for most women, is impossible without access to abortion.

In short, the protection of abortion rights is by far the more socially beneficial policy. Opponents accuse the advocates of abortion rights of placing the selfish desires of women above the good of society. In reality, it is they who are prepared to do untold damage to other people's lives for the sake of their own frequently irrational ends—such as promoting population growth or punishing women for sexual activity. Abortion is not just a right that women are entitled to claim for reasons related to their own personal well-being; it is also a social necessity.

Abortion and Men's Rights

What about men's rights in the context of abortion? Some people argue that to give women the unilateral right to decide whether or not to abort deprives men of their reproductive rights. Having a child, or not having one, may be as important to a prospective father as to a prospective mother; so why should the biological accident that pregnancies occur in the bodies of women be used to justify depriving men of an equal share in the decision process? Since it is impossible to "split the difference" when the prospective parents disagree about an abortion decision, why not turn the matter over to the courts for an impartial decision?[31]

The answer is that a prospective father's situation is simply not comparable with that of a pregnant woman. The abortion decision belongs to the woman because the pregnancy is a state of *her* body, not that of any other interested party. She alone must bear the physical burden, the pain, discomfort, and risk of death or permanent injury if she carries the pregnancy to term.

This is not to say that a prospective father does not sometimes have a right to participate in the making of an abortion decision (e.g., to be informed of the circumstances, to discuss them with the woman and her health care advisers, and to have his wishes given all due consideration). The extent of this right depends on the sorts of contracts or agreements that the man and woman may have made with each other in the past. Neither marriage nor voluntary participation in sexual intercourse constitutes, in itself, an agreement on the woman's part to bear children. But if she has voluntarily agreed to do so, in return for benefits that she has already received, then it would clearly be wrong for her to violate that agreement *for no good reason*. If she does, then in some cases the other party to the agreement may bring legal suit against her in an attempt to collect damages for the loss suffered. But no one has the right to use physical or legal coercion to force a woman to complete a pregnancy—or to terminate it, if the agreement was that she would *not* have a child.

Conclusions

If fetuses were persons, then abortion could be justified only in a rather limited range of cases. But in the ways that matter from a moral point of view, human fetuses are very unlike human persons, particularly in the early months of their development. First-trimester fetuses have not yet begun to develop a capacity for sentience and thus lack a necessary precondition for the possession of moral rights. That does not mean that one can do anything one likes with them, but it does mean that abortion is never a violation of fetuses' rights.

The fact that late-term fetuses probably do possess some capacity for sentience is a good reason for regarding them as having a somewhat different moral status than do presentient fetuses. Like sentient nonhuman beings, they should not be subjected to cruel treatment or harmed for no good reason. They are not, however, persons in the empirical sense, since a capacity for sentience, in the absence of rationality, self-awareness, and the other mental and behavioral capacities characteristic of persons, is not a sufficient condition of personhood. Nor is it appropriate to grant them the same (full and equal) moral status as human beings who are born, or later become, mentally handicapped in one way or another; for they differ from human beings who have already been born in that there is no way at present to treat them as persons with full and equal basic rights, without at the same time treating women as something *less* than persons with full and equal rights. Because women are persons, and because the basic rights of persons outweigh those of other sentient beings whenever there is an irreconcilable conflict between the two, it is women's right to choose that must be considered paramount.

Restrictive abortion laws not only violate women's most basic moral right; they are also socially counterproductive. Restrictive laws force women to resort to unsafe methods of abortion; aggravate overpopulation problems; increase the number of children born with severe medical problems, or to parents who cannot or will not care for them adequately; contribute to the inferior social status of women; and make outlaws of persons whose only crime is that they wish to exercise their reproductive role in a responsible manner or help others to do so. Denying women access to safe and legal abortion would be wrong even if it had no such tragic consequences. Yet it is worth emphasizing these consequences, in reply to those who say that women who seek reproductive freedom are ignoring their social obligations. Women's social obligation is *not* to bear children unless conditions are favorable to the latter's health and happiness and that of other persons.

Notes

1. Editor's note: On the specially persistent and controversial issue of abortion we include two discussions. One, by L. W. Sumner, surveys conservative, liberal, and moderate positions—defending the latter on the basis of a utilitarian moral viewpoint. The second, by Mary Anne Warren, developed from the standpoint of a rights theory and certain feminist concerns, defends a more permissive or liberal view. Instructors, of course, may wish to suggest essays defending more conservative views. For such defenses see the references at the end of Sumner's chapter to essays or books by Brody, Callahan, Donagan, Finnis, and Noonan.

2. The Supreme Court ruled that while neither first- nor second-trimester abortions may be prohibited, regulation of the conditions under which second-trimester abortions are performed—designed to protect the health of the woman—is permissible. Third-trimester abortions may be regulated even more strictly, in order to protect not only the woman but also the state's interest in the fetus as a potential life. (See "Majority Opinion in Roe v. Wade," in *Contemporary Issues in Bioethics*, ed. Tom L. Beauchamp and LeRoy Walters [Encino and Belmont, Calif.: Dickenson Publishing, 1978], 243–246.)

3. A feminist is one who advocates better recognition of women's rights to social and legal equality. Most feminists do *not* advocate female supremacy or a reversal of existing sex roles.

4. "Fetus" is here used to refer to the conceptus at any stage of its development from conception to birth. In more technical terminology, it is called a zygote in the earliest stages, and subsequently a blastocyst, a morula, and an embryo; and then finally a fetus.

5. Jane English, "Abortion and the Concept of a Person," in *Social Ethics*, ed. Thomas Mappes and Jane Zembaty (New York: McGraw-Hill, 1982), 30–37.

6. _____. "Abortion and the Concept of a Person," 34.

7. Judith Thomson, "A Defense of Abortion," *Philosophy & Public Affairs* 1 (Fall 1971): 47–66.

8. I do not mean to minimize or understate the frequency of rape, incest, sexual harassment, and other coercive sexual acts typically committed by men against girls or women; but it would be an exaggeration to hold that *most* heterosexual sex acts are overtly coercive.

9. "National tragedy" is a phrase used by President Ronald Reagan in calling for a Constitutional amendment banning abortion.

10. Biologists will point out that the process of conception occurs not in a moment but over a period of hours; but that is irrelevant for our purposes.

11. A zygote is a newly fertilized ovum, which has not yet developed into a blastocyst, or hollow ball of cells.

12. To say that a person has a certain capacity is not to say that he or she is able to exhibit that capacity at any time, under any circumstances. To be capable of speaking coherently, for example, is to be able to do so provided that the circumstances are not in some way incompatible with the exercise of such a capacity—that is, provided one is not asleep, drugged, emotionally overwrought, or the like. Thus, the fact that people sleep, and so on, is no objection to a definition of the empirical concept of a person based on the possession of certain mental and behavioral capacities: sleeping people are still people.

13. This is essentially the same list of mental and behavioral capacities given in my earlier article, "On the Moral and Legal Status of Abortion," *The Monist* 57 (January 1973): 43–61. That article, however, does not explore the distinction between the moral and empirical senses of the term "person."

14. Michael Tooley takes this ability to know oneself as a sentient being persisting in time as particularly central to the concept of a person. (See his "Abortion and Infanticide," *Philosophy & Public Affairs* 2 [Fall 1972]: 37–65.)

15. Some philosophers treat the capacity for moral autonomy (i.e., the capacity to regulate one's own behavior by moral rules or principles) as the central defining feature of personhood. Yet there are certainly some amoral persons, who possess normal intelligence yet who never learn, and perhaps

cannot learn, to be morally autonomous. Such individuals are sometimes called "sociopaths." They are persons in both the moral and empirical senses, even though it is often necessary to curtail their freedom in order to protect that of others.

16. Some writers have argued that trees and other nonsentient elements of nature ought to be given legal rights, much as corporations have been, in order that certain sorts of legal action could be taken against those who damage or endanger them. But such an assignment of legal rights—like the legal status of corporations as persons—would be a legal fiction, not a literal assignment of *moral* rights. (See Christopher Stone, *Should Trees Have Standing: Toward Legal Rights for Natural Objects* [Los Altos: William Kaufman, 1974].)

17. Eike-Henner W. Kluge, *The Ethics of Deliberate Death* (Port Washington, N.Y.: Kennikat Press, 1981), 91.

18. Or rather *some* of them do. It is estimated that perhaps 40 percent of human zygotes perish spontaneously before becoming implanted in the uterus, probably in most cases because of genetic abnormalities; and that 10 to 15 percent of implanted fetuses are spontaneously aborted.

19. Joel Feinberg, "Are Fertilized Eggs People?" (unpublished manuscript, 1982), 2.

20. This right, like most other rights, is not an absolute one. In desperate circumstances of overpopulation, for example, when all possible means of lowering the birth rate through voluntary contraceptive procedures have failed, democratically agreed-upon compulsory limitations on fertility may be justified.

21. See R. M. Hare, "Abortion and the Golden Rule," *Philosophy & Public Affairs* 4 (Spring 1975): 201–222.

22. See, for instance, Leonard Nelson, *System of Ethics* (New York: Oxford University Press, 1956).

23. Some writers assume that all invertebrate animals are nonsentient (L. W. Sumner, *Abortion and Moral Theory* [Princeton, N.J.: Princeton University Press, 1981] p. 143). This is implausible, since some invertebrates, such as insects and arthopods, have sense organs and central nervous systems and give every behavioral indication of being aware of their surroundings.

24. This is not an argument for the general moral legitimacy of eating meat, since we would not starve without it and might even be healthier on a vegetarian diet; we might also be able to provide better nutrition for people in impoverished parts of the world if food supplies suitable for human consumption were not used to raise meat-producing animals. (See Peter Singer, *Practical Ethics* [Cambridge: Cambridge University Press, 1979].)

25. See, for instance, Richard Werner, "Abortion: The Ontological and Moral Status of the Unborn," in *Today's Moral Problems*, 2d. ed., ed. Richard Wasserstrom (New York: Macmillan, 1979), 51–72; Sumner, *Abortion and Moral Theory*; and Kluge, *The Ethics of Deliberate Death*.

26. Sumner, *Abortion and Moral Theory*, p. 152.

27. See George J. Annas, "Forced Cesarians: The Most Unkindest Cut of All," *Hastings Center Report* 12 (June 1982): 16–17.

28. The best-known examples are cases in which parents who are Jehovah's Witnesses, and thus have strong religious objections to blood transfusions, have been required to permit their child to receive transfusions in order to save the child's life.

29. See Hilda Scott's account of the largely unsuccessful efforts by the governments of East European nations, earlier in this century, to raise the birth rate by reducing access to contraception and abortion (*Does Socialism Liberate Women?* [Boston: Beacon Press, 1974]).

30. James C. Mohr, *Abortion in America: The Origins and Evolution of National Policy, 1800–1900* (New York: Oxford University Press, 1978).

31. See, for instance, Wesley K. H. Teo, "Abortion: The Husband's Constitutional Rights," *Ethics* 85 (July 1975): 337–342.

CHAPTER V

The Treatment of Incompetents

Allen Buchanan

The aim of this chapter is to provide the elements of a moral theory of medical treatment decisions for those who are unable to decide for themselves.[1] The class of incompetents is large and diverse, including young children, mentally retarded and senile individuals, and those who have suffered brain damage from trauma.[2] There are four basic questions that such a theory must answer:

1. What principles should guide decisions made for incompetents?[3]
2. Under what conditions is it permissible or even obligatory to limit the rights and interests of the incompetent by consideration of the rights and interests of others?
3. Who should make treatment decisions for incompetents (who is the appropriate surrogate decision maker)?
4. Under what conditions should agents of the state or others intervene in the surrogate's decision making?[4]

Guidance Principles: Best Interest and Substituted Judgment

Two main principles have been advanced to guide decision making for incompetents: the Best Interest Principle and the Substituted Judgment Principle. The Best Interest principle states that the surrogate is to choose what will best serve the patient's interests. The qualifier 'best' signals two considerations that the surrogate is to take into account: first, some interests may be more important than others, in that they make a larger contribution to the patient's good; second, a particular decision may advance some of the patient's interests while frustrating others. Thus, the surrogate must try to determine the net benefit to the patient of each available option after assigning weights to reflect the relative importance of various interests and then subtracting costs or "dis-benefits" from benefits.

The Substituted Judgment Principle states that the surrogate is to choose as the patient would choose were he or she competent and aware of both the medical options and the facts about the condition, including his or her incompetence, at the time the decision is to be made. For example, a surrogate who must decide whether antibiotics should be given to an unconscious, terminal cancer patient might engage in the following thought-experiment: 'If the patient were miraculously to awaken from his coma for a few moments—knowing that he would soon lapse back into unconsciousness with no hope of recovery—what would he choose to do?'

The appeal of the Principle of Substituted Judgment derives from the widespread acceptance of the Principle of Self-Determination for *competent* patients. Both the law and the mainstream of work in medical ethics now acknowledge that a competent patient has the right to decide whether to accept or reject medical treatment, even life-saving treatment.[5] The same value that underlies the Principle of Self-Determination for competent patients—respect for individual autonomy—underlies the Principle of Substituted Judgment for incompetent patients. However, both the Principle of Self-Determination for competent patients and the Principle of Substituted Judgment for incompetents can also be seen as expressions of concern for the patient's well-being, not just respect for his or her autonomy, if it is assumed that the individual, when competent, is generally the best judge of what is in his or her best interest.

Recent court rulings have attempted to extend the right of self-determination for competent patients to incompetent patients.[6] Since the incompetent cannot exercise this right, the courts have held that the right must be exercised for him or her by a surrogate and that the principle the surrogate must employ is Substituted Judgment. If it is assumed—as the courts have apparently done—that a surrogate exercise of the right of self-determination is possible for all incompetents, then one will conclude that Substituted Judgment, not Best Interest, is the appropriate Guidance Principle. For if the right of self-determination is the right to choose even what is not in one's best interest, then the decision should be determined by the distinctive beliefs, preferences, and values of the particular patient when competent, not by an appraisal by others of his or her best interest.

THE SCOPE AND LIMITS OF SUBSTITUTED JUDGMENT

The assumption that a surrogate exercise of the right of self-determination can be achieved for all incompetents is, however, false. There are two types of cases in which this will not be possible. First, in many instances there will simply not be enough reliable evidence about the prior beliefs, preferences, and values of the patient when competent to warrant a conclusion that the patient if competent would or would not choose a particular treatment. In such cases, the appropriate Guidance Principle will be Best Interest. Second, some incompetents never possessed the cognitive capacities that the application of Substituted Judgment presupposes. The question of whether an individual, if competent, would choose a particular treatment can only be sensibly asked of one who at some time in the past had certain complex beliefs, values, and preferences and the conceptual framework that these presuppose. Consequently, for an infant or an individual who has been profoundly retarded for his or her entire life, there is no answer to the question of which treatment *that individual* would want, were *he or she* competent. Further, the very concept of self-determination and hence of a right of self-determination can only be sensibly applied to beings who have, or once had, rather sophisticated cognitive capacities, including the ability to conceive of the future, to discern alternative courses of action, to make judgments about their own good, and in general to conceive of themselves as agents. Because not all incompetents fit this description, the Principle of Substituted Judgment cannot be the sole Guidance Principle for decision making for incompetents.[7]

Even in cases in which Substituted Judgment can be sensibly applied, and in which there is sufficient evidence about the patient, when previously competent, to determine what the patient if competent would now choose, the moral authority of this principle may still be limited by two quite different considerations. The first is that Substituted Judgement can be viewed only as a second-best alternative to the informed choice of a competent patient. The moral authority of the Principle of Self-Determination for competent patients derives in part from a backdrop of assumptions about the communication process that occurs between physician and patient when the requirements of informed consent are duly satisfied. This process provides some protection against frivolous, imprudent, or uninformed exercises of the right of self-determination. Members of the health care team have the opportunity to offer opposing points of view and to question the competent patient's values and preferences, the reasons with which he or she supports them, and the factual beliefs on which they rest and to which they are applied.[8] This safeguard is not present in the case of Substituted Judgment, if the patient's decision must be constructed from evidence about his or her past. At best, others may probe the inferences the surrogate makes from evidence about the patient's former attitudes to a conclusion about what the patient, if competent, now would choose if confronted with concrete alternatives he or she may have never envisioned.

Another limitation on the moral force of Substituted Judgment becomes apparent when the distinction between using Substituted Judgment and implementing an "advance directive" is understood. The law now recognizes two basic types of advance directives: the living will, in which the individual, when competent, issues instructions as to what sorts of treatment, and under what conditions, he or she does not want undertaken; and durable power of attorney, wherein the individual, when competent, designates a surrogate to make decisions on his or her behalf, should he or she become incompetent.

It is important to understand that neither type of advance directive should be viewed as a form of Substituted Judgment: what an individual would now choose, were he or she competent (Substituted Judgment) need not be the same as the choice he or she made in the past about what treatment was desired in the future (the living will) nor to what would be chosen by the person designed in the past to be his or her surrogate.[9]

A bona fide advance directive of either type is something quite different from, and more morally weighty than, the prior expression of preferences upon which an application of the Substituted Judgment Principle is based, because an advance directive is *an act of will*, not a mere *expression of preference*. The distinction between an expression of preference and an act of will may be seen by contrasting the moral (and legal) significance of two different speech-acts that might be performed in uttering the same words in reply to the question "Will you take this woman to be your wife?" Under certain circumstances, one might take the question to be a straightforward factual inquiry about what one in fact will do at some time in the future. And absent any assumption of deceit or duress, the prediction one makes in answering "I will" might reasonably be taken as evidence of one's preferences for the woman in question. However, in other circumstances (when standing at the altar before witnesses) the same utterance ("I will") would not only express a preference but would also constitute an act of will—in this case the making of a promise—that has different moral implications. Similarly, while the competent person's statement that he or she would not wish to be sustained if severely brain-damaged may be an accurate expression of his or her preferences at that time, it may not have the same moral force as the clear act of will of a competent patient who, in the presence of witnesses and after serious discussion, explicitly chooses not to have a particular treatment. A mere expression of preference, as opposed to an act of will, may not be sufficient to waive a person's rights or release others from their duties to him or her.

Once the difference between Substituted Judgment and advance directives is understood, it becomes clear that even if the use of Substituted Judgment can be seen as the surrogate exercise of a right of self-determination, following an advance directive should not be so regarded. When we follow a patient's advance directive, we are simply giving effect to the choice he or she made through *his or her prior exercise of a right*—we are not now exercising the patient's right of self-determination for him or her.

Further, even if the patient when competent left explicit instructions that may be regarded as conclusive evidence of an act of will, the moral force of this advance directive still may be less than that of the choice a competent patient makes at the time a treatment decision must be made. For if questions arise about the application of prior instructions to the particular decision, problems of interpretation cannot be resolved by asking the patient.

So while neither Substituted Judgment nor an advance directive can be taken as the moral equivalent of the choice of a competent patient who chooses at the time the treatment is to be made, a bona fide advance directive will generally have greater moral weight than an exercise of Substituted Judgment. Even if a competent patient ought to be allowed to make a decision clearly contrary to his or her most basic interests, a surrogate should not be given such authority unless it can be shown that the surrogate is merely executing the explicit orders of the patient when competent and that the application of this directive to the circumstances at hand is wholly unambiguous.

It does not follow, however, that a decision should be made according to Substituted Judgment only if it yields a decision that is in the patient's *best* interest. To interpret Substituted Judgment in this way would be to abandon it entirely in favor of Best Interest. Instead, what is needed is a limitation on Substituted Judgment that is weak enough to allow the decision to be guided by evidence of the patient's own preferences when competent, yet strong enough to take into account the fact that Substituted Judgment is not the moral equivalent of the choice of a competent patient. Such a limitation might be expressed in either of two ways. On the one hand, it might be said that one is to choose what the patient if competent would choose unless doing so would pose a "clear and present danger" to the patient's fundamental interests. On the other hand, it might be said that Substituted Judgment is to be limited by a "reasonable person standard":[10] choose what the patient if competent would choose as long as this choice falls within the range of options that reasonable persons would choose. (Notice that the second strategy does *not* collapse Substituted Judgment into a Reasonable Person Standard, since it requires that the patient's own distinctive preferences should determine which of the "reasonable" options should be taken where there is more than one.) Both alternatives entail difficulties: the first requires a principled specification of "fundamental interests"; the second requires clarification of the relevant notion of reasonableness.

The second limitation on the moral authority of Substituted Judgment is more fundamental. It arises once we ask whether this Guidance Principle is to be applied only to decisions concerning the treatment of *living persons* or whether it is also to be used in decisions about medical procedures to be performed on beings that were, but no longer are, living persons. The question may be posed in another way. Does the right of self-determination whose surrogate exercise is to be achieved through Substituted Judgment accrue only to those who are living persons at the time the choice is to be made; or does this same right of self-determination also extend to choices about what is to be done to or with one's body after one is no longer a living person, though one's body or parts of it are still alive?

This question can be answered, granted the assumption that the surrogate exercise of right of self-determination derives from the competent individual's exercise of his or her own right of self-determination and that the right exercised by the surrogate is properly described as a right of self-determination. The right of self-determination exercised by the competent patient is best understood as the right of a living person to decide what medical procedures he or she will allow to be performed on him or her while he or she lives. If, as the courts have held, Substituted Judgment simply is that principle by which we achieve a surrogate exercise of this same right of self-determination, then Substituted Judgment by definition applies only to those incompetents who are still living persons.

We have just seen, however, that the right exercised through Substituted Judgment may be subject to certain restrictions (e.g., a reasonableness standard) that are not present when a competent patient exercises his or her right of self-determination. Thus it may be misleading, if not strictly speaking false, simply to say that the right exercised through Substituted Judgment is the *same* right as the right of self-determination exercised by a competent patient. Instead, it is more accurate to say either (1) that the incompetent's right of self-determination is a narrower and hence a *different* right than that of the competent patient, or (2) that it is the *same* right but that its *exercise* is more constrained than is the case of its exercise by the competent patient. In either case, the right of the incompetent that is to be exercised by Substituted Judgment is a right of self-determination, a right of a living person to determine which medical procedures shall be performed on the patient while he or she lives.

At this point, the theory of decision making for incompetents draws us into a dispute that pervades most of the important issues not only in bioethics but also in moral philosophy in general: the nature of personhood. According to the "cognitivist" concept of a person, the existence of certain psychological capacities—such as the ability to conceive of oneself as a subject of experience who persists through time, the ability to act for reasons and to have a conception of the good—is a necessary condition for being a person. In this view, an incompetent individual, even a temporarily comatose individual, still may be a living person, since personhood depends only on the existence of certain cognitive capacities, not their actual exercise.

According to the best neurophysiological theory, these cognitive capacities exist only when certain brain functions, located in the cerebral cortex in the upper brain, are intact. But in a patient who is in a persistent vegetative state, these higher brain functions have permanently ceased. Consequently, according to the "cognitivist" concept of personhood, the patient in a persistent vegetative state is not a living person. And if the right to self-determination accrues only to living persons, then these patients have no such right and hence no surrogate exercise of such a right (through the use of Substituted Judgment) is possible for them.

In contrast, proponents of the "whole-brain" concept of person-hood contend that a patient in a persistent vegetative state is still a living person because some activity remains in the lower part of the brain even though the functions of the cerebral cortex have perma-nently ceased. The life of the person has ended, according to this view, only when the whole brain is dead—that is, when there is no measurable electrical activity in any part of the brain, including the brain stem. If one accepts the whole-brain concept of personhood and the assumption that every living person has a right of self-deter-mination, then one cannot dismiss the idea of a surrogate exercise of the right of self-determination for those in a persistent vegetative state.

The main difficulty with the whole-brain concept is that it seems to be unable to meet a simple challenge: why draw the line at the permanent cessation of the functioning of the lower part of the brain? After all, there may still be measurable activity in other or-gans after the brain as a whole is dead; so why count the individual as alive if the brain shows some life, but dead if some activity per-sists in other organs such as the heart, but none in the brain? In other words, what is it about lower brain activity that makes it suffi-cient for personhood? It cannot be the fact that the lower brain con-trols and integrates various bodily functions such as respiration and digestion, since the same is true of the brains of lower animals that we do not regard as persons. Nor does the fact that an individual in a persistent vegetative state may breathe unassisted show that the person still exists, since lower animals that are not persons breathe without assistance.[11]

The best that can be said of the whole-brain concept of the death of a person is that it is superior to the traditional cardiopulmonary concept according to which a person is dead only if breathing and heartbeat have permanently ceased. The most obvious defect of the traditional cardiopulmonary concept is that it counts as a living per-son any human body in which the heart is pumping and the lungs are exchanging oxygen even if all that remains is a putrefying corpse on a respirator. Perhaps the most plausible argument in favor of the whole-brain concept as a superior replacement for the traditional cardiopulmonary concept relies on the premise that the person is dead when the necessary conditions for personal identity—the psy-chological characteristics that make this person the particular per-son he or she is—no longer remain. The second premise is that these conditions no longer exist when the whole brain is dead. The conclusion is that once these psychological characteristics no longer exist, continued breathing or beating of the heart is irrelevant.[12]

However, what this argument really shows is that heartbeat and respiration are not sufficient for the existence of a person, while the death of the whole brain is sufficient for the death of a person. The argument does not show that activity limited to the lower brain is sufficient for the existence of a person, nor that the death of the whole brain is necessary for the death of the person. Instead, what follows is that if *any* of the psychological characteristics that are necessary for personal identity depend for their existence on the functioning of the cerebral cortex, then the patient whose brain activity is limited to the lower brain is dead. As proponents of the whole-brain concept must acknowledge, the psychological characteristics that constitute personal identity include complex emotional and cognitive capacities, and these capacities depend in part on the higher brain centers, including the cerebral cortex. Consequently, a patient in a persistent vegetative state is dead—that person has ceased to be, even though a living (and perhaps breathing) organism persists. It seems, then, that the same reasoning that leads us to prefer the whole-brain concept to the traditional cardiopulmonary concept takes us beyond the whole-brain concept to the cognitivist concept.

However, in order to show that a patient in a persistent vegetative state has no right of self-determination, it is not necessary to show that such a being is not a person by defending the cognitivist concept of personhood. Instead, one can argue simply that even if those in a persistent vegetative state are living persons, they do not have a right of self-determination.

The right of self-determination—as distinct from the right to mere negative liberty or to freedom from interference—is a rather sophisticated right. It can be coherently ascribed only to individuals who not only are selves but also are selves capable of directing their own affairs, leading their own lives—agents who are conscious of their own agency and who can take an interest in determining what their interests are and shall be and how they are to be satisfied. Thus an individual might possess moral rights, such as the right not to be killed, that are so important that we would signal his or her membership in the moral community by calling him or her a person; and yet such an individual might lack the right of self-determination because he or she is not capable of self-determination. If so, then, regardless of which side we take in the dispute over personhood, it is a mistake to assume that the surrogate exercise of the right of self-determination by Substitute Judgment can be extended sensibly to all incompetents.

In arguing that a formerly competent person who is now in a persistent vegetative state no longer has a right of self-determination to be exercised by a surrogate, I am *not* saying that the patient's former status as a person is irrelevant to our current choices. For even if no exercise of a right of self-determination is now possible, it may still be possible to implement a choice that the patient previously made through exercising a right that he or she enjoyed when as a person and by virtue of his or her status as a person. In addition to the right of self-determination, the law and commonsense morality recognize the right of a competent individual to determine (within certain limits) what shall be done with his or her mortal remains. For example, one may issue instructions as to burial, or one may donate one's organs for transplantation. The same basic value that underlies the competent patient's right of self-determination—respect for individual autonomy—underlies this "right of disposal."

The right to dispose of one's mortal remains, however, is more akin to the right to bequeath one's property than to the right of self-determination.[13] Like the right to bequeath one's property, it is the right *of a self*, but not the right of a self to determine what shall be done *to that self*. Rather, the right of disposal is the right to determine what shall be done to *things* to which that self had special claims. It is reasonable to assume that the right of self-determination is in general a morally weightier right than the right of a self to determine what shall be done to its body after that self no longer exists. In part this is because determining what happens to one's self is usually a more important exercise of individual autonomy than determining what shall happen to things when the self no longer exists.

As we shall see later, this conclusion has important implications for one of the most urgent moral issues concerning decisions for incompetents: the problem of allocating scarce medical resources. Competing moral claims for the use of scarce resources may be sufficiently weighty to override the right of disposal even when they are not sufficient to override the right of self-determination. By neglecting to distinguish between the right of disposal and the right of self-determination and by failing to see that the right of self-determination cannot be sensibly ascribed to some incompetents, we only exacerbate moral dilemmas involving the rationing of scarce or costly medical resources.

THE SCOPE AND LIMITS OF THE BEST INTEREST PRINCIPLE

If for any of the reasons detailed above, the principle of Substituted Judgment cannot be employed, the presumption should be that the Best Interest Principle is to guide the surrogate's decision. There are, however, at least four serious problems that limit the usefulness of the Best Interest Principle as a Guidance Principle for decision making for incompetents.

The first problem concerns the concept of *interest* to be employed in the Best Interest Principle: is it to be understood in a purely objective way or in an at least partly subjective way? The distinction here is between a person's being interested in something, and something's being in a person's interest. An individual (whether competent or incompetent) may take an interest in something that is not in fact in his or her interest, or, he or she may fail to take an interest in something that is in his or her interest. Whether or not X is in A's interest depends on whether X in fact contributes (or at least can reasonably be expected to contribute) to A's good. But since A may be mistaken about what his or her own good is or about what will be conducive to it, what is in A's interest and what A takes an interest in may be distinct and even incompatible. According to the "objective" interpretation of Best Interest, the surrogate is to choose what is in fact in the patient's best interest, even if this diverges from that in which the patient takes an interest—even if it is contrary to the patient's expressed preferences.

Some writers, including many economists, have seemed to deny the distinction between maximizing the satisfaction of an individual's expressed preferences and achieving his or her good. This extreme subjectivist view would be defensible only if restricted to competent persons. After all, the entire enterprise of seeking principles to guide decision making for incompetents presupposes the commonsensical truth that the incompetent's own preferences are often not even a reliable guide to his or her good, much less definitive of it.

Nonetheless, there is a grain of truth in the extreme subjectivist view and it has troubling implications for the application of the Best Interest Principle to certain incompetents. The difficulty is this: if the good, and hence the interest, of a competent individual is at least *in part* subjectively determined, then the closer an incompetent lies to the threshold of competence, the harder it becomes to defend a purely objective application of the Best Interest Principle. In other words, as the incompetent more closely approximates competence, it becomes more difficult to justify a policy of disregarding his or her own expressed preferences and choosing according to an externally imposed conception of what is conducive to his or her good. The problem is especially acute in the case of adolescents or the mildly retarded or those who are intermittently incompetent because of senility.

The second difficulty in employing the Best Interest Principle is that of weighing current interests against future interests, including in some cases the interest in becoming a self-determining individual. For example, the surrogate may be faced with the awesome task of deciding how much pain and disruption of a child's family and social life may be imposed for the sake of extending his or her life or range of opportunities for future activities and enjoyments. Even if we could rationally assign relative weights to these competing goods, the problem seems all but intractable, at least in conditions of uncertainty regarding the probability of the various outcomes. This is so because there may be no consensus about what attitude toward risks one should adopt under such circumstances. This problem was raised in the highly publicized Chad Green case.[14] Although the court proceeded as though the only issue were that of determining the medically preferred treatment—Laetrile or orthodox chemotherapy—the child's mother raised this immensely difficult problem when she said it would be better for the child to have a short but relatively normal life than a longer one dominated by pain and isolation.

Two principles have sometimes been mistakenly regarded as alternatives to the Best Interest Principle, but these are best seen as ways of taking into account the conflict between present and future interests and the fact that interests change over time. Each has been proposed as a principle to guide paternalistic acts toward one important class of incompetents, namely children; but both are applicable to any incompetent, regardless of chronological age, who is expected to develop greater powers of judgment in the future, perhaps as a result of medical treatment. The first is the Future Consent Principle, the second the Primary Goods Principle.

The Future Consent Principle states that a decision for an incompetent who will later become competent is subject to the future approval of the incompetent once he or she becomes competent. Whether or not we regard Future Consent (or more accurately, Future Approval) as a necessary or sufficient condition for acceptable decisions, there are several serious objections to the proposal that this principle should play a major role in decision making for incompetents.

First, and most obviously, the principle is inapplicable in all cases in which the incompetent will not reach a state of maturity sufficient for approval. Second, there are certain cases, occurring with some frequency, in which it will be very difficult (if not impossible), to predict whether the individual, if he or she reaches maturity, will endorse the course others are now choosing for him or her. For example, whether or not an individual of normal intelligence who suffers from quadriplegia and permanent incontinence resulting from spina bifida (open spine syndrome) will later thank those who saved his or her life—or curse them—may not be predictable at the time the decision must be made. The third objection is that the idea that a prediction of future approval can justify present actions is most plausible in cases far removed from the typical instances of paternalism toward children (or others who may later become competent), and especially those decisions concerning medical treatment. If, for example, I physically prevent you from throwing a switch that unbeknownst to you will shut off the power for the entire building, I may justify my act by saying that I knew you would approve once I informed you of the error you were about to make. But in this sort of case, unlike many cases of decision making for incompetents, the future approval of the person interfered with is *independent* of the actions of the one who intervenes. We should be less eager to accept future approval as a justification for intervention in cases in which the future approval is caused or significantly influenced by the decision maker. The fact that I will come to thank the physician who performed psychosurgery on me or who subjected me to behavior control is not enough to justify the intervention if my gratitude is a product of his or her manipulation.[15]

The initial attraction of the Future Consent Principle may be its implicit assumption that there are certain goods that rational people in general find useful, regardless of what particular conception of the good they eventually come to espouse, and that our decisions concerning children and other incompetents who will become competent should be guided by an awareness of the special importance of such "primary goods."[16] But if there are such goods, then it seems plausible to drop the Future Consent Principle's requirement of the predictability of approval at some future time and instead justify our decisions by appealing to the idea that a rational person, because he or she would recognize the importance of primary goods, would accept our decisions.

A recent article on paternalism in the education of children employs this notion of hypothetical consent, advancing what I referred to earlier as the Primary Goods Principle.[17] The idea is that at least in our society basic education is a primary good—something that enhances one's opportunities for initially formulating, revising, and effectively pursuing a very broad range of conceptions of the good. To the extent that we subscribe to an ideal of the person as a self-determining being, a critical and autonomous chooser of goals, our treatment of children should be guided by the principle that every child should have at least some basic level of primary goods. Given the plausibility of this principle in education, it seems natural to extend it to the area of treatment decisions for children and other incompetents who are expected to become competent, since health is presumably one of the most important primary goods.

Although the notion of primary goods should play a role in treatment decisions for incompetents who are expected to become competent, there are at least two reasons to think that the Primary Goods Principle will be of more limited application in medical than in educational contexts. The first is that in many of the more dramatic and troubling cases of treatment decisions, in which there is little or no prospect that the incompetent will ever attain anything like normal functioning or will even survive, the appeal to primary goods will be irrelevant because the notion of autonomous agency or of freedom to choose a conception of the good is not applicable. Second, the Primary Goods Principle itself, because of its exclusive emphasis on the opportunity for future choices, appears to be incapable of giving sufficient weight to the *present suffering* of the incompetent. What is needed is some way of taking into account both a concern for the incompetent's future opportunities for autonomous choice and his or her current interest in avoiding suffering. This problem is likely to be much less pronounced in the application of the primary goods principle to education simply because the burdens educational interventions impose on the child typically are not severe. A plausible response to this second problem is to view the Primary Goods Principle not as a rival to the Best Interest Principle but rather as a reminder to give special weight to one exceptionally important future-oriented interest: the interest in being a critical and autonomous chooser of ends.

The third major difficulty besetting the Best Interest Principle is the issue of what we are to include among the patient's interests. There are two distinct issues here. First, should the interests to be maximized be limited to the patient's exclusively *self-regarding* interests or should they also include the patient's *other-regarding* interests—the interest the patient takes in the well-being of others? Second, in determining what is in the patient's best interest, how much weight should be given to the fact that what is in his or her best interest may be determined by the interest that others take in the treatment decision and the attitudes of others toward the patient?

Consider the first issue. An individual, even an incompetent individual, may care deeply about those with whom he or she is closely associated. For example, a retarded child may be deeply attached to his nonretarded sibling, who will die unless he receives a kidney from his retarded sibling. Since the mere fact of incompetence does not preclude the possibility that the individual takes a significant interest in the interests of others, it seems that in deciding what is in the incompetent patient's Best Interest we must consider not only his or her self-regarding but also his or her other-regarding interests. If one takes into account the interest the retarded individual takes in the well-being of his sibling, one might well conclude that the expected utility (for the incompetent) of saving the sibling's life outweighs the expected disutility (for the incompetent) of the operation.

The danger of taking into account the incompetent's other-regarding interests, however, is obvious. Interested parties may wrongly impute to the incompetent individual other-regarding interests that are at odds with his or her most basic self-regarding interests, including the interest in avoiding death and injury, or they may overestimate the strength of the incompetent's other-regarding interests. In order to minimize this danger, two safeguards might be considered. A higher standard of evidence could be required for evidence in support of the claim that the patient does take an interest in the well-being of others. And even when there is strong evidence that the incompetent patient takes an interest in the well-being of others who will be affected by the treatment decision, this evidence could be excluded from the determination of the patient's Best Interest if its inclusion would pose a serious threat to the incompetent's most basic self-regarding interests.

The second problem arises because the good of an individual, whether competent or incompetent, often is crucially dependent on the interests and preferences of others with whom he or she is closely associated, even if the person does not take an interest in their well-being. Given that this is so, there will be cases in which a particular decision would be in the incompetent's best interest but only because of the interest others take in that decision. For example, removing a kidney from child A to give to sibling B may be in A's best interest but only because of the fact that if the transplant were not undertaken, A's parents would behave toward A in psychologically damaging ways. Similarly, it might be said that psychosurgery or a massive dose of tranquilizer that reduces a patient to docility at the expense of personality is in the patient's best interest because they eliminate behavior that would lead to serious abuse or neglect by caretakers or retaliation by fellow patients. Finally, some would justify withholding life-sustaining treatment from a retarded newborn on the grounds that it would not be in his best interest either to live with parents who do not want him or in a state institution that is little more than a human warehouse.

The last two examples make vivid the enormous potential for abuse inherent in constructing the Best Interest Principle so as to include in the patient's interests the effects of the preferences and interests of others. It would be a tragic irony if adherence to a principle designed to protect the individual incompetent served only to perpetuate attitudes and social practices that systematically disadvantage incompetents as a class.

Finally, a fourth difficulty arises in the application of the Best Interest Principle to the incompetent who is in a persistent vegetative state—an individual who is expected never to regain even the most rudimentary consciousness. What result does the Best Interest Principle yield when applied to the question of whether to continue life support? Granted that the patient is in a persistent vegetative state and therefore will experience no pain from life-support procedures, it cannot be said that because the pain of treatment would outweigh any benefit to the patient, treatment would not be in his best interest. Instead, the Best Interest Principle would seem to require *perpetual* life support for *everyone* in a persistent vegetative state— unless one is willing to make the dubious claim that it is one's best interest to die, even though life can be preserved without suffering.

This unsettling result arises because of the unexamined assumption that the notion of interests relevant to the Best Interest Principle applies to the individual in a persistent vegetative state. If these individuals can be said to have interests at all, this is only because we are using the word 'interest' in a very attenuated sense. We may perhaps be operating with such an attenuated sense of the word when we speak of what is good or bad for rudimentary forms of animal life or plants. But if this is the only notion of interest that applies to an individual in a persistent vegetative state, then it is hard to see how discontinuing life support could ever be in that individual's best interest any more than refraining, from watering a plant could be said to be good for it. It seems, then, that application of the Best Interest Principle to this class of incompetents yields the very counterintuitive result that treatment should *never* be discontinued.

It might be suggested that as long as the probability is greater than zero that the prognosis is erroneous, there is a perfectly robust, unattenuated sense of interest that is applicable—namely, the interest in returning to a cognitive state in which one can lead a life, pursue goals, or at least reap satisfactions. If there is a chance of recovery, be it ever so slim, the Best Interest Principle appears to yield the same counterintuitive result as it does on the assumption that there is no chance of recovery at all. Given the tremendous value of the favorable outcome for the individual, acting in his or her Best Interest seems to require sustaining the patient indefinitely, as long as there is any hope at all. Such an application of the Best Interest Principle would exacerbate the already grievous dilemmas of allocating scarce medical resources, especially since advances in medical technology are making it possible to sustain larger numbers of individuals in a persistent vegetative state for longer periods of time.

There are two quite different ways to avoid this troubling result. We might simply acknowledge that, granted the scarcity of medical resources, concern for the best interests of the incompetent must sometimes give way to considerations of distributive justice. The trick, then, would be to devise a way of limiting the appeal to the incompetent's best interest without lapsing into a crude utilitarianism that subordinates the individual's good to the good of society without taking individual rights or interests seriously.

Or we might consider a more radical proposal. Instead of concluding that individuals who are in a persistent vegetative state are persons but do not have the same rights and interests as other persons, we might abandon our assumption that they are living persons. If we adopted a cognitivist conception of the death of a person, we would have a principled basis for excluding such individuals from the scope of the Best Interest principle as a Guidance Principle for decisions regarding incompetent persons, and the counterintuitive results encountered earlier would be avoided. Nevertheless, even if this approach were adopted, there would still be moral constraints on how we may treat such beings even if they are no longer living persons—just as there are moral constraints on our treatment of nonhuman animals.

The Constraints of Distributive Justice

The courts and most writers in the field have tended to exclude any explicit role for principles of distributive justice in decision making for incompetents, especially in life-or-death treatment decisions. This reluctance to face up to the fact that the rights and interests of others impose limits on the moral authority of the Best Interest and Substituted Judgment Principles is understandable and, up to a point, praiseworthy. The attraction of both principles is that they represent a serious effort to ensure that the rights and interests of an especially vulnerable class of individuals are not disregarded. In this respect, Best Interest and Substituted Judgment are superior to two other principles for guiding treatment decisions for incompetents that have been widely discussed and advocated: the Extraordinary Measures Principle and the Quality of Life Principle. Both of the latter principles contain profound ambiguities that encourage the surrogate to disregard the rights and interests of the patient or at least to blur the distinction between principles that respect the rights and interests of the patient and principles of distributive justice that limit their authority.

The Extraordinary Measures Principle states that a surrogate may decide to forgo extraordinary measures, defined variously as treatment that "would involve grave burdens" or that would serve no "meaningful purpose." The first formulation is ambiguous as long as it remains unclear *whose* burdens are to be considered.[18] If the burdens are restricted to those of the patient, then the Extraordinary Measures Principle collapses into the Best Interest Principle, assuming, as seems reasonable, that not just burdens but also benefits to the patient are to be considered and that treatment is to be foregone only if the burdens to the patient equal or exceed the benefits to the patient. If, however, "burdens" includes not only those of the patient but of others who will be affected by the decision as well, then the Extraordinary Measures Principle directs us to choose according to what will maximize social utility and gives no special weight, and hence no special protection, to the interests of the vulnerable incompetent patient. I will not rehearse here the well-known objections to the utilitarian principle as a principle for making treatment decisions in the case of competent individuals. Instead, I will note only that direct appeals to what will maximize social utility seem even less acceptable in the case of those who cannot defend or even articulate their own interests.

In the second definition of extraordinary measures, the ambiguity of the phrase "meaningful purpose" renders the principle just as dangerous. It could mean meaningful purpose so far as the patient's rights or interests are concerned or so far as the family or society at large is concerned. Those who invoke this second definition might reply that measures serve no meaningful purpose when they do not make possible a sufficient quality of life, but this collapses the Extraordinary Measures Principle into the Quality of Life Principle and merely shifts to another equally dangerous ambiguity.

The principle that we have no duty to sustain the life of an incompetent if his or her quality of life is sufficiently poor fails to provide genuine guidance as long as the notion of a "sufficient" level or degree of quality is left unspecified. This principle is also ambiguous because the phrase "quality of life" can be understood in at least three distinct ways. The first may be called the *intrapersonal comparison sense*. To make a judgment concerning quality of life in this first sense is to rank the value of this individual's life relative to the value of others, perhaps in terms of some notion of social contribution or productivity, for the purpose of calculating the costs and benefits of expending resources upon the person. In this interpretation, the Quality of Life Principle collapses into crude utilitarian calculation and is no more acceptable than the utilitarian interpretation of the Extraordinary Measures Principle.

The second sense of quality of life may be called the *intrapersonal (or noncomparative) sense*. To make a quality-of-life judgment of the intrapersonal sort is to estimate the value of the patient's life to or for that individual, regardless of how society or would-be calculations of social utility rank the value of that individual's life relative to some interpersonal standard. With this interpretation, the Quality of Life Principle is equivalent to the Best Interest Principle, depending on where the threshold of "sufficient quality" is set. There are only two alternatives. Either the threshold of quality is set at the "net benefit point," so that a life of sufficient quality is simply one in which benefits to the patient exceed costs to the patient, no matter by how small a margin; or the threshold is set higher, so that a life is of sufficient quality only if benefits exceed costs by some specified positive magnitude. If we are limited to a consideration of the value of the patient's life to or for the patient him- or herself, it seems difficult if not impossible to justify setting the threshold of sufficient quality higher than the net benefit point. But if so, then the Quality of Life Principle, on its only plausible interpretation, is equivalent to the Best Interest Principle and should not be considered as a rival to it.

There is, however, a third, quite different sense in which the idea of quality of life may be used in bioethical contexts, which may be called the "moral status" sense. When one asks whether a life is of sufficient quality in this third sense, one is asking whether the individual satisfies some threshold condition, in which attainment of the threshold constitutes one's membership in the primary moral community—the class of full-fledged persons. This third conception of quality of life is noncomparative in the following sense: if an individual satisfies the threshold condition for personhood, then he or she possesses at least a minimum of certain characteristics (such as a capacity for self-awareness); but the fact that others may possess those same characteristics to a greater degree or in a more developed form is irrelevant to the basic moral status the person possesses. Similarly, even if in order to be licensed to drive an automobile one must possess a minimum of certain skills, the fact that others may possess those same skills to a degree that exceeds that minimum is irrelevant to whether one satisfies the threshold of skills for being a licensed driver.[19] To ask whether an incompetent's life is of sufficient quality in the moral status sense is to ask a quite different and more basic question from the one asked when we apply the Best Interest Principle or the Substituted Judgment Principle.

I would now like to suggest that, in spite of their dangerous ambiguities, the Extraordinary Measures and Quality of Life principles express, albeit in a confused way, important moral limitations on the authority of the Best Interest and Substituted Judgment Principles. Both interpretations of Extraordinary Measures, which asks us to decide according to a calculation of the burdens a treatment would impose on all who would be affected by it, and the Quality of Life Principle, with its interpersonal comparison interpretation, show a recognition of the fact that the rights and interests of the incompetent are not absolute but must be limited by consideration of the rights and interests of others. Unfortunately, however, neither principle adequately protects the rights and interests of the incompetent. The Best Interest and Substituted Judgment principles exhibit precisely the opposite virtues and the opposite defects. Each of these principles, by focusing squarely on the patient, protects the incompetent from utilitarian calculations that threaten to sacrifice his or her rights and interests for the sake of others. But if either of these principles is regarded as having unlimited authority, it achieves this scrupulous protection of the patient by a ruthless feat of tunnel vision: we are to make treatment decisions for incompetents as though issues of distributive justice did not exist. What is needed, then, is a theory of decision making for incompetents that includes principles allowing us to sort out and give proper weight to the rights and interests of the incompetent, but also to limit the authority of these patient-centered principles with appropriate principles of distributive justice.

Although I will not attempt here to discharge this onerous task, I will conclude by sketching what I believe to be an important part of the appropriate structure for such a theory. My proposal is that the first step in integrating Guidance Principles for decision making regarding incompetents with the requirements of distributive justice is to recognize that some of what at first appear to be the most basic conflicts between the rights and interests of the incompetent and the rights and interests of others become much less difficult if we recognize that some who are now lumped together under the broad class of incompetents either are no longer living persons or no longer have a right of self-determination or no longer have interests in the sense of 'interest' relevant to the Best Interest Principle. If an individual in a persistent vegetative state is no longer a living person or if such an individual's interests are so attenuated that acting in his best interest is no longer morally required, then the decision to terminate support for such an individual in order to make medical resources available to others who are living persons or who have interests in a less attenuated and problematic sense does not raise the most fundamental and recalcitrant problems of distributive justice. Further, if we distinguish carefully between the right of self-determination and the right of disposal and recognize that the first is a much more basic right than the second, we can easily accommodate a significant limitation on the scope of the Principle of Substituted Judgment without having to defend the claim that the most basic rights of the individual must be subordinated to the good of others. In other words, by failing to make distinctions of moral status within the class of incompetents, by failing to clarify the relevant notion of interests in applying the Best Interest Principle, and by construing the right of self-determination so broadly that no distinction is made between the right to determine what is done to oneself and the right to determine what shall be done with one's mortal remains, we are driven to view every allocation decision as one involving a conflict of basic rights.

Nonetheless, even when the distinctions I have proposed are duly acknowledged, some decisions for incompetents do raise the most fundamental issues of distributive justice. However, it would be a mistake to assume that the issues here are in essence different from those that arise with respect to competent patients. Even when Substituted Judgment is properly applied as the instrument for the surrogate exercise of a living person's right of self-determination, and even when Best Interest is properly applied, to individuals who have interests in a nonattenuated sense, neither principle carries absolute moral authority. But this is equally true of the right of self-determination of a competent patient when the patient exercises that right. The right of self-determination of a competent patient is only the right to accept or refuse proffered medical treatment. It is not a positive or "welfare" right to be provided with health care.

Although there is considerable dispute regarding whether there is a positive moral right to health care, there is a broad consensus that if such a right exists it is a limited one, not a right to all health care that would be of any benefit (regardless of the cost to society). Such a limitation is required by a recognition of the fact that resources are scarce and that there are other goods besides health. If the right to health care, as a basic moral right, applies to individuals simply by virtue of their fundamental moral status as persons, then it applies equally to incompetent as well as competent persons. And if this is so, then the problem of reconciling the rights and interests of the individual person with the need to establish a right to health care for all persons is not a special problem for the theory of decision making for incompetents.

Notes

Acknowledgments: I would like to thank Deborah Buchanan for her detailed and perceptive criticisms and James Hallmark for several helpful comments on earlier drafts of this essay. I have also benefited from comments by Daniel Wikler on an earlier paper on this topic that I presented at the Conference on Government Paternalism, Lutsen, Minnesota, 1979, sponsored by the Liberty Fund.

1. In this chapter, I will focus on nonpsychiatric treatment decisions—psychiatric treatment decisions and decisions concerning experimentation will not be dealt with.
2. It is important to note that decision-making incompetence should be understood as incapacity to make a particular decision or set of decisions. An individual may be competent to make some decisions but incompetent to make others, depending in part on the complexity of the options. In particular, a child or a retarded or senile individual may be competent to make

some decisions but not others. For a detailed discussion of this selective notion of competence and a treatment of some of the problems of determining competence, see *Deciding to Forego Life-Sustaining Treatment*, Report of the President's Commission for the Study of Ethical Problems in Medicine and Biomedical and Behavioral Research (Washington, D.C.: U.S. Government Printing Office, 1983), especially chapter 4.

3. The primary purpose of this chapter is to develop sound *moral* principles for decision making for incompetents. Nonetheless, it will be fruitful to draw on legal principles, such as those of Substituted Judgment and Best Interest, since the law can be viewed as one very important attempt to provide reasonable answers to a variety of practical problems, many of which have a moral dimension.

4. For a discussion of some aspects of questions 3 and 4, see my "Medical Paternalism or Legal Imperialism: Not the Only Alternative for Handling Saikewicz-Type Cases," *American Journal of Law and Medicine* 5 (1979): 100–105.

5. The right of self-determination of a competent patient is not absolute: it is limited by the need to prevent harm to others, as in the case of the prevention of treatment of communicable disease.

6. In re Quinlan, 70 N.J. 10, 355 A. 2d 647, cert denied sub nom. Garger v. New Jersey, 429 U.S. 922 (1976); Superintendent of Belchertown State School v. Saikewicz, 373 Mass. 728, 370 N.E. 2d 417 (1977); In re Spring 1979 Mass. Adv. Sh. 1209, 405 N.E. 2d 115; and In re Eichner, 73 A.D. 2d 431, 426 N.Y.S. 2d 517 (1980), modified sub nom. Eichner v. Dillon, 52 N.Y. 2d 363, 420 N.E. 2d 64, 438 N.Y.S. 2d 266 (1981).

7. See my "The Limits of Proxy Decision-Making for Incompetent Patients," *UCLA Law Review* 29(1981): 391–396.

8. Unfortunately, medical professionals sometimes go further and act paternalistically toward competent patients by interfering with their decision making or by failing to inform them that there are decisions to be made. For examinations of attempted justification of medical paternalism, see my "Medical Paternalism"; Bernard Gert and Charles M. Culver, "Paternalistic Behavior," and Donald VanDeVeer, "The Contractual Argument for Withholding Medical Information" (all in *Medicine and Moral Philosophy, A Philosophy & Public Affairs Reader*, ed. Marshall Cohen, Thomas Nagel, and Thomas Scanlon [Princeton, N.J.: Princeton University Press, 1982]). For a book-length treatment, see James F. Childress, *Who Should Decide? Paternalism in Health Care* (New York: Oxford University Press, 1982).

9. Freedman, Benjamin, "On the Rights of the Voiceless," *The Journal of Medicine and Philosophy* 3 (Sept. 1978): 196–210.

10. Robert Veatch advances a "reasonableness" standard in "The Limits of Guardian Treatment Refusal: The Standard of Reasonableness" (unpublished manuscript). A major difference between Veatch's view and my own is that for Veatch the extent of the moral authority of Substituted Judgment is determined by the nature of the relationship between the surrogate and the patient: "bonded" (closely associated) surrogates are said to have greater

238 · ALLEN BUCHANAN

discretion than "nonbonded" (stranger) surrogates. In my opinion, this way of conceptualizing the issue is artificial, if not misleading, since the primary question in determining the moral authority of Substituted Judgment is not who employs it but rather how much reliable information is available about the patient's preferences when he or she was competent.

11. This criticism is applicable to the concept of death developed in *Defining Death: Medical, Legal and Ethical Issues in the Determination of Death*, Report of the President's Commission for the Study of Ethical Problems in Medicine and Biomedical and Behavioral Research (Washington, D.C.: U.S. Government Printing Office, 1981), 31–40.

12. Michael B. Green and Daniel Wikler, "Brain Death and Personal Identity," in *Medicine and Moral Philosophy, A Philosophy and Public Affairs Reader*, 49–77.

13. This is *not* to say that the relationship of a living person to his body, *while he lives*, is the same as his relationship to his clothing or furniture.

14. Custody of a minor, 375 Mass. 733, 379 N.E. 2d 1053 (1978).

15. For similar criticisms of the Future Consent Principle, see James F. Childress, *Who Should Decide? Paternalism in Health Care*, 92–97.

16. John Rawls introduces the concept of primary goods in chapter II of *A Theory of Justice* (Cambridge, Mass.: Harvard University Press, 1971).

17. Amy Gutmann, "Children, Paternalism, and Education," *Philosophy & Public Affairs* 9 (1980): 338–358.

18. For these and additional criticisms of the Extraordinary/Ordinary distinction and the Quality of Life Principle, see my "Medical Paternalism" (revised version), in *Paternalism*, ed. Rolf E. Sartorius (Minneapolis: University of Minnesota Press, 1983), 61–82.

19. Daniel Wikler, "Paternalism and the Mildly Retarded," in *Paternalism*, 83–99.

CHAPTER VI

Ill-Gotten Gains

Tom Regan

The Story

Late in 1981 a reporter for a large metropolitan newspaper (we'll call her Karen to protect her interest in remaining anonymous) gained access to some previously classified government files. Using the Freedom of Information Act, Karen was investigating the federal government's funding of research into the short- and long-term effects of exposure to radioactive waste. It was with understandable surprise that, included in these files, she discovered the records of a series of experiments involving the induction and treatment of coronary thrombosis (heart attack). Conducted over a period of fifteen years by a renowned heart specialist (we'll call him Dr. Ventricle) and financed with federal funds, the experiments in all likelihood would have remained unknown to anyone outside Dr. Ventricle's sphere of power and influence had not Karen chanced upon them.

Karen's surprise soon gave way to shock and disbelief. In case after case she read of how Ventricle and his associates took otherwise healthy individuals, with no previous record of heart disease, and intentionally caused their heart to fail. The methods used to occasion the "attack" were a veritable shopping list of experimental techniques, from massive doses of stimulants (adrenaline was a favorite) to electrical damage of the coronary artery, which, in its weakened state, yielded the desired thrombosis. Members of Ventricle's team then set to work testing the efficacy of various drugs developed in the hope that they would help the heart withstand a second "attack." Dosages varied, and there were the usual control groups. In some cases, certain drugs administered to "patients" proved more efficacious than cases in which others received no medication or

239

smaller amounts of the same drugs. The research came to an abrupt end in the fall of 1981, but not because the project was judged unpromising or because someone raised a hue and cry about the ethics involved. Like so much else in the world at that time, Ventricle's project was a casualty of austere economic times. There simply wasn't enough federal money available to renew the grant application.

One would have to forsake all the instincts of a reporter to let the story end there. Karen persevered and, under false pretenses, secured an interview with Ventricle. When she revealed that she had gained access to the file, knew in detail the largely fruitless research conducted over fifteen years, and was incensed about his work, Ventricle was dumbfounded. But not because Karen had unearthed the file. And not even because it was filed where it was (a "clerical error," he assured her). What surprised Ventricle was that anyone would think there was a serious ethical question to be raised about what he had done. Karen's notes of their conversation include the following:

Ventricle: But I don't understand what you're getting at. Surely you know that heart disease is the leading cause of death. How can there by any ethical question about developing drugs which *literally* promise to be life-saving?

Karen: Some people might agree that the goal—to save life—is a good, a noble end, and still question the means used to achieve it. Your "patients," after all, had no previous history of heart disease. *They* were healthy before you got your hands on them.

Ventricle: But medical progress simply isn't possible if we wait for people to get sick and then see what works. There are too many variables, too much beyond our control and comprehension, if we try to do our medical research in a clinical setting. The history of medicine shows how hopeless that approach is.

Karen: And I read, too, that upon completion of the experiment, assuming that the "patient" didn't die in the process—it says that those who survived were "sacrificed." You mean killed?

Ventricle: Yes, that's right. But always painlessly, always painlessly. And the body went immediately to the lab, where further tests were done. Nothing was wasted.

Karen: And it didn't bother you—I mean, you didn't ever ask yourself whether what you were doing was wrong? I mean. . .

Ventricle (interrupting): My dear young lady, you make it seem as if I'm some kind of moral monster. I work for the benefit of humanity, and I have achieved some small success, I hope you will agree. Those who raise cries of wrongdoing about what I've done are well intentioned but misguided. After all, I use animals in my research —chimpanzees, to be more precise—not human beings.

The Point

The story about Karen and Dr. Ventricle is just that—a story, a small piece of fiction. There is no real Dr. Ventricle, no real Karen, and so on. But there *is* widespread use of animals in scientific research, including research like our imaginary Dr. Ventricle's. So the story, while its details are imaginary—while it is, let it be clear, a literary device, not a factual account—is a story with a point. Most people reading it would be morally outraged if there actually were a Dr. Ventricle who did coronary research of the sort described on otherwise healthy human beings. Considerably fewer would raise a morally quizzical eyebrow when informed of such research done on animals, chimpanzees, or whatever. The story has a point, or so I hope, because, catching us off-guard, it brings this difference home to us, gives it life in our experience, and, in doing so, reveals something about ourselves, something about our own constellation of values. If we think what Ventricle did would be wrong if done to human beings but all right if done to chimpanzees, then we must believe that there are different moral standards that apply to how we may treat the two—human beings and chimpanzees. But to acknowledge this difference, if acknowledge it we do, is only the beginning, not the end, of our moral thinking. We can meet the challenge to think well from the moral point of view only if we are able to cite a *morally relevant difference* between humans and chimpanzees, one that illuminates in a clear, coherent, and rationally defensible way why it would be wrong to use humans, but not chimpanzees, in research like Dr. Ventricle's.

The Larger Context

That we cannot rationally avoid this challenge is an idea that has only recently taken root in some quarters. Cora Diamond, a philosopher at the University of Virginia, notes that a recent bibliography on society, ethics, and the life sciences was described by its publishers as "containing the most pertinent references on precisely such subjects as experimentation, containing nine pages on ethical and legal problems of experimentation, including, besides general material, sections specifically on experimentation on fetuses, prisoners, mental patients, and children"; the work includes *no* references to "the ethical problems of animal experimentation."[1] The explanation of this omission cannot be that there was, at that time, no (or not enough) literature on the topic, as even a cursory glance at Charles R. Magel's *A Bibliography on Animal Rights and Related Matters* will reveal.[2] By far the likelier explanation, as Diamond observes, is that "for many working in the field, the phrases 'ethical problems posed by research' and 'ethical problems posed by research *on human subjects*' are treated as simply interchangeable."[3] To treat them so is not to meet the challenge to give a clear, coherent, and rationally defensible basis for allowing research on animals that we would not allow on humans. It is, instead, symptomatic of the moral prejudices of those who persist in assuming that there is no ethical challenge to be met.

Because this book is concerned with issues in health care ethics, this chapter examines only the ethics of the use of animals in medical research. It is well to remind ourselves, however, of the magnitude and variety of animal use in scientific settings generally. Estimates of the total number of animals used for scientific purposes vary, some placing the total between twenty and forty million, others as high as 100 million, just for the United States, just for a single year. Worldwide, the totals frequently given are more than twice these. Of these totals, perhaps about a fourth are used in medical research, given any uncontorted meaning of the expression "medical research" and allowing, as before, that estimates vary and are difficult to verify with anything approaching certainty. The remaining animals are used for instructional purposes (for example, in lab sections in standard biology classes in high schools and universities), in toxicity testing (in which "animal models" are used to estimate the risks and levels of harm humans are likely to run by using, or by being exposed to, the ever-increasing array of therapeutic and nontherapeutic products, from oven cleaners to eyeshadow, from asbestos to interferon), and in other scientific contexts.

We would serve our purposes ill, moreover, if we failed to remind ourselves of the variety of research that falls within the category of medical research as well as the multiplicity of means used to conduct it. Burn experiments (immersion of a part or the whole of an animal's body in boiling water, use of hot plates and blow torches, and, with research on internal burns, such as burns to the esophagus, lye, are among the methods employed); radiation research (dogs and primates are common "animal models" who are studied after exposure to both small and large levels of radioactivity, an ongoing type of medical research conducted in connection with weapons development by the military); drumming (animals are placed in a revolving drum whose internal protuberances break bones and bruise the flesh as a preliminary to the study of traumatic shock); brain research (cats and primates are favorite test animals, with drugs, electrodes, and surgical alterations, for example, used to influence and manipulative behavior)—these are a sample of the types of research and methods current in medical research. When the scope and intent of the research are more psychological than physical, the methods employed vary accordingly. Punishment experiments (these commonly involve electrical shock administered to the feet, tail, tooth pulp, or brain of, for example, cats, dogs, rabbits, primates, rats, or mice); immobilization research (for example, dogs are suspended in so-called Pavlovian slings or chimpanzees are strapped in restraining chairs); blinding and other investigations of sensory deprivation (for example, on cats in the course of studying sexual behaviors); aggression research (here test animals are induced by researchers to fight among themselves); stress experiments (any and all of the above methods, or loud noises, or random blasts of air can be used to produce stress, the effects of which may then be studied scientifically)—these (and there are many more) alternative approaches are illustrative of psychological research and methods involving animals.

No doubt some will deny the propriety of including some of the foregoing in the general category of medical research. These sorts of disagreements are to be expected. However they are resolved, the differences in the methods used in medical research, as well as the differences in the specific form such research takes, should not obscure their similarities. All such research, we may assume, has as its goals the advancement of human knowledge and the improvement of public health. These are laudatory ends. Our interest in what follows lies in morally assessing some of the means used to achieve them. Our own "moral research" will use Dr. Ventricle's work on chimpanzees as its "model."

The Law

Among the difference between chimps and humans, one concerns their legal standing. It is against the law to do to human beings what Ventricle did to his chimpanzees. It is not against the law to do this to chimps. So, here we have a difference. But a morally relevant one?

The difference in the legal status of chimps and humans would be morally relevant if we had good reason to believe that what is legal and what is moral go hand in glove: where we have the former, there we have the latter (and maybe vice versa too). But a moment's reflection shows how bad the fit between legality and morality sometimes is. A century and a half ago, the legal status of black people in the United States was similar to the legal status of a house, corn, a barn: they were property, other people's property, and could legally be bought and sold without regard to their personal interests. But the legality of the slave trade did not make it moral, any more than the law against drinking, during the era of that "great experiment" of Prohibition, made it immoral to drink. Sometimes, it is true, what the law declares illegal (for example, murder and rape) is immoral, and vice versa. But there is no necessary connection, no pre-established harmony between morality and the law. So, yes, the legal status of chimps and humans differs; but that does not show that their moral status does. Their difference in legal status, in other words, is not a morally relevant difference and will not morally justify using these animals, but not humans, in Ventricle's research.

The "Right" Species

An obvious difference, one that is biological, not legal, is that chimps and humans belong to different species. Once more, a difference certainly; but a morally relevant one? Suppose, for the sake of argument, that a difference in species membership *is* a morally relevant difference. If it is, and if A and B belong to two different species, then it is quite possible that killing or otherwise harming A is wrong, while doing the same things to B are not.

Let us test this idea by imagining that Steven Spielberg's E.T. and some of E.T.'s friends show up on Earth. Whatever else we may want to say of them, we do not want to say that they are members of our species, the species *Homo sapiens*. Now, if a difference in species is a morally relevant difference, we should be willing to say that it is *not* wrong to kill or otherwise harm E.T. and the other members of his biological species in sport hunting, for example, even though it *is* wrong to do this to members of our species for this reason. But no double standards are allowed. If *their* belonging to a different species makes it all right to kill or harm them, then *our* belonging to a different species than the one to which they belong will cancel the wrongness of their killing or harming us. "Sorry, chum," E.T.'s compatriots say, before taking aim at us or prior to inducing *our* heart attacks, "but you just don't belong to the right species." As for us, we cannot lodge a whine of a moral objection if species membership, besides being a biological difference, is a morally relevant one. Before we give our assent to this idea, therefore, we ought to consider whether, were we to come face to face with another powerful species of extraterrestrials, we would think it reasonable to try to move them by the force of moral argument and persuasion. If we do, we will reject the view that species differences, like other biological differences (e.g., race or sex), constitute a morally relevant difference of the kind we seek. But we will also need to remind ourselves that no double standards are allowed: though chimps and humans do differ in terms of the species to which each belongs, that difference by itself is not a morally relevant one. Ventricle could not, that is, defend his use of chimps rather than humans in his research on the grounds that chimps belong to a different species from our own.

The Soul

Many people evidently believe that theological differences separate humans from other animals. God, they say, has given us immortal souls. Our earthly life is not our only life. Beyond the grave there is eternal life—for some, heaven, for others, hell. Animals, alas, have no soul, in this view, and therefore have no life after death either. That, it might be claimed, is the morally relevant difference between them and us, and that is why, so it might be inferred, it would be wrong to use humans in Ventricle's research but not wrong to use chimps.

Only three points will be urged against this position here. First, the theology just sketched (*very* crudely) is not the only one competing for our informed assent, and some of the others (most notably, religions from the East and those of many Native American peoples) do ascribe soul and an afterlife to animals. So before one could reasonably use this alleged theological difference between humans and animals as a morally relevant difference, one would have to defend one's theological views against theological competitors. To explore these matters is well beyond the limited reach of this chapter. It is enough for our purposes to be mindful that there is much to explore.

Second, even assuming that humans have souls, while animals lack them, there is no obvious logical connection between these "facts" and the judgment that it would be wrong to do some things to humans that it would not be wrong to do to chimps. Having (or not having) a soul obviously makes a difference concerning the chances that one's soul will live on. If chimps lack souls, their chances are nil. But why does that make it quite all right to use them *in this life* in Ventricle's research? And why does our having a soul, assuming we do, make it wrong *in this life* to use us? Many more questions are avoided than addressed by those who rely on a supposed "theological difference" between humans and animals as their basis for judging how each may be treated.

But third, and finally, to make a particular theology the yardstick of what is permissible and, indeed, supported by public funds in a pluralistic society such as we find in twentieth-century America is itself morally objectionable, offending, minimally, the sound moral, not to mention legal, principle that church and state be kept separate. Even if it had been shown to be true, which it has not, that humans have souls and animals do not, that should not be used as a weapon for making public policy. We will not, in short, find the morally relevant difference we seek if we look for it within the labyrinth of alternative theologies.

The Right to Consent

"Human beings can give or withhold their informed consent; animals cannot. That's the morally relevant difference." This argument is certainly mistaken on one count, and possibly mistaken on another. Concerning the latter point first, evidence steadily increases regarding the intellectual abilities of chimps and other primates (e.g., gorillas). Much of the public's attention has been focused on reports of studies involving the alleged linguistic abilities of these animals, when instructed in such languages as American Sign Language for the deaf (ASL). Washoe. Lana. Nim Chimpski. Individual chimps have attained international notoriety. But how much these animals do and can understand is very much up in the air at this point. Whether primates have sufficient ability to understand and use language and, if they do, whether they have sufficient ability to give or withhold their informed consent—these matters cannot be settled arbitrarily at this point in time. Possibly these animals lack these abilities. But possibly they do not. Those who trot out a doctrinaire position in this regard prove how little, not how much, they know.

Questions about the ability of chimps to give informed consent aside, it should be obvious that this ability is not the morally relevant difference we are seeking. Suppose that, in addition to using chimps, Ventricle also used some humans, but only mentally incompetent ones—those who, though they have discernable preferences, are too young or too old, too enfeebled or too confused, to give or withhold their informed consent. If the ability to give or withhold informed consent were the morally relevant difference we seek, we should be willing to say that it was not wrong for Ventricle to do his coronary research on these humans, though it would be wrong for him to do it on competent humans—those humans, in other words, who can give or withhold their informed consent.

But though one's willingness to consent to have someone do something to oneself may be, and frequently is, a good reason to absolve the other person of moral responsibility, one's inability to give or withhold informed consent is on a totally different moral footing. When Walter Reed's colleagues gave their informed consent to take part in the yellow fever experiments, those who exposed them to the potentially fatal bite of the fever parasite carried by mosquitoes were absolved of any moral responsibility for the risks the volunteers chose to run, and those who chose to run these risks, let us agree, acted above and beyond the normal call of duty—acted, as philosophers say, supererogatorily. Because they did more than duty strictly requires, in the hope and with the intention of benefiting others, these pioneers deserve our esteem and applause.

The case of human incompetents is radically different. Since these humans (e.g., young children and the mentally retarded) lack the requisite mental abilities to have duties in the first place, it is absurd to think of them as capable of acting supererogatorily; they cannot act "beyond the call" of duty, when, as is true in their case, they cannot understand that "call" to begin with. But though they cannot volunteer, in the way mentally competent humans can, they can be forced or coerced to do something against their will or contrary to their known preferences. Sometimes, no doubt, coercive intervention in their life is above moral reproach—indeed, is morally required, as when, for example, we force a young child to undergo a spinal tap to check for meningitis. But the range of cases in which we are morally permitted or obliged to use force or coercion on human incompetents in order to accomplish certain ends is not large by any means. Primarily it includes cases in which we act with the intention, and because we are motivated, *to forward the interests of that individual human being.* And that is not a license, not a blank check to force or coerce human incompetents to be put at risk of serious harm so that *others* might possibly be benefited by having *their* risks established or minimized. To treat the naturally occurring heart ailment of a human incompetent *is* morally imperative, and anything we learn as a result that is beneficial to others is not evil by any means. However, to intentionally bring about the heart attack of a human incompetent, on the chance that others might benefit, is morally out of bounds. Human incompetents do not exist as "medical resources" for the rest of us. Morally, Ventricle's research should be condemned if done on human incompetents, whatever benefits others might secure as a result. Imagine our gains to be as rich and real as you like. They would all be ill-gotten.

What is true in the case of human incompetents (those humans, once again, who, though they have known preferences, cannot give or withhold their informed consent) is true of chimps (and other animals like chimps in the relevant respects, assuming, as we are, that chimps cannot give or withhold their informed consent). Just as in the case of these humans, so also in the case of these animals, we are morally permitted and sometimes required to act in ways that coercively put them at risk of serious harm, against their known preferences, as when, for example, they are subjected to painful exploratory surgery. But the range of cases in which we are justified in using force or coercion on them is morally circumscribed. Primarily it is to promote *their* individual interests, as we perceive what is in their interests. It is *not* to promote the collective interests of *others*, including those of human beings. Chimpanzees are not our tasters, we are not their kings. To treat them in ways that put them at risk of significant harm on the chance that we might learn something useful, something that might benefit others (including other chimps!), something that just might add to our understanding of disease or its treatment or prevention—coercively to put them at risk of significant harm for any or all of these reasons is morally to be condemned.

To attempt to avoid this finding in the case of these animals, while holding on to the companion finding in the case of incompetent humans, is as rational as trying to whistle without using your mouth. It can't be done. As certain as it is that it would have been wrong for Ventricle to use human incompetents in his coronary research, it is at least as certain that it would have been wrong for him to use chimpanzees instead, despite the legality of using these animals and the illegality of using these humans, and notwithstanding the actual biological and alleged theological differences between these humans and animals. Whatever gains we might have harvested, for present or future generations of human beings, would have been ill-gotten.

The Indirect-Duty Response

People try to avoid this conclusion in a variety of ways. For example, some argue that we do not have any duties *to* animals (what philosophers call "direct duties"); rather, we have only duties *involving* animals (so-called "indirect duties"). Animals, in this view, have the same kind of moral status as redwoods, the Taj Mahal, and El Greco's *View of Toledo*. Few would deny that we have a duty to preserve these things, but most would deny that we have a duty *to them* to do so. Our duty, most people seem to think, is a duty *to other human beings*, both present and future generations, to preserve great works of art and the majesty of nature so that they, these other humans beings, might have an opportunity to see and appreciate them, thereby enriching the quality of their lives. Duties involving works of art and the majesty of nature, in short, are indirect duties to humanity.

The same is true, some people maintain, of our duties regarding animals. By all means, don't harm them unnecessarily, they say; but don't be misled into thinking that this is because we have duties directly to them. When animals are owned by others, we certainly ought not harm them unnecessarily because, after all, we have a duty to property owners not to harm their property. And when animals are not owned by anyone in particular, we still ought not harm them unnecessarily since people who do this to animals have a tendency to do the same sorts of things to human beings; since we *do* have a duty not to do this sort of thing to human beings, we therefore ought to avoid doing it to animals—not because we owe it to them, to be sure, but because we do owe it to one another.

If our duties regarding animals were indirect duties, one might then argue that Ventricle's research would have been wrong if done on human incompetents, but morally permissible if done on chimpanzees. If our duties regarding animals are indirect duties to humanity, then the morality of how we treat them is to be decided by what promotes human interests, and it is certainly possible that our interests would be promoted more by allowing animal research like Ventricle's than if we banned it.

But what about human incompetents? What type of duty do we have in their regard—direct or indirect? If one affirms direct duties in their case, while denying direct duties owed to chimpanzees, then, once again, one will want to be told what is the morally relevant difference between these humans and animals, something that, as we know, has not been established by the arguments so far considered. Moreover, one cannot say that the morally relevant difference simply is that the duties owed to human incompetents are direct, while those involving chimps are indirect, since this view presupposes that a morally relevant difference exists between the two. This view, therefore, cannot itself specify what that difference is.

The second option is to hold that our duties involving human incompetents, like our duties regarding chimpanzees, are indirect. This option at least has the merit of being consistent. Its principal defect is that it is false. Morally, it is preposterous to maintain that the reason why we ought not torture little children, for example, or kill their senile grandparents is because of the interests of others —for example, the children's parents or other elderly, more lucid people who, learning of the fate that befalls the senile, will live out their last years in wretched anxiety. It *is* wrong to torture children. But it is wrong to do this because in doing it we violate a duty we have directly to individual children *quite apart* from what their parents (or anyone else) happen to think or feel. And the same is true in the case of other harms we might visit upon other human incompetents. We owe it to them directly not to harm them. If others benefit in the bargain when we do as duty requires, they may count themselves lucky. But whether or not others benefit as a result of our refusal to harm human incompetents is, strictly speaking, morally irrelevant to whether we have duties to them. Our duties regarding human incompetents are not indirect duties to other people.

Of the two options, therefore, the second (that we have direct duties to human incompetents) is the one we should accept. Not to do so would be to distort, rather than illuminate, the moral status of these humans. Once more, however, we cannot consistently regard the moral status of chimpanzees any differently than that of these humans, if we are unable to cite a morally relevant difference. In other words, since our duties regarding human incompetents are direct duties, since we have duties regarding chimpanzees, and assuming we are unable to cite and defend a morally relevant difference between these animals and humans, then our duties regarding chimpanzees are likewise direct, not indirect, duties—*duties we owe directly to them, considered as individuals.* In particular, therefore, we owe it to these animals themselves not to harm them. Any further moral thinking about these animals must both take this into account and be able to account for it, and any treatment of chimpanzees that rests on a view about these animals that is deficient in these respects cannot be rationally satisfactory. One cannot, therefore, defend the gains others might have received from Ventricle's research on chimps, but condemn any gains stemming from such research if done on human incompetents, by claiming that our duties to these animals are indirect, while those involving these humans are direct. If one end is ill-gotten, then so is the other.

The Contractarian Response

Contractarianism is a second position that might seem to support research on chimps but not on incompetent humans. Roughly speaking, contractarians view morality as consisting of a set of mutually agreed-upon constraints on everyone's behavior. Each party to these agreements (or "the contract"), we are to suppose, seeks to maximize what is in his or her individual self-interest. Each party soon realizes, however, that to achieve this objective, others must be limited in what they may do. For example, it is self-defeating for Friday to work to secure food and a place to live if Crusoe is at liberty to steal his property. Since no one has any self-interested reason to limit the pursuit of his or her self-interest unilaterally, such limits can come into being only if enough people agree to abide by them and, relatedly, agree to impose appropriate sanctions (e.g., fines or other punishments) on those who fail to cooperate.

Contractarians have important intramural differences. Some believe that present-day morality can be traced to an actual historical agreement ("the original contract"); others interpret the notion of a contract ahistorically. These and other internal differences to one side, it should be clear that animals, chimps included, can find a precarious home at best within standard versions of contractarianism. As far as we know, human beings are the only terrestrial creatures capable of entering into contracts. That being so, what duties, if any, we have regarding animals must depend on what these human contractors judge to be in *their* (human) self-interest. If most of these humans agree that it is in their individual self-interest to allow Ventricle-like research on chimps, while forbidding analogous research on human incompetents, then the former, but not the latter, research would be justified. In this way, then, contractarianism might seem to provide an adequate moral basis for Ventricle's research.

But contractarianism, at least given one of its expressions, could justify far more than research on animals. If enough people happen to believe that it would be in their self-interest to suppress or oppress the members of a given minority (e.g., a racial or religious minority), when it comes to such vital matters as access to medical care, education, or career opportunities, then such policies, if mutually agreed upon by the majority, could not be morally condemned, given this version of contractarianism. That approach to morality, in other words, has the undesirable feature of legitimating the philosophy that might, understood as the collective judgment and power of the majority, makes right. Few, if any, will find this a congenial moral philosophy, since it would justify the most extreme expressions of racial and other forms of oppression. To have recourse to this philosophy as a defense of Ventricle-type research on chimps, therefore, is like trying to keep one's moral position afloat by drilling a hole in it. Our (human) might does give us the power to use animals in research, just as the might of the majority gives it the power to exploit the members of racial or religious minorities. But in neither case does might make right.

One could, it is true, endeavor to retain the spirit of contractarianism while altering the letter somewhat. Instead of allowing the parties to the contract to know, for example, their race, sex, religion, and nationality, one might ask them to imagine that they stand "behind a veil of ignorance," a veil that is thick enough to preclude their knowing the particular details of their life, thereby ensuring that they will select principles of justice impartially rather than on narrow, partisan grounds. As was explained in the introduction to this book, such a view can be found in John Rawls's influential work, *A Theory of Justice*. This is not the occasion to offer a full account or lengthy assessment of Rawls's version of contractarianism. Here it must suffice to note that Rawls, while insisting that the veil of ignorance keeps his contractors in the dark about, for example, what race or sex they will be, allows them to know that they will be members of the human race. Small wonder, then, that Rawls's view implies that we do have duties directly to one another but not to animals. The cards, as dealt by Rawls, are stacked against ensuring an impartial judgment of the moral status of animals. Though his theory has much to recommend it, we will not find in it a rationally satisfying basis for defending research like Ventricle's.

The Utilitarian Response

A third view worthy of consideration concedes that chimpanzees are on all fours, so to speak, with human incompetents, when it comes to their respective moral status: both are owed the same basic duty owed to those humans who are competent (that is, who have the ability to give or withhold their informed consent and, in having this ability, have all those other cognitive abilities thereby presupposed). That duty is twofold: first, to consider their interests and second, to count equal interests equally. The interests in question are what individuals prefer or would rather do without —what they like or dislike, love or hate, what they are "for" or "against." In the case of every individual with interests, then, we must first take the time and trouble to ask what his or her interests are before we can decide what, morally speaking, we ought to do. More than this, however, we must also weigh or count equal interests equally. If Jack and Jill both want to go up the hill, and if they both want to do so equally, then we must count their interests in going up the hill as being equal in importance. Rationally, we cannot discount the importance of Jill's interest on the grounds that "she's only a girl" or Jack's because "he's a dumb jock." To treat Jack and Jill fairly, to treat them equitably, to treat them as equals, requires that we consider their respective interests and count their like interests as of like importance. Let us refer to the principle that demands equal consideration and weighting of like interests as the *equality of interests principle* or *equality principle*.

The equality of interests principle is one part of a currently fashionable view called "preference utilitarianism." Utilitarianism, very roughly speaking, requires that we act in order to bring about the optimum aggregate balance of good over bad consequences for all those affected by what we do. If we think of "the good" as involving the satisfaction of individual preferences, and "the bad" as involving the frustration of such preferences, then the close connection between the principles of utility and equality should be clear. As preference utilitarians, what we aim to bring about is the best aggregate balance of the satisfaction of preferences over their frustration for all affected by what we do. To aim at this objective, however, we must first consider who has what preferences (interests) and count equal interests equally; we must, that is, first rely on the equality of interests principle.

Some preference utilitarians think that preference utilitarianism would condemn Ventricle's research on chimpanzees. The arguments these thinkers give, however, are far from convincing. Essentially, what they come to is the claim that allowing research on the chimps while forbidding it on human incompetents must violate the equality of interests principle, a principle that, given preference utilitarianism, it is always wrong to violate. But those who argue in this way are confused. Suppose both Clint Eastwood and Clyde (the chimp in the movie *Any Which Way You Can*) have the same interest in avoiding the excruciating pain associated with a heart attack. As preference utilitarians, we certainly must take the interests of both into account, and, assuming their equality, we must count them as being of equal importance. It does not follow from our having done this, however, that we must now approve of doing only those things to Clint that we would approve of doing to Clyde, and vice versa. What we ought to do to either, assuming we have observed the strictures of the equality principle, is now to be determined by appeal to the principle of utility. And there is no reason why *the consequences for others* (namely all those who will be affected by the consequences of our acts) will be the same if we do only the same things to Clyde as we would be willing to do to Clint. In particular, it is certainly possible that the aggregate balance of good over bad for all affected by the outcome would be better if Ventricle did his research on Clyde than if he did it on Clint.

It does not follow from this that preference utilitarians cannot condemn research such as Ventricle's when done on chimps. What follows is, first, that they cannot condemn it on the ground that it must violate the equality of interests principle (for it need not), and, second, that they must acknowledge that whether or not they have grounds on which to condemn it depends on their having knowledge of the relevant consequences of Ventricle-like research. What consequences, then, are relevant? In the nature of the case, these must deal with the degree to which the interests (preferences) of all those affected by the outcome of the research are satisfied or frustrated. This requires more than our knowing how Clyde's interests would fare. There are also Ventricle's interests to take into account, as well as those of his staff, plus those who build the tools of the medical researcher's trade (e.g., cages, restraint chairs), plus those who have an economic interest in the development of new drugs, plus our vital interest in health, and so on. There are, in a word, numerous interests to take into account and assess equitably before anyone could plausibly claim, with any degree of credibility, that the consequences of not allowing Ventricle to do his research on chimps would not bring about the best aggregate balance of preference satisfaction over frustration for all those affected by the outcome. Indeed, given that what we are being asked to do is compare the interests of relatively few chimpanzees against the not unimportant (e.g., economic, scientific, and health) interests of many more human beings, the utilitarian case seems to bode ill for the chimps. On the face of it, there is a very strong presumptive utilitarian case to be made in favor of Ventricle's research when done on chimpanzees.

This might seem to be good news for those who favor such research. It isn't. Preference utilitarianism does more than offer a way to justify Ventricle-type research when done on animals. It will also justify similar research done on human incompetents or, for that matter, on human competents, even without or against their informed consent. Granted, in cases involving humans, just as in cases involving animals, we must take pains to consider everyone's interests and count equal interests equally. Having done this, however, there is no reason why, in this or that case, the aggregate consequences for others might not be "the best" if we allowed research to be done on the humans in question. If we agree that research involving these humans is wrong, then we shall certainly want a moral principle that will not sanction it. That being so, we shall certainly want to avoid preference utilitarianism. It is no rational defense of Ventricle-type research on chimpanzees, therefore, to note that preference utilitarianism will, or very likely will, allow it. That view will, or very likely will, allow a great deal that is wrong. To show that preference utilitarianism would sanction research on chimpanzees is far from showing that such research is morally tolerable.

Perfectionist and Utilitarian Views of Value

Thus far we have advanced a controversial moral thesis—namely, that research like Ventricle's, when done on chimpanzees, cannot be justified by appealing to the benefits others do or might receive. And we have also considered, only to reject, various responses that seek to refute this thesis. Even if this thesis and its defense to this point are sound, much philosophical work remains to be done. A controversial thesis like the one before us does not stand on its own two feet. One must not only defend it against likely objections, a task to which we have attended, if incompletely, in the foregoing; one must also attempt to identify and defend the moral grounds on which the thesis stands, a task we have thus far failed to undertake. When, as now, we turn our attention to this item on our agenda, we must anticipate that the full weight of this challenge cannot be borne here.

Although preference utilitarianism is not the adequate position its advocates suppose, the emphasis it places on treating individuals as equals is an important corrective to less egalitarian visions of morality. The ancient Greek philosopher Aristotle, for example, offers a perfectionist moral theory: people are better (and so deserve more) than others if they have a certain cluster of intellectual and artistic excellences (virtues). Indeed, some people are so lacking in the favored virtues that Aristotle thinks they are born to be the slaves of those who are more generously endowed. Perfectionism of the Aristotelian sort must strike us as morally offensive, and it is one of the virtues of utilitarianism, because of the importance it places on treating relevantly similar individuals as equals, that it disassociates itself from perfectionism.

But the *type* of equality we find in preference (and other forms of) utilitarianism is easily misunderstood. For the preference utilitarian (to limit our attention to this version of utilitarianism), it is not individuals that count as equals but rather their mental states—their preference satisfactions and frustrations. Individuals are *receptacles* of value, things "into which," so to speak, what has value can be "poured," like liquid in a cup. But it is the liquid in the cup (that is, the mental states of satisfaction or frustration) that have value, whether positive or negative. The cup (that is, the individual human being or, for that matter, the individual chimpanzee), though "containing" what has value, has no value of its own.

To view humans or chimps in this way is to offer a theory of their value (or, more precisely, their lack of it) that can legitimate using them as medical and other sorts of resources, when this theory of value is coupled with the utilitarian injunction to act in order to bring about the best aggregate balance of good over bad for all affected by the outcome. If we consider the interests of all those who will be affected, if we count equal interests equally, and if, having done this, we can bring about the best aggregate balance of good over bad for all affected by doing medical research on chimps (or on human incompetents, or, indeed, on unwilling competent human beings), then our research is justified. The gains others secure, on this view, are *not* ill-gotten. To maintain, as we have, that such gains *are* ill-gotten is thus implicitly to reject preference utilitarian approaches to questions about the justification of medical research. More deeply and, for present purposes, more important, it is also to reject standard utilitarian theories of value. According to these theories, as noted, it is what "goes into" the individual, what the individual "contains"—for example, the mental state of satisfaction —that has value, not the individual. Our controversial thesis about using animals such as chimps in research such as Ventricle's thus

ILL-GOTTEN GAINS · 257

turns out to involve a different vision, neither perfectionist nor utilitarian, of the value of the individual.

The Value of the Individual

This alternative vision consists in viewing certain individuals as themselves having a distinctive kind of value, what we will call "inherent value." This kind of value is not the same as, is not reducible to, and is not commensurate either with such values as preference satisfaction or frustration (that is, mental states) or with such values as artistic or intellectual talents (that is, mental and other kinds of excellences or virtues). We cannot, that is, equate or reduce the inherent value of an individual to his or her mental states or virtues, and neither can we intelligibly compare the two. In this respect, the three kinds of value (mental states, virtues, and the inherent value of the individual) are like proverbial apples and oranges.

They are also like water and oil: they don't mix. It is not only that Clint's inherent value is not the same as, not reducible to, and not commensurate with *his* satisfaction, pleasures, intellectual and artistic skills, etc. In addition, *his* inherent value is not the same as, is not reducible to, and is not commensurate with the valuable mental states or talents of *other* individuals, whether taken singly or collectively. Moreover, and as a corollary of the preceding, the individual's inherent value is in all ways independent both of his or her usefulness relative to the interest of others and of how others feel about the individual (for example, whether one is liked or admired, despised or merely tolerated). A prince and a pauper, a streetwalker and a nun, those who are loved and those who are forsaken, the genius and the retarded child, the artist and the philistine, the most generous philanthropist and the most unscrupulous used car salesman—all have inherent value, according to the view recommended here, and all have it equally. Decidedly nonperfectionist in letter and spirit, this vision of value is decidedly nonutilitarian as well.

What Difference Does It Make?

To view the value of individuals in this way is not an empty abstraction. To the question, "What difference does it make whether we view individuals as having equal inherent value, or, as utilitarians do, as lacking such value, or, as perfectionists do, as having such value but to varying degree?"—our response to this question must be, "It makes all the moral difference in the world!" Morally, we are *always* required to treat those who have inherent value in ways that display proper respect for their distinctive kind of value, and though we cannot on this occasion either articulate or defend the full range of obligations tied to this fundamental duty, we can note that we fail to show proper respect for those who have such value whenever we treat them as if they were mere receptacles of value or as if their value was dependent on, or reducible to, their possible utility relative to the interests of others. In particular, therefore, Ventricle would fail to act as duty requires—would, in other words, do what is morally wrong— if he conducted his coronary research on competent human beings, without their informed consent, on the grounds that this research just might lead to the development of drugs or surgical techniques that would benefit others. That would be to treat these human beings as mere receptacles or as mere medical resources for others, and though Ventricle might be able to do this and get away with it, and though others might benefit as a result, that would not alter the nature of the grievous wrong he would have done. And it would be wrong, not because (or only if) there were utilitarian considerations, or contractarian considerations, or perfectionist considerations against his doing his research on these human beings, but because it would mark a failure on his part to treat them with appropriate respect. To ascribe inherent value to competent human beings, then, provides us with the theoretical wherewithal to ground our moral case against using competent human beings, against their will, in research like Ventricle's.

Who Has Inherent Value?

If inherent value could nonarbitrarily be limited to competent humans, then we would have to look elsewhere to resolve the ethical issues involved in using other individuals (for example, chimpanzees) in medical research. But inherent value can only be limited to competent human beings by having recourse to one arbitrary maneuver or another. Once we recognize that we have direct duties to competent and incompetent humans as well as to animals such as chimpanzees; once we recognize the challenge to give a sound theoretical basis for these duties in the case of these humans and animals; once we recognize the failure of indirect duty, contractarian, and utilitarian theories of obligation; once we recognize that the inherent value of competent humans precludes using them as mere resources in such research; once we recognize that perfectionist vision of morality, one that assigns degrees of inherent value on the basis of possession of favored virtues, is unacceptable because of its inegalitarian implications; and once we recognize that morality simply will not tolerate double standards, then we cannot, except arbitrarily, withhold ascribing inherent value, to an equal degree, to incompetent humans and animals such as chimpanzees. All have this value, in short, and all have it equally. All considered, this is an essential part of the most adequate total vision of morality. Morally, none of those having inherent value may be used in Ventricle-like research (research that puts them at risk of significant harm in the name of securing benefits for others, whether those benefits are realized or not). And none may be used in such research because to do so is to treat them as if their value is somehow reducible to their possible utility relative to the interests of others, or as if their value is somehow reducible to their value as "receptacles." What contractarianism, utilitarianism, and the other "isms" discussed earlier will allow is not morally tolerable.

Hurting and Harming

The prohibition against research like Ventricle's, when conducted on animals such as chimps, cannot be avoided by the use of anesthetics or other palliatives used to eliminate or reduce suffering. Other things being equal, to cause an animal to suffer is to harm that animal—is, that is, to diminish that individual animal's welfare. But these two notions—harming on the one hand and suffering on the other—differ in important ways. An individual's welfare can be diminished independently of causing her to suffer, as when, for example, a young woman is reduced to a "vegetable" by painlessly administering a debilitating drug to her while she sleeps. We mince words if we deny that harm has been done to her, though she suffers not. More generally, harms, understood as reductions in an individual's welfare, can take the form either of *inflictions* (gross physical suffering is the clearest example of a harm of this type) or *deprivations* (prolonged loss of physical freedom is a clear example of a harm of this kind). Not all harms hurt, in other words, just as not all hurts harm.

Viewed against the background of these ideas, an untimely death is seen to be the ultimate harm for both humans and animals, such as chimpanzees, and it is the ultimate harm for both because it is their ultimate deprivation or loss—their loss of life itself. Let the means used to kill chimpanzees be as "humane" (a cruel word, this) as you like. That will not erase the harm that an untimely death is for these animals. True, the use of anesthetics and other "humane" steps lessens the wrong done to these animals, when they are "sacrificed" in Ventricle-type research. But a lesser wrong is not a right. To do research that culminates in the "sacrifice" of chimpanzees or that puts these and similar animals at risk of losing their life, in the hope that we might learn something that will benefit others, is morally to be condemned, however "humane" that research may be in other respects.

The Criterion of Inherent Value

It remains to be asked, before concluding, what underlies the possession of inherent value. Some are tempted by the idea that life itself is inherently valuable. This view would authorize attributing inherent value to chimpanzees, for example, and so might find favor with some people who oppose using these animals in research. But this view would also authorize attributing inherent value to anything and everything that is alive, including, for example, crabgrass, lice, bacteria, and cancer cells. It is exceedingly unclear, to put the point as mildly as possible, either that we have a duty to treat these things with respect or that any clear sense can be given to the idea that we do.

More plausible by far is the view that those individuals have inherent value who are *the subjects of a life*—who are, that is, the experiencing subjects of a life that fares well or ill for them over time, those who have *an individual experiential welfare*, logically independent of their utility relative to the interests or welfare of others. Competent humans are subjects of a life in this sense. But so, too, are those incompetent humans who have concerned us. And so, too, and not unimportantly, are chimpanzees. Indeed, so too are the members of many species of animals: cats and dogs, monkeys and sheep, cetaceans and wolves, horses and cattle. Where one draws the line between those animals who are, and those who are not, subjects of a life is certain to be controversial. Still there is abundant reason to believe that the members of mammalian species of animals do have a psychophysical identity over time, do have an experiential life, do have an individual welfare. Common sense is on the side of viewing these animals in this way, and ordinary language is not strained in talking of them as individuals who have an experiential welfare. The behavior of these animals, moreover, is consistent with regarding them as subjects of a life, and the implications of evolutionary theory are that there are many species of animals whose members are, like the members of the species *Homo sapiens*, experiencing subjects of a life of their own, with an individual welfare. On these grounds, then, we have very strong reason to believe, even if we lack conclusive proof, that these animals meet the subject-of-a-life criterion.

If, then, those who meet this criterion have inherent value, and have it equally relative to all who meet it, chimpanzees and other animals who are subjects of a life, not just human beings, have this value *and* have neither more nor less of it than we do. (To hold that they have less than we do is to land oneself in the inegalitarian swamp of perfectionism). Moreover, if, as has been argued, having inherent value morally bars others from treating those who have it as mere receptacles or as mere resources for others, then any and all medical research like Ventricle's, done on these animals in the name of possibly benefiting others, stands morally condemned. And it is not only cases in which the benefits for others do not materialize that are condemnable; also to be condemned are cases, such as the research done on chimps regarding hepatitis, for example, in which the benefits for others are genuine. In these cases, as in others like them in the relevant respects, the ends do not justify the means. The *many millions* of mammalian animals used each year for scientific purposes, including medical research, bear mute, tragic testimony to the narrowness of our moral vision.

Conclusions

This condemnation of such research probably is at odds with the judgment that most people would make about this issue. If we had good reason to assume that the truth always lies with what most people think, then we could look approvingly on Ventricle-like research done on animals like chimps in the name of benefits for others. But we have no good reason to believe that the truth is to be measured plausibly by majority opinion, and what we know of the history of prejudice and bigotry speaks powerfully, if painfully, against this view. Only the cumulative force of informed, fair, rigorous argument can decide where the truth lies, or most likely lies, when we examine a controversial moral question. Although openly acknowledging and, indeed, insisting on the limitations of the arguments in this chapter, these arguments make the case, in broad outline, against using animals such as chimps in medical research such as Ventricle's. Various challenges to this position have been considered and judged inadequate, and the deeper philosophical grounds that stand beneath the surface of this controversy, grounds that concern alternative theories of the value of the individual (or lack of it), have been, if not thoroughly excavated, at least turned over. That does not bring thinking about value to an end, but it is something of a beginning.

Those who oppose the use of animals such as chimps in research like Ventricle's and who accept the major themes advanced here, oppose it, then, not because they think that all such research is a waste of time and money, or because they think that it never leads to any benefits for others, or because they view those who do such research as, to use Ventricle's words, "moral monsters," or even because they love animals. Those of us who condemn such research do so because this research is not possible except at the grave moral price of failing to show proper respect for the value of the animals who are used. Since, whatever our gains, they are ill-gotten, we must bring an end to research like Ventricle's, whatever our losses. A fair measure of our moral integrity will be the extent of our resolve to work against allowing our scientific, economic, health, and other interests to serve as a reason for the wrongful exploitation of members of species of animals other than our own.

Notes

1. Cora Diamond, "Experimenting on Animals: A Problem in Ethics," in *Animals in Research: New Perspectives in Animal Experimentation*, ed. David Sperlinger (New York: John Wiley & Sons, 1981), 345. The bibliography to which Diamond refers is S. Sollitte and R. M. Veatch, *Bibliography of Society, Ethics, and the Life Sciences, 1979–80* (Hastings-on-Hudson, N.Y.: The Hastings Center).

2. Charles R. Magel, *A Bibliography on Animal Rights and Related Matters* (Washington, D.C.: University Press of America, 1981).

3. Diamond, "Experimenting on Animals," 345.

Suggestions for Further Reading

The argument against using animals in medical research, sketched in the preceding essay, is developed at length in my *The Case For Animal Rights* (Berkeley, Calif.: University of California Press, 1983). For fuller discussions of indirect duty views, see chapter 5, especially 5.5 and 5.6; of contractarianism, see 5.3 and 5.4; of preference (and other forms of) utilitarianism, see 6.2, 6.3, and 7.7; of perfectionism, see 7.1; and of inherent value, the subject-of-a-life criterion, and the fundamental duty to treat those having inherent value with respect, see the whole of chapter 7. These discussions do greater justice to the subtleties of such views as contractarianism and utilitarianism than is possible in an essay with the dimensions of this one. The same is true of the cumulative argument for viewing mammalian animals as sophisticated mental creatures, set forth in chapters 1 and 2 in *The Case for Animal Rights*. The immorality of using these animals for scientific purposes, including medical research in both human and veterinary medicine, is discussed in 9.4.

There is a steadily growing body of literature devoted to exploring the ethical foundations of our treatment of animals. By far the most extensive, helpful bibliography is Charles R. Magel, *A Bibliography on Animal Rights and Related Matters* (Washington, D.C.: University Press of America, 1981). Less extensive bibliographies are Charles R. Magel, "An Updated Bibliography," in Henry S. Salt, *Animals' Rights*, (Clarks Summit, Pa.: Society for Animal Rights, 1980) and Charles R. Magel and Tom Regan, "Animal Rights and Human Obligations: A Select Bibliography," *Inquiry* 22 (1979), reproduced in my *All That Dwell Therein: Essays on Animal Rights and Environmental Ethics* (Berkeley, Calif.: University of California Press, 1982).

Among the works that survey the general moral terrain regarding our treatment of animals, in addition to those already cited, the following should be examined.

Frey, R. G. *Interests and Rights: The Case Against Animals*. Oxford: Oxford University Press, 1980.
Godlovitch, Stanley and Roslind, and Harris, John, eds. *Animals, Men and Morals*. New York: Taplinger, 1972.
Morris, Richard Knowles, and Fox, Michael W., eds. *On the Fifth Day; Animal Rights and Human Ethics*. Washington, D.C.: Acropolis Press, 1978.
Paterson, D.A., and Ryder, Richard, eds. *Animals' Rights: A Symposium*. London: Centaur Press, 1979.
Regan, Tom, and Singer, Peter, eds. *Animal Rights and Human Obligations*. Englewood Cliffs, N.J.: Prentice-Hall, 1976.
Singer, Peter. *Animal Liberation*. New York: Avon Books, 1975.
Sperlinger, David, ed. *Animals in Research: New Perspectives in Animal Experimentation*. New York: John Wiley & Sons, 1981.

Although most of the books cited above include discussions of the use of animals in science, including their use in medical research, the following works are especially relevant to this topic.

Diner, Jeff. *Physical and Mental Suffering in Experimental Animals*. Washington, D.C.: The Animal Welfare Institute, 1974.

Jamieson, Dale, and Regan, Tom. "On the Ethics of the Use of Animals in Science." In *And Justice For All: New Introductory Essays in Ethics and Public Policy*, ed. Tom Regan and Donald Van DeVeer. Totowa, N.J.: Rowman & Littlefield, 1982.

Magel, Charles R. "Humane Experimentation on Humans and Animals, or Muddling Through." Chicago: National Anti-Vivisection Society, 1981.

Pratt, Dallas. *Alternatives to Pain in Experiments on Animals*. New York: Argus Archives, 1982.

Rollin, Bernard. *Animal Rights and Human Morality*. Buffalo: Prometheus Books, 1982.

Rowan, Andrew. "Alternatives to Laboratory Animals: Definitions and Discussions." Washington, D.C.: The Institute for the Study of Animal Problems, 1980.

Ryder, Richard. *Victims of Science*. London: Davis-Poynter, 1975.

Smyth, David H. *Alternatives to Animal Experimentation*. London: The Scholar Press, 1978.

Vyvyan, John. *The Dark Face of Science*. Levittown, N.Y.: Transatlantic Arts, 1972.

It should not be inferred that the authors of any of the works cited here necessarily would agree with the position set forth in the preceding essay. Names and addresses of major organizations working to limit or abolish the use of animals in science, including their use in medical research, are listed in Magel's *A Bibliography on Animal Rights and Related Matters* (above).

CHAPTER VII

The Value of Life

Michael D. Bayles

Though often not consciously considered, the value of life is involved in decisions that many people make every day. Deciding whether to fly or drive to another city involves different risks to one's life, risks that lead some people never to fly, though the risks of injury and death are greater in driving. Whenever one decides to engage or not to engage in some risky activity, the value of one's life may be a factor. Many people also make daily decisions that implicitly or explicitly place a value on the lives of others. Decisions about building highways and skyscrapers and about allocating funds to health care lead to more or fewer people dying. These decisions are often made without explicitly considering their effect on whether or not people live, let alone taking the value of their lives into account. Yet sometimes this is considered, and surely it should be. The continued existence of other people is a morally relevant factor in deciding for one option rather than another.

Moreover, many decisions appear to value people's lives inconsistently.[1] For example, the risk of death in agriculture is much higher than in other fields, yet much less money is spent to prevent deaths in agriculture. Similarly, in the health care field, much more money is spent to provide renal dialysis per year of life saved than on other, preventive measures. It appears to be inconsistent, irrational, and unfair to spend much more money to save the lives of some people than those of others. Are people's lives really of such different value, some being worth twenty times those of others? Or are other considerations involved?

To speak of the value of a person's life is ambiguous. One must specify to whom it is valuable. The *personal value* of a life is its value to the person whose life it is. The *social value* of a person's life is its value to other people. The *total value* of a person's life is then the sum of its personal and social values, that is, its value to everyone. These distinctions are important, because when people hear about valuing lives, they often think only of social value. They then become upset and object to all talk of the value of a person's life because they mistakenly think that the individual is ignored and that only the value of a person's life to others is meant.

Much discussion in ethics is confusing because people start from different fundamental assumptions. Although it is not possible to defend them here, it is appropriate to state the moral assumptions underlying the following discussion. The fundamental assumption is that correct moral principles are those that rational persons would accept for a soceity in which they expected to live.[2] To be rational, one must have all relevant, publicly ascertainable information and use logic and scientific method. Rational persons do not have irrational desires—that is, desires that they would not have were they to reflect on all relevant available information using logic and scientific method.

What type of moral code or theory rational people would accept is a separate and open question. The value of life is the value of a state of affairs that can be affected by actions. It is relevant to determining the correctness of actions, as long as the consequences are relevant. Thus, it is quite important for such consequentialist theories of ethics as utilitarianism. However, for the value of life to be morally relevant, the rightness or wrongness of actions need not depend solely on their consequences. Other, nonconsequentialist considerations could also be relevant.

Thus, this discussion is not concerned with whether it is right or wrong, everything considered, to save or take lives.[3] It is concerned only with trying to place a value on what is saved or lost. For example, even if the same number of lives or amount of valuable life would be saved, one might consider it morally preferable to cure a disease that affects men and women equally, rather than one that affects only men. Other possible considerations concern how deaths come about, either by causing them or failing to prevent them, causing them intentionally or negligently, and so forth.

Finally, this discussion is not concerned with the value of bringing lives into existence, that is, whether it is valuable to beget a child and what the value of that child's life might be. Although this issue is interesting and tangentially relevant, it is too complex to discuss adequately in the confines of this chapter.

Life, Length of Life, or Quality of Life

The first task in considering the personal value of life is to determine what makes a life valuable to the one who lives it. Some possible moral principles, for example, that physicians should always prolong life if they can, assume that it is biological life itself that is valuable. Such a view is not acceptable. Suppose one were to become irreversibly comatose. Would one's biological life then be of any value to one? The answer is obviously no. Being unconscious, one would be incapable of valuing anything, so one's life would not have any personal value. Consequently, consciousness, not constant consciousness, but at least intermittent consciousness, is a necessary condition for life having personal value.

One might, then, contend that what has personal value is the amount of (years of) conscious life. The longer one is consciously alive, the more valuable life is. One could then determine the personal value of people's lives by their number of years of conscious life. People's conscious lives would be equally valuable. A period of conscious life for one person would have the same personal value as an equal period of conscious life for another person.

Unfortunately, on reflection, good reasons exist to reject the view that mere conscious life is what is personally valuable. One must distinguish two senses of a 'valuable life.' In one sense, a valuable life is one that can have value, but the value can be positive or negative. In the other sense, a valuable life is one that is good. The concern here is with what makes life good or bad. Consciousness makes life capable of having value, but it does not necessarily make it good. If it did, conscious life would be equally valuable whatever happened to one. Even if one's spouse died a horrible death, one lost one's money, and one was ill and racked with pain, one's life would be just as good as if none of these things had happened. The actual value of one's life surely varies with what happens. For example, I found life better in 1979 than in 1980. Whereas 1979 was a very good year for me, 1980 was a very bad one. Any view that denies that the personal value of life can vary is mistaken.

Moreover, the personal value of life might be negative (bad). Some people, for example very seriously injured and dying persons, do not find their life good at all and would prefer an early death to prolonged life. It is not plausible to claim that if these people had more information, or used logic and scientific method, they would change their minds. Any theory of the value of life must allow for it to have both positive and negative value, to be good or bad.

If the value of conscious life can vary, then it must depend on some characteristics or qualities of life that can vary. A number of views contend that the value of life depends on some capacities besides that for consciousness, such as the capacities to think, or to give and receive love, or to feel pleasure and pain. However, these capacities, like consciousness, pertain to the capability of life having value; their existence does not make life good or bad. One can have the same capacity to think or to express and receive love over a period of time but the value of one's life during that period might vary. Although the value of my life varied between 1979 and 1980, my abilities to think and to express and receive love did not vary significantly between those two years. Whether or not I thought, gave and received love, and experienced pain did vary. It is not the mere existence of these capacities that makes life good or bad, but how they are exercised.

The personal value of life then depends on the characteristics of the *experiences* one has, which may be called the quality of one's life. Utilitarian theorists have generally held that pleasure and pain, or happiness and unhappiness, are the qualities that make life good or bad. Clearly, although they are relevant, physical pleasure and pain are not the only factors. Many people, for example some victims of arthritis, suffer physical pain without compensating physical pleasures, yet find their lives valuable or good. The classical utilitarians used the words 'pleasure' and 'pain' in broader senses to include mental satisfaction and dissatisfaction. 'Happiness' and 'unhappiness,' perhaps, are better terms. Even they are probably inadequate. Either they are used as simple equivalents for "finds experience good (bad)" or people can positively value their lives even though they are unhappy.

Some people find life *good* but are *not very happy*. Some philosophers, scientists, and others work very hard to complete projects but are unhappy even if successful. They think that they have accomplished something and that their sacrifice of happiness was worthwhile. Nor is it plausible to suggest that either they must be happy when successful or they are irrational. Often, success simply leads to another project. Nor is it clear that these people lack some information or have reasoned incorrectly. To establish that happiness is not the sole determinant of the value of life, one need only show that the value of life to rational persons does not vary in proportion to their happiness. Consequently, one can reasonably conclude that at least two different factors affect the personal value of life—the *happiness* it involves and the pursuit or accomplishment of one's *projects.*

Although capacities are not the sole determinants of the value of life, they are relevant. In medicine, judgments of the potential quality or value of a person's life are often made on the basis of physical and mental capacity and likely pain. These can be rough indicators of the likely value of life to an individual. Physical and mental capacity and pain are relevant to the possibility of accomplishing projects and achieving happiness. However, capacities only set limits to possible value. With few capacities, the possibility of value in life is limited; but with greater capacities, the possibility of disvalue is also increased.

The *personal value* of life, then, is a function of the *length* and *quality* of conscious life. The basic unit for the personal value of life can be specified as quality-adjusted life years. This unit allows for variation over time as the value of life fluctuates due to happiness, projects, and other possible factors.[4]

Self-Sacrifice

Can one rationally trade or sacrifice length of life for something else? To answer this, it is instructive to consider the argument that life is of infinite monetary value because no rational person would sacrifice his or her life for any amount of money.[5] The value of life could be considered the amount of money that would compensate a person for losing his or her life. Were death to be immediate and no bequests permitted, then no amount of money could compensate one.

There are a number of difficulties with this argument. First, the argument is not correct unless one rules out people whose lives have such disvalue that they would prefer to be dead. Thus, at best, the argument shows that if life has positive value, then it has infinite monetary value. Second, as the death is to be immediate, the individual has no time in which to enjoy anything. As one lengthens the time before death, compensation becomes more and more plausible and the amount necessary decreases. For example, a twenty-year-old person might settle for $100,000 now in exchange for not living beyond age seventy. One might reply that the person has no guarantee of living that long anyway. Nonetheless, the general point is that people might well trade length of life for quality of life. If the standard of personal value is quality-adjusted years of one's life, then one can increase that sum by increasing quality at the expense of length.

Third, the argument assumes that no bequests can be made. This rules out any compensation after one's death or benefits for others. One might trade one's life for benefits for others. Soldiers who throw themselves on hand grenades and many other people who die to save others do so. One might also sacrifice one's life for financial benefits for others, such as money for one's family. One might even sacrifice one's life for some rather "selfish" benefit, such as publication of one's collected works. Of course, one could not experience or see the publication, but one might well trade one's life for its guarantee.

The argument for the infinite monetary value of life thus proves nothing. It asks whether money could compensate one by increasing the personal value of one's life given that there is no life to enhance. Of course, the answer is no. The question it asks is really the following: Given that one wants to live and expects one's future life to be good, is there any instantaneous experience money could buy that one would value more?

More generally, this discussion has shown that one might rationally trade one's life, or better, the rest of one's life or part of the rest of one's life, for a variety of things. One can rationally trade some of its length for an increase in its quality. Money could be spent to increase happiness or to accomplish projects. One could even trade length of life for the completion of projects after one is dead. Thus, one might trade one's remaining years for the education of one's children or the publication of one's books. However, completion of some projects, such as a book one is writing, requires one's continued existence. If someone else completed the book, it would not be one's own book, but at best a coauthored one. Most people have several projects at one time, so they might trade their lives and the failure to complete projects involving their existence for a guarantee that other projects not requiring their existence be completed. The upshot is that people reasonably can sacrifice part of their lives for any of a variety of other things, including money, if they have some time to use the money or can direct the use to which it is put after their death.

Social Value

The social value of a person's life is somewhat easier to conceptualize than its personal value. Overall, social value is likely to be significantly less than personal value. Usually, a life means more to the one who lives it than it does to others. The social value of a life can be divided into at least three elements. One element is its emotional or psychological value. Other people are often emotionally involved with a particular individual. No one else can take that person's place. One usually thinks of people who love the individual, but people may hate a person as well, in which case the individual's life has a *social disvalue* to them. A second element can be called personal services—things that only a particular individual can do. For example, only Doe can paint Doe's pictures. Many of the services people provide others, such as fixing plumbing, are not thus personal; they can be performed by others. In those cases, the services really belong to the third element, the economic value of a person's life to others. An individual's life has economic value to financial dependents and others. A person's life can also be an economic disvalue; the life of an incapacitated invalid can be an economic cost to others.

The general purpose of determining the value of life is to be able explicitly to take it into account in making decisions. To make decisions about their own lives, individuals do not need a very precise concept or set of principles. If decisions affect only them, they need only to judge which course of action has most value to them. Of course, if they are to be rational, they do need to try to be consistent in such judgments. Sometimes individuals consider the social as well as personal value of their lives. A terminally ill patient might think that his or her continued life would have personal value but, because of its social disvalue, ask not to be resuscitated or to have heroic measures taken to preserve life. People sometimes make such decisions in order not to expend their family's wealth on medical treatment. Although their continued life might have positive emotional value for their family, its economic disvalue might outweigh that element. In addition, the emotional loss could only be postponed a few days or weeks. It is not irrational for an individual to trade some positive quality-adjusted life years to avoid social disvalue.

Many people consider it wrong for others to make similar decisions for an individual. The heart of such an objection must be that only the individual should be permitted to make such a decision. As no *conceptual* difficulty exists about trading personal value for social value of a life, any objection must be a moral one based on factors other than the value of the life in question. It is not because life has absolute value or a value that cannot be compared with other values.

It is not even plausible to claim that one should not trade the personal value of another's life for social value. Indeed, it is impossible for a world to operate without such decisions. If the government funds one type of health care rather than another—for example, renal dialysis rather than heart transplants—different people will live. Suppose Jones has heart disease. Then a decision not to fund heart transplants, assuming Jones is a likely candidate for one, means that his life, and its personal value, is traded for the personal value of another person's life. But from Jones's perspective, the value of another person's life is its social value.

The distinction between personal and social value is a relative one depending on which life or lives one considers. In the final analysis, all social value reduces to the personal value of other persons' lives. If one sums up all the personal value of all the lives lived, one has taken account of all the value of all the lives that are lived. There is no extra social value. One can see this by simply noting that the elements of social value—emotional, personal service, and economic—contribute to the personal value of the lives of other people.

Consequently, when decision makers are choosing between projects that will mean life or death for different people, they are actually choosing between the personal value of different lives. Conceptually, they are working with the same units—namely, quality-adjusted life years—for different people. They cannot avoid such trades, for whatever decision they make will affect the personal value of some lives differently from others. It is pointless to claim they ought not do what they cannot avoid doing. The difficulty, if there is a difficulty, is in obtaining an adequate measure of quality-adjusted life years so that one can compare those of one person with those of another.

Levels of Governmental Decisions

At this point, it is useful to distinguish three rough levels of social decisions in which the value of life may enter. For sake of simplicity, it is easiest to look at government funding of health care, although similar decisions arise in other types of programs and in nongovernmental decisions, such as the safety of products manufactured by private corporations.

The first and most general level of decision making concerns how much money to allocate to health care rather than education, agriculture, and so forth. At this level, the choice situation is amorphous because not all health care—related activities fall within a health budget. For example, school lunches or food stamps can have important implications for health in a society but not fall within a broadly defined health budget. It is also difficult to get any clear notion of the benefit to be expected from different areas of spending. One reason is simply the inability to predict the success of programs. Another difficulty is that some areas will primarily extend life while others might do little to extend life but might enhance its quality (e.g., home mortgages).

The second level of decision making concerns the allocation of resources among programs. For example, within the health care budget, one must decide on the relative priority of programs of prevention, research, and health care delivery. This level is not a simple one but comprises many sublevels of decisions depending on what the programs are. Even within the category of health care delivery, for example, one must choose between providing neonatal intensive care units and burn centers. Within research, one must decide whether to fund research on cancer or arthritis, or how much to fund each. Different people will be benefited depending on which programs are funded or the relative levels of funding, and some programs (e.g., arthritis research) may do little to prevent death but will primarily affect quality of life.

A third level of decision making primarily concerns choices between individuals or groups of individuals to receive the benefits of programs. For example, given limited intensive care facilities, one must decide which types of patients or which individual patients should be admitted. Another similar problem, cne which the Canadian Medical Association is studying, is the priority of patients for elective surgery.[6] Because not all patients can receive elective surgery when they would like, some system is needed to determine priorities among them. In deciding this type of question, one element that seems relevant is to determine which lives are more valuable. Such a suggestion raises fears among many people.

Identifiable Versus Statistical Lives

One of the fears raised is that doctors would be deciding to treat or not to treat patients by their (the physicians') estimates of the value of their patients' lives. People generally abhor the idea of determining that known or identifiable people's lives are not worth saving, or are not as worth saving as other people's. Society appears to spend more to save the lives of known or identifiable individuals than it does unidentifiable or statistical lives. Thousands of dollars' worth of medical care will be provided to extend the life of one gravely ill or injured person, but a comparable expenditure will not be made to reduce the risk of injury or death to a group of individuals. Often this is dramatically shown by mine disasters. Once a cave-in or explosion occurs, thousands of dollars are spent to rescue trapped miners, but comparable expenditures are not made to improve mine safety, although those expenditures might save even more lives.

One factor that might account for this difference of treatment between known and statistical lives is emotional identification with the victims. One knows who the individual is; one can identify with that person as well as the person's family. Think how difficult it might be to tell an individual that his or her life is not worth saving. It is much easier to tell a group of people that an increased level of safety for them is not worthwhile.

While this emotional involvement or psychological identification with known victims might explain differential expenditures to save known and statistical lives, it does not justify it. A rational person would try to vividly imagine the consequences of various options, including the pain and suffering of those who would likely die and of their families.[7] Consequently, the difference in emotional attachment is not a rational basis for deciding that statistical lives are worth less. Although this consideration suggests that known and statistical lives should be treated the same, it does not indicate which of the present social attitudes is best. Perhaps statistical lives should be weighted more heavily. Yet emotional involvement and identification may lead to an undue weighting of known lives that should be weighted less than they are presently.

Another argument to justify greater expenditures for saving known lives is its symbolism of the social value of not abandoning members of society.[8] Military patrols take extra chances to bring back wounded soldiers. This is an expression of social solidarity and protects people from the thought and fact of having coworkers, friends, family, and others abandon them to their fate. This consideration, however, does not indicate that known lives are more valuable than unknown or statistical ones. Rather, it imports another consideration into the decision making.

Moreover, it is not clear that the symbolic significance of not abandoning known individuals can withstand critical scrutiny. If people realized that society is willing to spend considerably more to save them once they are in dire straits than to prevent their getting into dire straits, there might be little symbolic importance. The message is that society will not spend much money to prevent one's being killed, as in a mine disaster, but if there should be a disaster and one survives the initial effects, society will spend a lot of money to extricate one. People would find little comfort, symbolically or otherwise, in such a message.

Yet another argument has been suggested for emphasizing known lives over statistical ones.[9] Suppose one has a choice between policies A and B. Their overall benefits are the same, except that policy A involves the death of five known individuals out of 10,000, whereas policy B involves the death of .05 percent of the 10,000 people (i.e., five statistical lives). One might prefer policy B over A. The randomness of who shall die makes it more fair than policy A. Thus, it appears that statistical lives should be valued less than known lives.

There are at least two problems with this argument. First, even if randomness has something to be said for it—for example, that it is more fair— it does not show that the statistical lives are worth less. Instead, the appeal is to another consideration, fairness, that might decide when the value of lives is the same. Second, if randomness does have an independent value, then it also provides a reason for preferring the saving of statistical lives over known lives. In saving known lives, all the resources are devoted to five specific people and others get nothing from the expenditure. Fairness as randomness would indicate that others should also have an opportunity to have their lives saved.

The upshot of this discussion is that known and statistical lives should be valued similarly.[10] Any differences in preferring one to the other in specific circumstances should stem from considerations based on their equal value, for instance, preferring more known to fewer statistical lives. Even if the suggested arguments for different allocations of expenditures to save known rather than statistical lives were sound, they would not show a difference in the value of the lives. Instead, they would provide other reasons for saving known rather than statistical lives. However, that known and statistical lives should be valued equally does not necessarily indicate which of society's present practices more accurately reflects the value of lives. It is likely that statistical lives should be valued more than they are and that they are valued less because of an inability to psychologically grasp the value involved. Yet it is also likely that more funds than appropriate are spent to save known lives because of undue weighting of symbolism and avoidance of unpleasant tasks.

Cost-Effectiveness and Cost-Benefit

The purpose of clarifying the value of life is to be able to take it more explicitly into account in making decisions. It is useful to consider whether and how this could be done at the different levels of decision making. At the level of decisions between broad categories of programs, nothing very explicit can be done. The primary reason is that the implications of decisions for quality and length of life are unclear. To what extent funds allocated to health care might improve the quality or length of life depends on which programs are funded. The same applies to other areas of funding. Consequently, decisions at this level must be based more on general principles and judgments, such as whether there is an adequate health care system, judicial system, and so on. That is, one must rely on prior evaluations of the programs within the various areas, increasing support for more beneficial programs and decreasing it for less beneficial ones.

At the second level, considerations of the value of life can be more explicitly included.[11] Here one is given a sum of money to spend, and the choices are between various programs. Even so, the implications are often unclear. For example, if the decision is simply between percentages of available funds to be allocated to research, prevention, and health care delivery, net effects on quality-adjusted life years will still depend crucially on which specific programs are funded. As one is presented with more concrete choices, the value of life can be taken more explicitly into account.

One common objection to considering the value of life in making decisions is the claim that one cannot tell where else the money might be spent.[12] If money is not spent on neonatal intensive care units, then it might be spent on something much less valuable, such as funding government tea tasters to ensure the quality of imported tea. This argument appeals to many people, but often it is unsound. For example, a provincial health agency in Canada's governmental health insurance may face a choice between more neonatal intensive care units or more general beds or other services. The funds will not revert to a more general budget. Thus, the choice is between a finite set of programs with a given number of dollars. Similar choices are often confronted in hospitals.

When choices of this sort are confronted, the value of life can be explicitly considered. Given a certain number of dollars, one can make reasonable estimates of which programs will contribute most to quality-adjusted life years. Essentially, one calculates the number of quality-adjusted life years to be expected from each program and then chooses that program producing the most quality-adjusted life years.[13] This method is a form of cost-effectiveness evaluation. Given a desired outcome (quality-adjusted life years) and a fixed sum of money, one can evaluate different programs to determine which will produce more of the desired outcome for the money. This approach can even be used to compare programs in quite different areas, such as an increased safety program in agriculture versus a hospital CAT scanner.

This type of cost-effectiveness evaluation has a number of complexities, only a few of which can be noted here. First, one must be able to evaluate outcomes in terms of quality-adjusted life years. Often it is possible to obtain reasonably reliable evaluations of life years saved. For example, fairly good statistics are available regarding saving lives by spina bifida closure, kidney transplant, and coronary bypass operations. Evaluating the quality of life is more difficult, yet this aspect can be crucial. Some programs contribute primarily to quality of life, (e.g., the provision of prosthetic devices). Some programs may save lives but allow only a very poor quality of life afterward, and thus may be less desirable than other programs that save fewer lives but allow for a higher quality of life. For example, the death rate from infants with spina bifida whose backs are closed and heads shunted (if need be) is lower than for low-birth-weight and highly premature infants (say, those between twenty-four and twenty-six weeks gestation and below 750 grams birth weight). However, the level of ability and quality of life is probably much higher for surviving low-birth-weight infants than spina bifida infants. The latter are certain to have physical disabilities and have a good chance of mental retardation, while the percentage of handicapped surviving low-birth-weight infants is quite similar to that for more mature and higher-birth-weight infants (1,000–1,500 grams), perhaps around 15 percent.

Although one cannot have precise calculations of quality of life, precision is perhaps not crucial. All one needs is a relative comparison of quality of life between the two groups. That is, one need only be able to make general judgments that spina bifida survivors have half or three-fourths or whatever of the quality of life of low-birth-weight survivors. Given different costs per life saved, one can also determine exactly how much relatively more quality of life low-birth-weight infants need have before more benefit comes from treating them. Although the quality of life depends on a large variety of factors, as discussed earlier, people's incapacities can limit their possible quality of life. Consequently, one is apt to be reasonably close in determining relative quality of life by considering comparative physical and mental capacities and known sources of pain, such as needed operations. Other factors that affect quality of life, such as accidents, may be about the same across both groups. As their employment opportunities are generally fewer, wealth is likely to be less for more handicapped persons, roughly proportional to the handicap.

A second complication of cost-effectiveness evaluation is that one should not merely look at which type of program will have the most benefit. Often the choice is not between this program or that one, but between greater or lesser funding of this program and that one. Even so, one can still estimate the marginal benefit gained per dollar spent on each program. Ideally, one would fund both programs so that the expectable benefit of quality-adjusted life years from an extra dollar spent is the same. Of course, in practice it is not possible to be this precise.

Third, one must remember that the value of life need not be the only consideration in funding one program rather than another. Other types of considerations may also be important, such as fairness of distribution. For example, cost-effectiveness calculations of quality-adjusted life years tend to favor programs for younger people over those for older persons, because if the lives of younger people are saved, they have more years to live. One might then decide that considerations of fair distribution support funding some health care measures for older persons even though more quality-adjusted life years could be gained by funding programs aimed at younger persons. What cost-effectiveness considerations do is indicate how much value of life one is sacrificing for considerations of fairness or justice.

In sum, then, cost-effectiveness analysis by quality-adjusted years of life allows one to consider more explicitly the value of life in decisions to allocate given amounts of resources among alternative programs. It does not require absolute (cardinal) evaluations of quality of life, only comparative or proportional ones. These can sometimes be roughly calculated by considering the amounts of handicap. One can allocate resources to programs so that the amount of benefit per given unit of resource is roughly equal between programs. Finally, although the above discussion was in terms of dollars allocated, one need not use that unit of measurement. One can use amounts of staff time or other factors to determine costs. The units of cost (dollars) and of benefit (quality-adjusted life years) need not be the same, but the same cost and benefit units must be used for the different programs.

Although cost-effective analysis enables one to make many comparative judgments between programs affecting the value of life, it does not enable one to make all the judgments one might wish to make. In particular, in some cases one might contend that the benefits are not worth the costs. Although it is highly controversial, many people think that such judgments are correct about treating some severely defective newborns (e.g., some infants severely affected with spina bifida). Cost-effectiveness analysis does not necessarily enable one to make that judgment, because it does not require that costs and benefits be measured in the same units. To claim that the costs of some program are not worth the benefits, the costs and benefits must be expressed in the same units. It is unlikely that one could devise a way to express costs in terms of quality-adjusted life years. Consequently, the most plausible approach is to try to express the value of life in dollar terms. Many costs are expressed in dollar terms, and money is the most pervasive unit of expressing value in society.

The Monetary Value of Life

Some people object to trying to express the value of life in monetary terms. One cannot, it is claimed, put a dollar value on life. To do so is to degrade life, to lose the respect and dignity of life.

This objection is unclear. First, it might mean that one cannot in fact find a correct money equivalent for the value of life. That might be true, but then it must be argued for after examining various methods that attempt to establish this equivalent, not assumed to be true before examining them.

Second, it might mean that one cannot in principle express the value of life in monetary terms, that the value of life cannot be compared with money. However, for this to be true, there would have to be an element of the quality of life that (1) cannot be part of the economy, (2) cannot be equivalent to any combination of other elements that can have a monetary value, and (3) does not have causes or conditions that can have a monetary value. Requirement (2) means that the element would have absolute value. It is difficult to conceive what it would be, since life itself does not qualify. Freedom, justice, privacy, and well-being do not meet these three conditions. Moral integrity might be thought to be such an element, but one would have to either be willing to sacrifice any amount of others' lives, freedom, and well-being to preserve one's integrity, or not care for others, which calls into question one's morality if not integrity. Consequently, in principle, there can be a monetary expression of the value of life.

Finally, the objection might mean that one ought not express the value of life in monetary terms. If one *can* do so, however, it is unclear why it would be wrong *to* do so. People do and rationally can trade length of life for quality of life, and even personal value for social value. If such judgments and trade-offs are rational and sometimes morally praiseworthy (consider soldiers throwing themselves on grenades), then why is it morally wrong to try to make them more explicit and rational? Perhaps more morally defensible decisions will result. For example, perhaps the lives of mine workers have been undervalued in decisions about mine safety, and this analysis will lead to a higher and more appropriate valuing of lives.

Economists have suggested many ways of expressing the value of life in monetary terms.[14] It is not possible here to go through all of them or any of them in detail. The best that can be done is to indicate the two major approaches and a few of their difficulties. These two approaches are the human capital approach and the willingness-to-pay approach.

HUMAN CAPITAL

This approach is the simpler of the two and probably the most used in practice. Essentially, the value of a human life is taken to be a person's expectable future lifetime earnings (e.g., a thirty-five-year-old university professor's lifetime earnings might be $1,000,000). Usually, one then corrects this figure for inflation and discounts it at some real interest rate. The resulting figure is the current value of the individual's life.

This approach has some obviously undesirable distributional aspects. For example, net lifetime earnings vary with age. Young adults have the highest expectable lifetime earnings. Older people have fewer remaining work years and so lower expectable earnings.

Infants and young children are net consumers for a number of years, and this cost is subtracted from total earnings. Moreover, there are differences between sexes and races, because women and blacks generally hold lower-paying jobs. Indeed, housewives do not earn any income, and even if one values their work at the wages of domestic servants, housewives are still given a low value. All of these factors point to an underlying defective assumption—namely, that value of life varies directly with income produced. The personal value of life, which is usually greater than social value, is unlikely to do so. Although studies indicate that the rich are on average happier than the poor, it is doubtful that the difference in happiness and value of life is directly proportional to income.

One might reply that even if the personal value of the lives of high-income people is not much greater than that of low-income people, their social value is greater. But this considers only economic social value. The emotional value of a low-income worker to family and friends is not captured in lifetime earnings. Nor is the social value of personal services, though the economic value of such services might be. The human capital method simply omits value that is not already part of the monetary economy.

Moreover, lifetime earnings may overestimate social economic value. The assumption is that if this individual dies, then the economy loses this individual's productivity. In an economy with high unemployment, this is not true. If a university professor dies, someone else will take his or her job. In the end, an unemployed person will become employed. All the people who thus benefit will increase their lifetime earnings, so the loss of the university professor is not a net loss to the economy. It means only that an unemployed Ph.D. will have an opportunity to work and produce. Indeed, in many cases total productivity would be increased by the death of some university faculty members and their replacement by others. (Readers can perhaps supply names.) What could not be replaced is the emotional and personal service value of the professor, such as love and the books or articles he or she might have written.

Finally, this approach underestimates the personal value of life. It assumes that the personal value of life is the monetary value of goods and services consumed, which in turn is determined by wealth plus income.[15] This is a materialistic emphasis. Just as emotional elements of social value are not included in earnings, neither are emotional elements in the personal value of life encapsulated in consumption. Indeed, many people find less expensive activities more valuable than expensive ones, such as playing cards with friends versus flying an airplane. In short, nonconsumptive activities can contribute to the personal value of life but are not included in the human capital approach.[16]

WILLINGNESS TO PAY

The second approach is based on how much people are willing to pay for an increase in safety or how much they would want to be paid for an increased risk of death. This can be done by seeing what people actually pay or request, or by questionnaires. It does not directly evaluate the value of life, but the value of a risk of life. The value of a life is then calculated by multiplying the value of some risk in order to obtain a certainty of death. For example, suppose a person is willing to pay fifty dollars for a decreased risk of one in 10,000 of dying. Then the value of that individual's life is $500,000, the figure arrived at by multiplying fifty dollars by 10,000.

This approach has difficulties at high levels of risk. For example, an individual might pay almost all of his or her money to avoid a 50 percent chance of death. Consequently, the person would not be able to pay much more to avoid an 80 percent chance of death. Similarly, if one looks at compensation for a risk, as one reaches greater and greater risks, the person will want much more compensation. Indeed, as was discussed earlier, no amount of money would directly compensate the person for a certainty of immediate death if that person could not specify the money's use after his or her death. Note also the asymmetry between what someone would pay and what someone would take as compensation. How much a person would pay is limited by how much the person has, but there is no theoretical limit, save all the money in the world, to possible compensation.

This approach leads to several difficulties. First, the results will be biased by wealth. Because they have more than the poor, the wealthy will probably pay more for a given amount of increased safety. Consequently, the lives of wealthy people will be valued more than those of poor persons. However, personal value of life (happiness) does tend to vary with income or wealth. If people's willingness to pay is not directly proportional to wealth, the willingness-to-pay approach will not be as inaccurate a measure of personal value of life as the human capital approach, which makes personal value equivalent to consumption. Some lives are more valuable to those who live them, and there is some general relation to wealth. If this is unjust, it is not because of the willingness-to-pay approach, and the cure is a more equal distribution of wealth. The willingness-to-pay approach can also be modified to discount differences of wealth.[17]

Another alleged difficulty with willingness to pay is that it uses an *ex ante* rather than *ex post* measure. That is, it uses what a person takes to be the likely loss as modified by his or her expectation of that loss rather than the value that person actually places on loss of life. To evaluate the latter, it is alleged, one should consider what the person will pay to avoid immediate death or take as compensation for immediate death. Now if one allows bequests or directions for the use of money after death, some people might trade their immediate death for money. It is certainly clear that there is a limit to how much people would pay to avoid such death: namely all they have or can get. However, it is not clear that the *ex post* measure is the one desired. One wants to know how much people value their remaining lives. Perhaps a more appropriate method would be to ask how much a person would pay for an extra year of life, or take as compensation for one less year of life. The answer would indicate the trade-off that person is willing to make between length and quality, so it would come close to giving an average value for one quality-adjusted life year. The personal value of remaining life is simply that value times the number of remaining years.

Nonetheless, there is a difficulty with this change that pervades the willingness-to-pay approach. Generally, the last year of one's life is apt to be of lower quality than earlier years. For example, many elderly people suffer chronic, debilitating illnesses. So the value of the last year of life is not likely to be the average. More generally, how much people are willing to pay for increased safety varies with age, with older people typically not willing to pay as much (except for their likely increased wealth). This is not necessarily a defect, because what one is concerned with measuring is quality-adjusted life years.

None of the difficulties considered thus far appears to be a catastrophic objection to the willingness-to-pay approach. Wealthy people will pay more than poor ones, but there is some reason to believe that quality of life varies with wealth, at least within moderate limits, and gross distortions can be taken into account. Asking about decreased risk of death comes reasonably close to an evaluation of average value per quality-adjusted life year. And variable responses by age simply adjust for possible lower quality.

Thus, willingness to pay rather accurately captures the personal value of life, but it does not directly capture social value. Social value is captured only if the individual considers the benefit of his or her life to others, such as family, and even then it leaves out benefits to persons the individual does not think about. A better picture would emerge were spouse and friends asked what they would pay to decrease the risk of death to that person or to prolong that person's life by a year. After this figure was established it could be combined with the individual's willingness to pay. The total value of the person's life would equal the total of these two figures. Although in practice it might be difficult to arrive at this final amount, this approach does theoretically solve the problem of a general monetary measure of the value of life.

However, this is a global amount and hides factors that might be important for specific policy choices. What a person is willing to pay depends on the context. It includes the individual's evaluation of risks. People's aversions to risk vary with more than probability of death; they include other factors, such as whether the death results from a voluntarily undertaken risk, as in mountain climbing, or an involuntary risk, as from a nuclear power plant. In short, people are willing to pay different amounts to avoid the same chance of death from different causes.

A willingness-to-pay approach can take this consideration into account by asking how much an individual is willing to pay to avoid a risk of death from one cause, such as heart attack. More generally, one can ask how much an individual is willing to pay for a 10 percent reduction in deaths resulting from heart attack. This last change, however, is significant. One is no longer getting an indication of the individual's value of his or her own life. The person might also be considering that the life saved might be that of a spouse or other loved one. Indeed, an individual beyond reproductive years might be willing to pay some amount for a reduction in deaths to infants (e.g., low-birth-weight infants). By combining everyone's willingness to pay, one has a measure of society's value of the reduction of risk of death from some given cause. This evaluation will take into account distributional considerations and other factors. In short, one no longer has an evaluation of the value of life as merely one consequence of a choice, but rather an evaluation that takes into account all the different considerations as people in society judge them.

This is not necessarily a bad thing. The reason for considering the value of life was to help clarify decision making. The value of life was taken as only one of many factors that might be considered in deciding whether or not to undertake a program, and its limited scope can be thought to be a virtue; it does not try to do everything. What this last version of the willingness-to-pay model has provided, although perhaps not completely accurately, is the monetary value of a particular type of program, including its effect on the value of life. But this might be more useful than a merely monetary figure for the value of life, since the latter must still be balanced with various other considerations, such as distributive justice. The monetary value resulting from this version of willingness to pay has taken all these other factors into account. Thus, it can be directly compared with the total monetary costs of the program. It provides more of an answer than originally sought.

Nonetheless, there are difficulties with this approach. First, questionnaires and surveys of practice are perhaps not good ways of getting people's true views. People have considerable difficulty adequately appreciating small probabilities, such as a reduction of a one in 10,000 chance of dying from heart attack. Second, when asked about specific programs separately, people may be willing to spend more than in aggregate. For example, a person might be willing to spend five dollars for a reduction in heart attacks, five dollars for a reduction in deaths from renal failure, and so on for a large variety of causes of death. But if asked whether he or she would be willing to spend the total, the person might say no. This is only another version of the common problem of spending a few dollars here, a few there, and not considering what it all adds up to.

Third, one who accepts this approach is committed to accepting the existing moral views of the people in society. If people are not very benevolent, they will not be willing to spend much money to save the lives of others. People might not be willing to spend money to save the lives of persons affected by rare diseases, and those likely to be affected by them might not have enough money to pay for them. This is a problem in the drug industry, where the expectable income from discovering drugs to treat rare diseases, so-called orphan drugs, will not pay for the costs of their development. Perhaps people should be more concerned for others than they are. The response is that, in a democracy, one should not force people to pay for things from which they will not benefit; these decisions must rest on the will of the people, which the willingness-to-pay model encapsulates. The alternative is a moral dictatorship. This issue leads far beyond the scope of this chapter and cannot be pursued here.

Conclusions

Getting clear about the value of life might enable people to make better decisions affecting life and death. The fundamental unit of concern is quality-adjusted years per life. Individuals do, reasonably, trade length of life for quality of life, and the value of life to a person can be negative. Self-sacrifice, of life or of length of life, need not be irrational. Besides the personal value of life (the value to the one who lives it) one must also consider the social value of life (the value of the life to others). This includes at least three elements—emotional, personal service, and economic value—and can also be positive or negative.

The value of life can be relevant to decisions at three levels. One is the general allocation of resources between various types of programs, such as health and education. Decisions at this level cannot be much aided by considerations of the value of life, because it is unclear what the implications will be until specific programs are determined. The second level involves deciding between various programs given a sum of money. The third level concerns decisions between individuals, or groups of individuals, to be offered a program or existing services, such as intensive care.

Although society generally seems to value known or identifiable lives more than statistical lives, the arguments for such a differential valuing are not sound. This does not indicate which, if either, is correct, and it is plausible to believe that known lives are overvalued and statistical lives undervalued.

Cost-effectiveness analysis can be used to help decide allocations of funds between particular types of programs. Funding can be adjusted until benefits in quality-adjusted life years from different programs are roughly equal per unit of resource spent. It helps provide rational consistency between programs, but it cannot determine whether a program is worth pursuing at all. To determine this, one needs to use a cost-benefit analysis, for which it is practically necessary to express the value of lives in dollars.

Two major approaches have been developed to value lives in dollars. The human capital approach basically measures expectable future lifetime earnings. However, it omits a number of elements of social value as well as of personal value, and it probably overestimates economic social value.

The willingness-to-pay approach depends on how much people might pay for a given reduction in risk of death, or accept as compensation for an increased risk of death. It can provide a useful measure of personal value, but its use to include social value is difficult practically. A variation of this approach asks how much people would be willing to pay to have the risk of death from a given cause reduced by a specific amount. This version no longer measures the value of the individual's life, but rather the individual's willingness to spend for a specific program. It can reasonably reflect the actual desires or preferences of people, which seems to be appropriate in a democratic society, but it also might include moral judgments that are mistaken.

Neither version of the willingness-to-pay method is perfect. But they can both be used to provide information that can improve social decision making. Human lives have a finite value, and a reasonably good measure of that value is possible. To fail explicitly to obtain and use such information in making social decisions is irrational, and as the quality-adjusted length of people's lives will not be appropriately considered, it is also immoral.

Notes

Acknowledgments: This chapter benefited from the comments of Bruce Chapman and Benjamin Freedman on an earlier draft.

1. Jonathan Glover, "Assessing the Value of Saving Lives," in *Human Values*, ed. Godfrey Vesey (Atlantic Highlands, N.J.: Humanities Press, 1978), 210.

2. See generally, Richard B. Brandt, *A Theory of the Good and the Right* (Oxford: Clarendon Press, 1979).

3. In general, cost-effectiveness and cost-benefit analyses, of which the economic value of life is a part, should not be the sole determinants of health care decisions. See Office of Technology Assessment, *The Implications of Cost-Effectiveness Analysis of Medical Technology: Summary* (Washington, D.C.: U.S. Government Printing Office, 1980), 4,8.

4. A technical addition is needed for an adequate conceptual measure of the personal value of life. Because unconscious life is of no personal value, the Roman stoic philosopher Lucretius argued that death is nothing to one, for when one is dead, one does not experience. Consequently, it seems that if someone dies prematurely, no harm has been done to the person. The person does not experience disvalue. so long as one focuses on the time after the person is dead, no harm or injury is involved. Moreover, if one merely says that valuable life has been lost, then that valuable life might be replaced. Assuming the same average quality of life, there would be the same amount of personally valuable life if one person lived to age seventy as if two people lived to age thirty-five.

From a personal perspective, it does make a difference to me, to the value of my life, whether I live to age seventy or only to age thirty-five and am replaced by someone who has the same value of life for thirty-five years as I would have had. This point can be captured by using as the basic conceptual measurement of the personal value of life the quality-adjusted years per life. Thus, what makes life valuable to one who lives is the number of quality-adjusted years of that life. It follows that it is better for those who live, assuming equal quality of life, that there be one generation that lives to age 70 rather than two that each live to age 35. This addition, however does not make any difference if considerations are limited, as they are in this chapter, to people who are already alive.

5. John Broome, "Trying to Value a Life," *Journal of Public Economics* 9 (1978): 92.

6. Geoffrey York, "Doctors Will Study Rationing of Services," Toronto *Globe and Mail*, 1 June 1982, 1–2.

7. See Jonathan Glover, *Causing Death and Saving Lives* (New York: Penguin Books, 1977), 211–212.

8. See, for example, Philip B. Heymann and Sara Holtz, "The Severely Defective Newborn: The Dilemma and the Decision Process," *Public Policy* 23 (1975): 403.

9. This argument was suggested to me by a discussion in an unpublished paper by John Broome.

10. For a more detailed criticism of valuing known and statistical lives differently, see Charles Fried, "The Value of Life," *Harvard Law Review* 82 (1969): 1,415–1,437.

11. See Office of Technology Assessment, *Implications of Cost-Effectiveness Analysis*, 12.

12. See, for example, Heymann and Holtz, "The Severely Defective Newborn," 401.

13. See Richard Zeckhauser and Donald Shepard, "Where Now for Saving Lives?," *Law and Contemporary Problems* 40 (1976): 5–45, esp. 19–32, for examples of this approach.

14. For a more detailed survey, see Jan Paul Acton, "Measuring the Monetary Value of Lifesaving Programs," *Law and Contemporary Problems* 40 (1976): 46–72.

15. Glover mistakenly claims that it completely omits personal value ("Assessing the Value of Saving Lives," 224). It does not; it merely uses an implausible method of calculating it.

16. Joanne Linnerooth, "The Value of Human Life: A Review of the Models," *Economic Inquiry* 17 (1979): 64.

17. See my "The Price of Life," *Ethics* 89 (1978): 31–32.

Suggestions for Further Reading

Acton, Jan Paul. "Measuring the Monetary Value of Lifesaving Programs." *Law and Contemporary Problems* 40(1976): 46–72.

Bayles, Michael D. "The Price of Life." *Ethics* 89 (1978): 20–32.

Broome, John. "Trying to Value a Life." *Journal of Public Economics* 9 (1978): 91–100.

Fein, Rashi. "On Measuring Economic Benefits of Health Programs." In *Ethics and Health Policy*, ed. Robert M. Veatch and Roy Branson, 261–287. Cambridge, Mass: Ballinger Publishing, 1976.

Fried, Charles. "The Value of Life." *Harvard Law Review* 82 (1969): 1,415–1,437.

Glover, Jonathan. "Assessing the Value of Saving Lives." In *Human Values*, ed. Godfrey Vesey, 208–227. Atlantic Highlands, N.J.: Humanities Press, 1978.

———. *Causing Death and Saving Lives.* New York: Penguin Books, 1977. Chaps. 16–17.

Jones-Lee, M. W. *The Value of Life.* Chicago: University of Chicago Press, 1976.

Mishan, E. J. *Cost-Benefit Analysis.* Expanded ed. New York: Praeger Publishers, 1976. Chap. 45.

Office of Technology Assessment. *The Implications of Cost-Effectiveness Analysis of Medical Technology: Summary.* Washington, D.C.: U.S. Government Printing Office, 1980.

Schelling, T. C. "The Life You Save May Be Your Own." In *Problems in Public Expenditure Analysis*, ed. Samuel B. Chase, Jr., 127–162. Washington, D.C.: The Brookings Institution, 1968.

Zeckhauser, Richard; and Shepard, Donald. "Where Now for Saving Lives?" *Law and Contemporary Problems* 40 (1976): 5–45.

CHAPTER VIII

Justice and
Health Care

Norman Daniels

Introduction

MICRO AND MACRO

Medical ethics in general has focused on the *micro* or individual level of moral decision making. This focus is not surprising, for here dramatic issues abound. Should aggressive treatment be stopped for a terminal patient with metastasized bone cancer? Should a hydrocephalic newborn with spina bifida be treated at all? Which of several medically eligible patients with biliary atresia should receive the life-saving liver transplant? Should a leukemic child's parents be allowed to switch him from chemotherapy to Laetrile? Is a geriatric patient with Alzheimer's disease competent to agree to amputation of his foot and commitment to a nursing home? Should a physician tell one of his female patients that her finacé, who is also his patient, is homosexual or sterile? It is easy to imagine having to face these dilemmas as a patient, family member, or practitioner, which may explain their grip on us.

But there is a social or *macro* level of decision making that has been much less discussed by philosophers, even though it has an even greater impact on our health. The macro level concerns the scope and design of *basic health care institutions.* Most visible among these institutions is the complex system for delivering and financing the *personal medical services* that comprise acute care. This includes our system of high-technology hospital and clinic-based medicine, the training institutions for physicians, nurses, and allied professionals, and the research institutions supporting these forms of health services. Less visible among health care institutions are the various *public health agencies* concerned with preventive programs. Included here are the laws and agencies responsible for the control of infectious disease, drug and food protection, consumer product safety, and the regulation of health hazards in the environment, including the workplace. Health care also involves the institutions responsible for *social support* and *personal care services* needed by the mentally and physically disabled. Together, all these institutions distribute well over 10 percent of the total goods and services included in the U.S. gross national product.

JUSTICE AND MACRO DECISIONS

Macro decisions determine (1) what kinds of health care services will exist in a society, (2) who will get them and on what basis, (3) who will deliver them, and (4) how the burdens of financing them will be distributed. These decisions affect the *level* and *distribution* of the risks of our getting sick, the likelihood of our being cured, and the degree to which others will help us when we become impaired or dysfunctional. Because these macro decisions critically affect the level and distribution of our well-being, they involve issues of social justice.

No less than individual medical decisions, these important public policy decisions should be made in accord with acceptable moral principles. Such principles should serve as a public and final basis for resolving conflicts about how basic institutions, such as health care institutions, should be designed. These principles can thus serve as a framework within which planners and legislators can make more specific public policy decisions, about which there is often controversy because of conflicting interests.

A natural way to seek such principles of justice for regulating health care institutions is to examine different general theories of justice. Libertarian, utilitarian, and contractarian theories, for example, each support more general principles governing the distribution of rights, opportunities, and wealth, and these general principles may bear on the specific issue of health care.[1] But there is a central difficulty with this strategy. In order to apply such general theories to health care, we need to know what kind of a social good health care is. An analysis of this problem cannot be provided by appeal to the theories of justice themselves. One way to see the problem is to ask whether health care services, say personal medical services, should be viewed as we view other *commodities* in our society. Should we allow *inequalities* in the access to health care services to vary with whatever economic inequalities are permissible according to more general principles of distributive justice? Or is health care "special" and not to be assimiliated to other commodities, like cars or personal computers, whose distribution we allow to be governed by market exchange among economic unequals?

The strategy to be followed in this chapter will be to focus first on answering the question, "Is health care *special?*" To answer it, we will have to analyze the notion of health care *needs* and distinguish needs from *mere preferences*. Health care needs, it will be argued, are specially important because of their effects on *opportunity*. This result suggests that a general principle of justice governing the distribution of opportunity can be extended to include the regulation of health care institutions. Before taking up these theoretical issues, it will be useful to examine how public controversy about health care delivery focuses on the question of whether health care is special.

Current Public Policy Issues

Issues of distributive justice lie at the center of much current debate about health care delivery. They underlie demands for more equal access to personal medical services, for more rational planning of medical and other health care resources, and for more effective regulation of health care providers to ensure cost control and quality accountability. These demands interact in complex ways.

Access to Health Care

The issue of access to health care is really two issues: access for whom? and access to what? To many, the first question has a very simple answer. There should be access to medical services for anyone in *medical need*. Specifically, nonmedical features of individuals—their race, sex, geographical location, or ability to pay—should not determine whether or not they have access to care. Sometimes the point is asserted as a claim of right: individuals have a right to health care and a wrong is done to them if their medical needs are not met. Minimally, what is demanded is that certain nonmedical barriers to care should be eliminated (i.e., society has an obligation to provide medical services on the basis of medical need, regardless of the ability to pay).

To support such a view, some offer what we may call the "argument from function":

1. The function of medical services is to meet medical needs.
2. The sole rational basis for distributing a good that functions to meet certain needs is in proportion to those needs.
3. Therefore, the sole rational basis for distributing medical services is to meet medical needs.
4. Therefore, health status should determine access to medical services.[2]

But this argument will not do as it stands. The *function* of food processors is to meet vegetable slicing needs. But no one insists that the willingness to pay for food processors is an inappropriate basis for distributing them and that access to them should be subsidized for those who cannot pay. Similarly, no one insists on a "right" to Cuisinarts. Clearly, if the argument from function has any merit, it is only with regard to a special class of needs and things that function to meet them. Similarly, if there is a right to health care, it is because of the kind of social good health care is, the *kind* of needs it meets. We are back to our question, "Is health care special?"

It is important to put this recent concern about access to health care in historical perspective. Before the emergence of scientific, efficacious medicine, medical care had relatively little effect on health.[3] Access to it was clearly less important or urgent. But the increased scientific and technological basis for medical services also increased its costs dramatically, so access to it became far more difficult beginning in the middle part of this century. A rational way to distribute the burden of facing such expensive but important services is to pool the risks and costs through public or private insurance schemes. In the United States, private, third-party payer schemes, largely in the form of tax-sheltered group insurance plans for employees, thus grew after World War II to replace a system of direct patient payments to physicians and hospitals.[4] By the mid-1960s, it became clear that major gaps existed in insurance coverage, and thus in access to care. If financial barriers to care were to be reduced, large public subsidies would be needed. Medicaid and Medicare were established to guarantee health care financing to the very poor and the elderly, two of the largest groups without private insurance coverage. Important "coverage gaps" remain, notably among those temporarily out of work who fail to meet state eligibility re-

294 · NORMAN DANIELS

quirements for Medicaid. Indeed, a full twenty-five million Americans have *no* insurance coverage at all![5] Still, these public programs, along with efforts to bring providers to "medically underserved" areas through urban neighborhood health centers and rural programs, had a significant impact in reducing inequalities in the rates of use of personal medical services, though recent budget cutbacks threaten to reverse the trend.

But as public policy has moved in the direction of reducing some —if not all—barriers to access to care, it has had to face more directly the question, "Access to what?" Health care services are *nonhomogeneous*. Some services save or extend lives; others improve the quality of life. Some functions are more important, more basic, or more urgent than others. Should we guarantee access to *all* the services offered anywhere in our health care system? Or should we provide only a key set of services, defined by reference to some central or basic function, regardless of their availability within our system? Is there a social obligation to provide access to all services or only to a basic minimum? Mrs. Bow, a welfare mother in Boston's Bromley Heath housing project, is not fed or sheltered as well as Mr. Arrow, a hospital administrator living in expensive Chestnut Hill. Should Medicaid guarantee that her access to health care be equal to his? This is another form of the question, "Is health care special?"

RESOURCE ALLOCATION AND RATIONING

The question, "Access to what?" already raises some questions about resource allocation and rationing, but the issue is more general. So far, in inquiring about access, we have taken the medical services provided in our health care system as a given. But we can ask an even more basic question: What kinds of services should the system provide? And, if not all services can be provided because resources are restricted, then which are the most important to provide? Should we concentrate on delivering a liver transplant to little Jamie Fisk or Brandon Hall and an artificial heart to Barney Clark? Or should we restore recent cuts in funding for prenatal and maternal care? Or should we revitalize enforcement of existing workplace health-hazard regulations governing lead, asbestos, and cotton dust, which has been lax because of the antiregulation stance of the Reagan administration?

In general, many critics of our health care system have argued that it is biased in favor of high-technology, acute care and ignores preventive measures, which are of comparable or greater importance, even if less glamorous or profitable. Others complain of a similar bias in favor of acute care over other kinds of personal health care and social support services. Thus, Mr. Styx, dying of colon cancer, has had the full range of exotic, hospital-based care his physician has ordered for his seventy-eight-year-old-body, but Mrs. Frail, who is seventy-five and partially disabled, faces a critical absence of adequate long-term care or home care services. Even if we decide that access to health care should be based on need for services, which needs should we meet when we cannot meet all? Here we need guidance in deciding which health care services are more special than others. This question is not faced squarely by current proposals to control Medicare costs by increasing the proportion of "cost sharing" or out-of-pocket payments. Mrs. Angst, who was hospitalized twice last year for brief periods, is frightened that she will be forced to "stick it out" at home when the next episode of her illness strikes.

PROVIDER RESPONSIBILITIES AND AUTONOMY

Just as there is no "free lunch," and whatever health care society provides must be paid for by someone, so too it must be prepared by someone. Issues of access and demands about resource allocation both have a bearing on the traditional roles and responsibilities of health care providers. If society believes it must guarantee access to medical services to the rural and inner-city poor, then some physicians, nurses, and technicians must be there to deliver them. If society insists that certain medical services must be made available— say, more primary care for the elderly—then some physicians will have to have geriatric training and forego other specialties. If society believes that diagnostic and therapeutic services must be delivered in a cost-effective fashion, and it insists that physicians take such costs into account in their medical decision making, then we may have to modify the traditional view that physicians should do everything possible to pursue their patients' best interests. These examples point to possible conflicts between the traditional liberties, privileges, and responsibilities of providers and the requirements of justice. It is the problem of the "specialness" of health care that forces us to examine the reasons we have for extending to providers their traditional autonomy and power.

BASES OF CONTROVERSY

Some of the controversy about these issues reflects a simple conflict of interest between providers and consumers. Providers have vested interests in a system that traditionally has guaranteed enormous power and autonomy, as well as healthy incomes and profits. The introduction of considerations of justice and the social controls they involve presents a clear threat to those interests. Some of the controversy over these issues reflects a conflict of class interests: If redistributive financing of health care is a social obligation, it is the middle- and upper-income groups who will bear the burden of increased costs.

But these sources of economic and political conflict are also interwoven with clear moral disagreements. Much of the controversy in this area reflects conflicting views about the nature of health care as a social good: Namely, how special is it? And some of the controversy mirrors more general disagreements about the demands of social justice. It is to these matters that we now turn by attempting to develop a theory of health care needs. Such a theory must come to grips with two widely held judgments: First, that there is something important about health care, and second, that some kinds of health care are more important than others. In various ways, these judgments have influenced our public policy concerning access and resource allocation in health care. The philosophical task is to assess, explain, and justify or modify distinctions we make about the importance of different wants, interests, and needs.

Can We Avoid Talking About Needs?

Consider the following "argument from fair shares,"[6] which is intended to show we can avoid talk about health care needs. Suppose we agreed on a theory of distributive justice and knew that we each had a *fair income share* according to that theory. Suppose further that there was a *competitive medical market* in which a variety of insurance schemes could be bought, much as some employees have a choice between enrolling in one of several prepaid group plans, (such as health maintenance organizations, or HMOs) or various traditional insurance schemes (e.g., Blue-Cross/Blue Shield, Aetna). Then we could protect ourselves against the risk of needing health care through voluntary purchase of insurance. We would each be responsible for buying insurance at the level of protection we desired. No one (except children or the congenitally handicapped) would have a *claim* on *social* resources to meet health care needs. Each would be entitled—whatever his needs—only to what he was prudent enough to purchase from his fair income share (though charity might intervene to keep people from dying in the streets). In this market (so the argument assumes), demand, understood as our preferences for different insurance packages, will be *efficiently* matched to supply, understood as resources and services.[7]

Such a system would provide protection against expensive but rare needs for health care, for which relatively inexperience insurance can be bought. Similarly, common but inexpensive services can either be risk shared through insurance or paid for out of pocket without great sacrifice, whichever is preferred. But expensive and potentially common "needs"—for example, to be provided with artificial hearts or dialysis—would not become a drain on social resources. Individuals who wanted protection against facing these "needs" would have to buy expensive insurance out of their own fair shares. This way of meeting individual preferences for health services would not create a bottomless pit into which we are forced to drain all available social resources. No one could claim a right to have extravagant "needs" met—unless he had already bought appropriate insurance. Most important, we would need no general theory about which health care needs we have social obligations to meet. The scheme allows individual preferences to resolve all resource allocation questions through a medical market.

The argument from fair shares fails to show that we can do without a theory of health care needs. Suppose we define a *reasonable* health care insurance package as one that meets the health care needs or risks it is rational for prudent persons to insure against. Though we know little else about "fair income shares," it seems plausible to insist that an income share is "fair" only if it is adequate to permit the purchase of a reasonable insurance package. If an income share is too small to cover the premium for a reasonable insurance package, then the share is inadequate: it is unfair that whoever has it cannot buy reasonable insurance. So, to know whether income shares are fair, we must know that they can buy reasonable coverage. But to know what coverage is reasonable, we need to know what health care needs it is prudent to insure against. Thus we must talk about health care needs after all. We cannot reduce the problem of just health care distribution to the problem of just income distribution, for the latter presupposes income adequate to meet reasonable *needs*.

A theory of health care needs is implicit in the insurance scheme approach in yet another way. The approach puts health care needs on a par with other wants and preferences, allowing them to compete for resources within a medical market. But this stance *is* a view of health care needs: It treats them as one kind of preference among many, with no special claim on social resources except that which derives from *strength of preference* (or willingness to pay for insurance). To be sure, where strength of preference is high, needs may be met, but strength of preference may vary in ways that fail to reflect the importance we ought to (and usually do) ascribe to health care. Such a market view needs justification, and it is not a justification simply to point to the existence of such a market.

Needs and Preference

NOT ALL PREFERENCES ARE CREATED EQUAL

The conclusion of the preceding argument is that we must talk about health care *needs* if we are to give an account of distributive justice for health care. But the concept of needs is slippery. Without abuse of language, we refer to the means necessary to reach any of our goals as *needs*. To reawaken memories of Miller's, the neighborhood delicatessen of my childhood, I *need* only the smell of pickles in a barrel. To stay at Cape Cod next weekend, I *need* a motel reservation. Since the concept of needs is so expansive, the problem of the importance of needs seems to reduce to the problem of the importance or urgency of preferences or wants in general (leaving aside the fact that not all the things we need are even expressed as preferences).

Just as not all preferences are on a par—some are more important than others—so too not all the things we say we need are equally important. It is possible to pick out various things we say we need, including needs for health care, which play a special role and are given a special weight in a variety of moral contexts. If I appeal to my friend's duty of beneficence in requesting $100, I most likely will get a quite different reaction if I tell him I need the money to get a root-canal than if I tell him I need the money to go to the Brooklyn neighborhood of my childhood to smell pickles in a barrel. Indeed, it is not likely to matter in his assessment of *obligations* that I strongly *prefer* to go to Brooklyn. Nor is it likely to matter that I insist I feel a great *need* to reawaken memories of my childhood—I am overcome by nostalgia. Of course, he might give me the money for either purpose, but if he gives it so I can smell pickles, we would probably say he is not doing it out of any duty at all, that he feels no obligation, that it is just friendly generosity.

Part of what is going on here is that in certain contexts we use an *objective* rather than a *subjective* criterion in assessing well-being.[8] A *subjective* criterion uses the individual's own assessment of how well-off he is with and without the claimed benefit to determine the importance of his preference or claim. An *objective* criterion invokes a measure of importance independent of an individual's own assessment (i.e., independent of the individual's strength of preference for the benefit). But it is important to see that it is not just a question of rejecting subjective criteria in favor of objective ones, say on the grounds that we can have better knowledge of them. What counts is the *kind* of objective criterion we invoke.

Suppose we adopted a view central to utilitarian (and egoist) theory, that how well-off an individual is depends on the level of satisfaction of *all* his various preferences. How well-off someone is depends on how much of what he wants in life he has gotten. The view requires that we be concerned with the *full* or *complete* range of an individual's preferences and their satisfaction. Suppose further that we could agree intersubjectively on how satisfied individuals are: we agree, that is, on a "social utility function." Such a "full range" standard would be *objective* and not merely subjective. But that objectivity would not be sufficient grounds for using the *complete* scale to assess the importance of certain preferences or to measure the relevant notion of well-being in various moral contexts. Indeed, in our actual moral practice, especially where we are concerned with issues of distributive justice, we do not use any such full-range or complete scale of well-being.

What is distinctive about the scale we do use for measuring well-being and assessing the importance of an individual's preference is that it does not include or reflect the full range of kinds of preferences people have. Rather, we use a *truncated* or *selective* scale.[9] The satisfaction of preferences falling into certain categories (e.g. the satisfaction of certain needs) weighs heavily in the truncated scale; the satisfaction of certain other preferences may not be counted or viewed as relevant at all. It is sensitivity to the use of this truncated scale that would lead me to admit that the root-canal, but not the smell of pickles in a barrel, is something I *really* need (assuming the dentist is right). It is a need and not a "mere desire." My admission is an awareness that some of the things we claim to need fall into special categories that give them a weightier moral claim in contexts involving the distribution of resources, depending, of course, on how well-off we already are within those categories of need.[10]

So far I have not shown that we *ought* to use such a truncated scale. I have only claimed that our moral practice uses one in favor of a full-range or complete scale of well-being. That is, I have said something about what our moral practice is, not what that practice ought to be. Later, I shall return to argue more directly in favor of the appropriateness of a selective scale, but it first will be helpful to continue our examination of the concept of needs already embodied in these moral practices. Our philosophical task will be to characterize the relevant categories of needs in a way that *explains* two central properties they have. First, they are *objectively ascribable*. We can ascribe them to someone even if he does not realize he has them or even if he denies he does because his preferences run contrary to his needs. Second, and of greater interest to us, these needs are *objectively important*: we attach a special weight to claims based on them in a variety of moral contexts. Our task is to characterize the class of things we need that has these properties and to do so in a way that explains their importance.

NEEDS AND SPECIES-TYPICAL FUNCTIONING

One plausible suggestion for distinguishing the relevant needs from all the things we can come to need is David Braybrooke's distinction between "course-of-life needs" and "adventitious needs." *Adventitious needs* are the things we need because of the particular contingent projects (which may be long-term ones) on which we embark. Their relative importance will reflect many idiosyncratic facts about our personal choice of a plan of life. *Course-of-life needs* are those needs that people "have all through their lives or at certain stages of life through which all must pass." They include food, shelter, clothing, exercise, rest, companionship, a mate (in one's prime), and so on. Such needs are not themselves deficiencies, for example, when they are anticipated. But a deficiency with respect to them "endangers the normal functioning of the subject of need, *considered as a member of a natural species*."[11] Thus course-of-life needs are important when we abstract from many particular choices and preferences individuals might make or have.

Our hypothesis, then, is that the needs that interest us are necessary to achieve or maintain species-typical normal functioning. Do such needs have the two properties noted earlier? Clearly they are objectively ascribable, assuming we can come up with the appropriate notion of species-typical functioning. (So, incidentally, are adventitious needs, assuming we can determine the relevant goals by reference to which the adventitious needs become determinate.) Are these needs objectively important in the appropriate way? In a broad range of contexts, we do treat them as such—a claim I shall not trouble to argue. What is of interest is to see *why* being in such a need category gives them their special importance.

A tempting first answer might be this: whatever our specific chosen goals or tasks, our ability to achieve them (and consequently our happiness) will be diminished if we fall short of normal species functioning. So whatever our specific goals, we need them whatever else we need. For example, it is sometimes said that whatever our chosen goals or tasks, we need our health, and so we need appropriate health care. But this claim is not, strictly speaking, true. For many of us, some of our goals, perhaps even those we feel are most important to us, are not necessarily undermined by failing health or disability. Moreover, we can often adjust our goals—and presumably our levels of satisfaction—to fit better with our dysfunction or disability. Coping in this way does not necessarily diminish happiness or satisfaction in life.

Still, there is a clue here to a more plausible account. Impairments of normal species functioning reduce the range of opportunity we have within which to construct "plans of life" or "conceptions of the good." Life plans we are otherwise suited for and have a reasonable expectation of finding satisfying or happiness-producing are rendered unreasonable by impairments of normal functioning, as when, say, a ballerina is paralyzed or a mechanic loses a hand. Similarly, if persons have a higher-order interest in preserving the opportunity to revise their conceptions of the good through time, then they will have a pressing interest in maintaining normal species functioning by establishing institutions—such as health care systems—that do just that. So the kinds of needs picked out by reference to normal species functioning are objectively important because they meet this high-order interest persons have in maintaining a normal range of opportunities. I shall try to refine this admittedly vague answer, but first I want to characterize health care needs more specifically and show that they fit within this more general framework.

Health Care Needs

DISEASE AND HEALTH

To specify a notion of health care needs, we need clear notions of health and disease. I shall begin with a narrow, if not uncontroversial, "biomedical" model of disease and health. The basic idea is that health is the absence of disease, and disease (I here include deformities and disabilities that result from trauma) are *deviations from the natural functional organization of a typical member of a species.*[12] The task of characterizing this natural functional organization falls to the biomedical sciences, which must include evolutionary theory, since claims about the design of the species and its fitness to meeting biological goals underlie at least some of the relevant functional ascriptions. (Thus the concept of disease is not merely a statistical notion—such as deviation from the statistical norm.) The task is the same for man and beast, with two complications. For human beings, we require an account of the species-typical functions that permit us to pursue biological goals as social animals. So there must be a way of characterizing the species-typical apparatus underlying such functions as the acquisition of knowledge, linguistic communication, and social cooperation. Moreover, adding mental disease and health into the picture, which we must do, complicates the issue further, most particularly because we have a less well-developed theory of species-typical mental functions and functional organization. The biomedical model clearly presupposes that we eventually can supply the missing account and that a reasonable part of what we now take to be psychopathology would show up as disease.[13]

The biomedical model has controversial features. First, some insist it too narrowly defines health as the absence of disease, a narrowness that encourages too much focus on acute care. In contrast, some—as in the World Health Organization's definition[14]—view health as an idealized level of well-being. But health is not happiness, and confusing the two overmedicalizes social philosophy. Nor does a "narrow" view of disease mean that we should ignore its social etiology. Second, some insist the concept of disease is not descriptive, as in the biomedical model, but normative: a disease is a deviation from a social norm.[15] But even if some conditions or behaviors have historically been *viewed* as diseases—for example, "drapetomania" (the running-away disease of slaves) or masturbation—such views do not *make* them diseases. Nor does the fact that many diseases are discovered and treated only when people complain about them make their complaints a necessary feature of having a disease. The biomedical model, of course, allows us to make normative judgments about diseases (such as which ones are undesirable) and justify our entering a "sick role." These normative judgments yield the normative notion of illness, not the theoretically more basic notion of disease (which thus departs from looser ordinary usage.)[16]

Some pure forms of the biomedical model also involve a deeper claim, namely that species-typical functional organization can itself be characterized without invoking normative or value judgments. Here the debate turns on hard issues in the philosophy of biology.[17] Fortunately, these need not detain us, since our discussion does not turn on so strong a claim. It is enough for our purposes that the line between disease and the absence of disease is, for the general run of cases, uncontroversial and ascertainable through publicly acceptable methods, such as those of the biomedical sciences. It will not matter if there is some relativization of what counts as a disease category to some features of social roles in a given society, and thus to some normative judgments, provided the core of the notion of species-typical functioning is left intact. The model, I presume, would still count infertility as a disease, even though some or many individuals might prefer to be infertile and seek medical treatment to render themselves so. Similarly, unwanted pregnancy is not a disease. Again, dysfunctional noses are diseases, since noses have normal species functions and anatomy. If the dysfunction or deformity is serious, it might warrant treatment as an illness. But deviation of nasal anatomy from individual or social conceptions of beauty does not constitute disease.[18]

Thus the modified biomedical model allows us to draw a fairly sharp line between uses of health care services to prevent and treat diseases and uses to meet other social goals. The importance of such other goals may be different and may rest on other bases, as in the cases of induced infertility or unwanted pregnancy. My intention is to show which principles of justice are relevant to distributing health care services where we can take as fixed, primarily by nature, a generally uncontroversial baseline of species-typical functional organization.

Although I have deliberately selected a rather narrow model of disease and health, at least by comparison with some fashionable construals, health care needs emerge as a broad and diverse set. Health care needs will be those things we need in order to maintain, restore, or provide functional equivalents (when possible) to normal species functioning. They can be divided into:

1. Adequate nutrition and shelter.
2. Sanitary, safe, unpolluted living and working conditions.
3. Exercise, rest, and other features of healthy lifestyles.
4. Preventive, curative, and rehabilitative personal medical services.
5. Nonmedical personal (and social) support services.

Of course, we do not tend to think of all these things as included among health care needs, partly because we tend to think narrowly about personal medical services when we think about health care. But the list is constructed not to conform to our ordinary notion of health care but rather to point out a functional relation between quite diverse goods and services and the various institutions responsible for delivering them.

DISEASE AND OPPORTUNITY

I have argued that not all preferences are of equal moral importance and that when we judge the importance of meeting someone's preferences we use a restricted or truncated measure of well-being. Among the kinds of preferences to which we tend to give special weight are those that meet certain "important" categories of need. I have argued that the important needs include those necessary for maintaining normal functioning for individuals, viewed as members of a natural species. Health care needs fit prominently into this characterization of important needs because they are things that we need if we are to prevent or cure diseases, which are deviations from normal functional organization.

But we now need to fill an important gap in this argument: why give such moral importance to health care needs, and the somewhat broader class of needs within which they fall, merely because they are necessary to preserve normal species functioning? What is so important about normal species functioning? To answer this question, I shall develop the remark made earlier about the relationship between species-typical functioning and opportunity. We shall need to introduce the notion of a normal opportunity range.

The *normal opportunity range* for a given society is the array of life plans reasonable persons in it are likely to construct for themselves. The range is thus relative to key features of the society—its stage of historical development, its level of material wealth and technological development, and even important cultural facts about it. Facts about social organization, including the conception of justice regulating its basic institutions, will of course determine how that total normal range is distributed in the population. Nevertheless, that issue of distribution aside, normal species-typical functioning provides us with one clear parameter relevant to determining what share of the normal range is open to a given individual. However, the share of the normal range open to an individual is also *determined to a significant extent by his talents and skills.* (Thus, individual shares are not in general *equal*, even if they are *fair* to the individual.) So impairment of normal functioning through disease (and disability) constitutes a fundamental restriction on individual opportunity *relative to that portion of the normal range his skills and talents would ordinarily have made available to him.*

Of course, we also know that skills and talents can be undeveloped or misdeveloped because of social conditions (e.g., because of adverse family situations or racist educational practices). So, if we are interested in having individuals enjoy a fair share of the normal opportunity range, we will want to correct for special disadvantages here, too, say through compensatory educational programs. Still, restoring normal functioning through health care shares has a particular and limited effect on an individual's share of the normal range. It lets him enjoy that portion of the range to which his full range of skills and talents would give him access, assuming that these too are not impaired by special social disadvantages. There is, however, no presumption of eliminating individual differences: *these act as a baseline constraint on the degree to which individuals enjoy the normal range.*

Two points about the normal opportunity range need emphasis. First, some diseases constitute more serious curtailments of opportunity than others relative to a given range. But because normal ranges are defined by reference to particular societies, the same disease in two societies may impair opportunity differently and so have its importance assessed differently. For example, dyslexia might be less important to treat (suppose we could cure it with brain surgery) in an illiterate society than in a literate one. Thus the social importance of particular diseases is a notion we ought to relativize between societies.

Second, within a society, the normal opportunity range abstracts from important individual differences in what might be called *effective opportunity.* From the perspective of an individual who has a

306 · NORMAN DANIELS

particular plan of life and who has developed certain skills accordingly, the effective opportunity range will be only a part of his fair share of the normal range. Suppose a college teacher and a skilled laborer each finds his manual dexterity impaired by disease. The impairment of the effective opportunity range for the skilled laborer may be greater than for the college teacher, but if both originally had comparable dexterity, their shares of the normal range would be equally affected by the disease. By measuring the effect on opportunity by reference to (share of) the normal range and not the effective range, I abstract from the special effects that derive from an individual's conception of the good. This level of abstraction seems appropriate given our search for a measure of the social importance, for claims of justice, of impairments of health.[19]

My conclusion is that we should use impairment of the normal opportunity range as a fairly crude measure of the relative importance of health care needs at the macro level. In general, it will be more important to prevent, cure, or compensate for those disease conditions that involve a greater curtailment of normal opportunity range. Of course, impairment of normal species functioning has another distinct effect. It can diminish satisfaction or happiness for an individual, as judged by that individual's conception of the good. Such effects are important at the micro level—for example, to individual decision making about health care utilization. But I am here seeking the appropriate framework within which to apply principles of justice to health care at the macro level. So we shall need to look further at considerations that weigh against appeals to satisfaction at the macro level.

Toward a Distributive Theory

"SATISFACTION" AND SOCIAL HIJACKING

I have been describing and explaining certain features of our moral practice: in many moral contexts, including those of justice, we use a scale of well-being that is selective or truncated. It gives more weight or importance to certain kinds of preferences over others. These "importance" preferences or needs, including health care needs, seem to be necessary for maintaining normal species functioning. In turn, such normal functioning affects an individual's share of the normal opportunity range. But this effect allows us to explain why people treat such needs as special and important: people have a fundamental interest in protecting their share of the normal range of opportunities. This description and explanation fall short of giving us a normative account in two ways, which now need to be addressed.

One issue was left hanging in our earlier discussion. Should we, for purposes of justice, use the objective, truncated scale of well-being we happen to use rather than a more complete measure of satisfaction? This question is a general one that takes us beyond the scope of this chapter. Moreover, considering the health care context alone is not likely to yield a conclusive case for or against either scale. For example, a utilitarian might argue that any social application of a satisfaction scale would depend on the general tendencies of types of health care needs to improve levels of satisfaction, and that such an approach would be roughly equivalent to seeing the ways in which health care needs affect opportunity.[20] Still, it is worth suggesting some considerations that weigh against the use of a satisfaction scale.

Consider a special case in which our moral judgment inclines us against using a complete satisfaction scale, namely the case of "social hijacking" by persons with expensive tastes.[21] Suppose we judge how well-off someone is by reference to the full range of individual preferences in a satisfaction scale. Suppose further that *moderate* people adjust their tastes and preferences so that they have a reasonable chance of being satisfied with their share of social goods. *Extravagant* people, however, form exotic and expensive tastes, and they are desperately unhappy when their preferences are not satisfied. Since the extravagants are so unhappy compared with moderates, should we increase their shares? It seems unjust to deny the moderates equal claims on further distributions just because they have been modest in forming their tastes. Rather, it seems reasonable to hold people responsible for their unhappiness when it results from extravagant preferences that could have been otherwise.[22]

THE SCOPE OF JUSTICE

A more general division of responsibility is suggested by this hijacking case. John Rawls urges that we hold *society* responsible for guaranteeing the individual a fair share of basic liberties, opportunity, and all-purpose means, like income and wealth, needed for pursuing individual conceptions of the good. But we should hold *indi-*

viduals responsible for choosing their ends in such a way that they have a reasonable chance of satisfying them under just arrangements.[23] Consequently, the special features of a person's own system of preferences do not give rise to special claims of justice on social resources—despite levels of dissatisfaction.

This suggestion about a division of responsibility is actually a fundamental claim about the *scope* of theories of justice. Just arrangements are supposed to guarantee individuals a reasonable share of certain basic or primary social goods—and these primary goods constitute for Rawls the relevant, truncated scale of well-being *for purposes of justice.* (We shall come shortly to the problem of fitting together Rawls's scale and my talk about needs.) The immediate object of justice is not, then, happiness or the satisfaction of desires, though just institutions provide individuals with an acceptable framework within which they may pursue happiness. But in this pursuit, individuals remain responsible for the choice of their ends, so there is no injustice in not providing them with means sufficient to reach extravagant ends.

A full defense of this claim about the scope of justice and the social division of responsibility, and thus for the restriction to a truncated scale of well-being, cannot rest on isolated moral intuitions like those appealed to in the hijacking example. Thus, Rawls's full argument for his view depends on showing that adopting a satisfaction scale commits us to an unacceptable view of the nature of persons. It forces us to view them as mere "containers" for satisfaction. Such a view departs significantly from acceptable views of moral agents or persons.[24] I must be content here to suggest that there are deep problems facing attempts to abandon our moral practice, with its truncated scales of well-being, in favor of a complete scale.

FAIR EQUALITY OF OPPORTUNITY AND HEALTH CARE

In this chapter, we set out to answer the question, "Is health care special?" Our analysis suggests that health care has a direct impact on the opportunity enjoyed by individuals. If we could show that justice required guaranteeing fair equality of opportunity, then we could complete our justification of the importance we attribute to meeting health care needs. We would then be able to assert that the social obligation to meet health care needs derives from the more general social obligation to guarantee fair equality of opportunity. Unfortunately, showing that justice requires guaranteeing fair equality of opportunity would take us into difficult problems at the heart of the general theory of justice. Still, a few remarks about equality of opportunity will be helpful.

Liberal political philosophy has relied on what is essentially a *procedural* notion, equality of opporunity, to justify a system in which unequal *outcomes* are thought morally acceptable. It is all right that there are winners and losers, provided the race is fair. Since the major rewards in our socioeconomic system derive from jobs and offices, the competition for securing these positions must be "fair." Specifically, certain irrelevant features of persons—race, religion, ethnic origin, sex—must not be the basis on which people are selected for positions. Rather, their talents and skills, at least those relevant to the positions being sought, should determine who is selected and ultimately rewarded. In Rawls's theory, for example, inequalities are justified on the grounds that it would be irrational to rule out inequalities that work to the benefit of the worst-off individuals. But a proviso is included: competition for positions must be fair, and a fair equality of opportunity principle is given high priority in the theory of justice.

Even this narrow notion of equal opportunity is both problematic and controversial. It is conceptually problematic for several reasons. Some claim it is illusory: irreducible differences between persons will always make opportunity greater for some in competitive situations. We cannot "level" people down to bare personhood. Suppose that we accept some irreducible differences in talents and skills as a natural baseline, as was suggested when we defined normal opportunity range. Some will argue that any such baseline is morally arbitrary. Others will cite the ineliminable effects of family influences on the development of talents and skills. This suggests that the goal of equal opportunity is unrealizable—unless, that is, we threaten liberty by interfering with parental autonomy in drastic ways. This conflict with liberty suggests another reason that equality of opportunity is controversial: some construe it as a negative constraint, requiring that we refrain from imposing certain barriers; others insist it imposes a positive obligation to correct for all the influences that interfere with equal opportunity. Distributive theories differ dramatically on these issues, and resolving them would take us far beyond our task here.

We shall have to settle for less, and in particular for a weaker, conditional justification. Specifically, *if* an acceptable theory of justice includes a principle that requires basic institutions to provide for fair equality of opportunity, then health care institutions should be among those governed by it. This weaker claim does not depend on the acceptability of any particular theory of justice. For example, a principle of fair equality of opportunity might be part of a system of principles, a moral code, general compliance with which would produce at least as much utility as any alternative code. We would then have a utilitarian theory of justice that supported the principle. That utilitarian theory could then be extended to health care through the analysis in this chapter. In fact, the main theory that has incorporated a fair equality of opportunity principle is John Rawls's contractarian theory of justice as fairness. In the next section, I shall suggest how Rawls's theory can be extended to health care, through its fair equality of opportunity principle. But this exercise is intended to clarify how such a general theory can be made to fit with the analysis we have been offering. It is not an endorsement of Rawls's theory; nor does the weak, conditional claim depend on the acceptability of justice as fairness.

EXTENDING RAWLS'S THEORY TO HEALTH CARE

Rawls's *index of primary social goods*—his truncated scale of well-being used by parties "contracting" to choose principles of justice —includes five types of social goods:

1. A set of basic liberties.
2. Freedom of movement and choice of occupations against a background of diverse opportunities.
3. Powers and prerogatives of office.
4. Income and wealth.
5. The social bases of self-respect.

Actually, Rawls uses two simplifying assumptions when using the index to assess how well-off representative individuals are. First, income and wealth are used as approximations to the whole index. Thus the two principles of justice[25] require basic structures to maximize the long-term expectations of the least advantaged, estimated by their income and wealth, given fixed background institutions that guarantee equal basic liberties and fair equality of opportunity. Second, the theory is *idealized* to apply to individuals who are "normal, active, and fully cooperating members of society over the course of a complete life."[26] *There is no distributive theory for health care because no one is sick.*

This simplification seems to put Rawls's index at odds with the thrust of my earlier discussion, for the truncated scale of well-being we in fact use includes needs for health care. Rawls's index of primary goods seems to be *too* truncated a scale, once we drop the idealizing assumption that all people are normal. People with equal indices will not be equally well-off once we allow them to differ in health care needs. Moreover, we cannot simply dismiss these needs as irrelevant to questions of justice as we did when we said people should be held responsible for their tastes and preferences (we are supposing that individuals are not responsible for the disease they have, a simplification we return to later). But if we simply build another entry into the index, we raise thorny issues about how to weight the index items.[27] Similarly, if we treat health care services as a distinct primary social good, we abandon the useful generality of the notion of a primary social good: we risk generating a long list of such goods, one to meet each important need.[28] Finally, as I argued earlier, we cannot just finesse the question of whether there are special issues of justice in the distribution of health care by assuming fair shares of primary goods will be used in part to buy decent health insurance. A constraint on the adequacy of those shares is that they permit one to buy reasonable protection—so we must already know what justice requires by way of reasonable health care.

The most promising strategy for extending Rawls's theory simply includes health care institutions among the basic institutions involved in providing for fair equality of opportunity.[29] Because meeting health care needs has an important effect on the distribution of opportunity, the health care institutions are regulated by a fair equality of opportunity principle.[30] Once we note the special connection of normal species functioning to the opportunity range open to an individual, this strategy seems the natural way to extend Rawls's view noted earlier, about the *scope* of theories of social justice. Health care institutions will help provide the framework of liberties and opportunities within which individuals can use fair income shares to pursue their own conceptions of the good.

Including health care institutions among those that are to protect fair equality of opportunity is compatible with the central intuitions behind wanting to guarantee such opportunity. Rawls is concerned primarily with *the opportunity to pursue careers*—jobs and offices—that have various benefits attached to them. So equality of opportunity is *strategically* important: a person's well-being will be measured for the most part by the primary goods that accompany placement in such jobs and offices. Rawls argues that it is not enough simply to eliminate formal or legal barriers to persons seeking such jobs—for example, race, class, ethnic, or sex barriers. Rather, positive steps should be taken to enhance the opportunity of those disadvantaged by such social factors as family background.[31] The point is that none of us *deserves* the advantages conferred by accidents of birth—either the genetic or social advantages. These advantages from the "natural lottery" are morally arbitrary, and to let them determine individual opportunity—and reward and success in life—is to confer arbitrariness on the outcomes. So positive steps, such as through the educational system, are to be taken to provide fair equality of opportunity.[32]

But if it is important to use resources to counter the advantages in opportunity some get in the natural lottery, it is equally important to use resources to counter the natural disadvantages induced by disease. (Since social conditions, which differ by class, contribute significantly to the etiology of disease, we are reminded that disease is not just a product of the natural component of the lottery.) But this does *not* mean we are committed to the futile goal of eliminating or "leveling" all natural differences between persons. Health care has normal functioning as its goal: it concentrates on a specific class of obvious disadvantages and tries to eliminate them. That is its limited contribution to guaranteeing fair equality of opportunity.

The approach taken here allows us to draw some interesting parallels between education and health care, for both are strategically important contributors to fair equality of opportunity. *Both address needs that are not equally distributed among individuals.* Various social factors, such as race, class, and family background, may produce special learning needs; so too may natural factors, such as the broad class of learning disabilities. To the extent that education is aimed at providing fair equality of opportunity, provision must be made to meet these special needs. Thus, educational needs, like health care needs, differ from other basic needs, such as the need for food and clothing, which are more equally distributed among persons. The combination of their *unequal distribution* and their *great strategic importance* for opportunity puts these needs in a separate category from those basic needs we can expect people to purchase from their fair income shares, like food and shelter.

There is another point of fit worth noting between my analysis and Rawls's theory. In Rawls's contract situation, a "thick" veil of ignorance is imposed on contractors choosing basic principles of justice: they do not know their abilities, talents, place in society, or historical period. In selecting principles to govern health care resource allocation decisions, we need a thinner veil, for we must know about some features of the society, such as its resource limitations. Still, using the normal opportunity range and not just the effective range as the baseline for measuring the importance of health care needs has the effect of imposing a suitably thinned veil. It reflects basic facts about the society—since the normal range is socially relative—but it keeps facts about an individual's particular ends from unduly influencing *social* decisions. Ultimately, defense of a veil depends on the theory of the person underlying the account. The intuition here is that persons are not defined by a particular set of interests but are free to revise their life plans. Consequently, they have an high-order interest in maintaining conditions under which they can revise such plans, which makes the normal range a plausible reference point.

Subsuming health care institutions under the opportunity principle can be viewed as a way of keeping the system as close as possible to the original idealization under which Rawls's theory was constructed, namely, that we are concerned with normal, fully functioning persons who enjoy a complete life span. One important set of institutions thus works to make the idealization more plausible: it minimizes the likelihood that there will be departures from the normality assumption. These institutions include those which provide for public health, environmental cleanliness, preventive personal medical services, occupational health and safety, food and drug protection, nutritional education, and educational and incentive measures to promote individual responsibility for health lifestyles. A second layer of institutions corrects departures from the idealization. It includes those institutions that deliver personal medical and rehabilitative services that restore normal functioning. A third layer, when feasible, attempts to maintain persons in a way that is as close as possible to the idealization. Institutions involved with more extended medical and social support services for the (moderately) chronically ill and disabled and the frail elderly would fit here. Finally, a fourth layer involves health care and related social services for those who in no way can be brought closer to the idealization. Terminal care and care for the seriously mentally and physically disabled fit here, but they raise serious issues that may not be issues of justice at all. Indeed, by the time we get to the fourth layer, moral virtues other than justice become prominent.

DIFFICULTIES WITH THE FAIR EQUALITY OF
OPPORTUNITY APPROACH

Several difficulties with the approach adopted here should be noted.
Some are specific to Rawls's theory, used as an illustration of the approach. Others are problems with the approach itself. One problem
with appealing to Rawls's theory has already been noted: his principle of fair equality of opportunity is narrowly concerned with access
to jobs and offices, but my notion of normal opportunity range is far
broader. Even on a narrow equal opportunity principle, health care
turns out to be an important social good. But it is implausible that
the Rawlsian principle would yield an adequate account of justice
for health care. Disease impairs opportunity in fundamental aspects
of our lives that go beyond access to jobs or offices, for example, in
ways that affect family life or the opportunity to pursue and complete important avocational projects. Moreover, job opportunities
are important primarily in our middle years, but health care is important throughout our lives. Adopting the narrow principle risks
making the account of health care age-biased.

The broader notion of normal opportunity range yields a fair
equality of opportunity principle that avoids these problems. It
more readily accommodates the broad impact of health care on our
lives. Also, normal opportunity range can be age-relativized. At each
stage of life there is a normal opportunity range that reflects basic
facts about the life cycle and a society's response to it. Consequently, diseases may have different effects on the young and the elderly, and their importance will be assessed differently. A prudent
society would assure individuals that resources were distributed
over their lifetime in a way that guaranteed fair equality of opportunity at each stage of life. I cannot here discuss this extension of the
broader equal opportunity approach, but I do so elsewhere.[33]

But if the broader view of opportunity has some advantages, it also
has some drawbacks. Rawls's arguments for his narrow fair opportunity principle turn on the strategic importance of job opportunities,
for job placement determines access to other social rewards. These
arguments do not directly carry over into less competitive contexts
in which opportunity is important. So the price of modifying
Rawls's equal opportunity principle is that we have less of an idea of
how to justify the modified principle. We must sidestep this problem here. Another drawback is that the broader opportunity principle is less clear than the narrow one about its limits: we have a fairly
clear idea what impediments there are to equal opportunity in job-

related contexts and we can estimate their costs and make social policy accordingly. But the broader opportunity principle threatens to be too expansive.

In response to this complaint, it is important to see that health care needs are defined by reference to a narrowly construed notion of disease. Here the natural baseline of restoring normal functional organization exerts a restraint on the scope of health care institutions. Other constraints are imposed by the fact that health care institutions must compete for resources with other institutions that have an effect on opportunity. Deciding which needs are to be met and what resources are to be devoted to doing so requires careful moral judgment about how various institutions and their services affect opportunity. Similarly, the resources required to provide for fair equality of opportunity must be weighed against what is needed to finance other important social institutions. Health care institutions that are capable of protecting fair equality of opportunity can be maintained only in societies whose productive capacities they do not undermine. Individual entitlements to health care, it should be noted, will depend on the overall structure of the health care system, not on any fundamental individual right to have all health care needs met when they impair opportunity.

Finally, throughout this discussion, we have spoken about social obligations to promote health, not individual obligations to do so. Indeed, the fair equality of opportunity approach seems to assume that diseases are not things people are responsible for having (they are unlike preferences). But much recent literature focuses on the major impact of lifestyle choice on health status. Nothing in the fair equality of opportunity approach is incompatible with encouraging people to adopt healthy lifestyles; but the account is silent on the fashionable issue of how we should distribute the burdens when people "voluntarily" incur extra health risks.

Application to Public Policy Issues

Earlier, we saw how the question, "Is health care special?" was at the focus of public policy debate about access to health care, resource allocation, and provider responsibilities and autonomy. We have tried to answer the question by urging that health care is special because of its impact on opportunity. We can now look briefly at some implications of the account developed here for current public policy debates.

ACCESS TO HEALTH CARE

The fair equality of opportunity account has several important implications for the issue of equitable access.[34] First, the account is
compatible with, though it does not imply, a multitiered health care
system. In contrast, some proponents of "market" approaches to
health care (at least medical care) are committed to a two-tier system in which public programs provide a "decent minimum" to the
very poor and other health care is sold to consumers (e.g., through
insurance schemes). My account shares with the market approach
the view that health care services serve a variety of functions, only
some of which may give rise to social obligations to provide them.
But the approaches draw lines in different places. The basic tier in
my account would include health care services that meet health
care needs, or at least important health care needs—as judged by
their impact on opportunity range. Other tiers, if they are allowed,
might involve uses of health care services to meet less important
health care needs or to meet other needs and wants—such as preferences for cosmetic surgery. My account leaves open the possibility
that other tiers of the system might also be important enough to be
given special precedence over other uses of social resources; but if
they are, it will be for reasons different from those that give such
precedence to the basic tier.

Second, the fair equality of opportunity account provides a way of
characterizing the health care services that fall in the socially guaranteed tier. They are the services needed to maintain, restore, or
compensate for the loss of normal functioning. In turn, normal functioning is a central determinant of the opportunity range open to individuals. This account is, to be sure, abstract. It requires moral
judgment in its application. Still, it provides a principled basis for argument about what is included in the basic tier. In many public policy contexts we get no such principled way of characterizing the
health care society is obliged to provide: it is often labeled a "decent
basic minimum," but what is delivered depends on the vagaries and
whims of state legislatures.

Third, whichever way the upper tiers of the health care system are
to be financed, there should be no obstacles—financial, racial, geographical, and so on—to access to the basic tier. The importance of
such equality of access follows from basic facts about how health
care needs are determined. The "felt needs" of patients are at best
only initial indicators of the presence of real health care needs.
Structural and other process barriers to initial access—for example,

lack of a regular physician—compel people to make their own determinations of how important their symptoms are. Of course, every system requires some such assessment, but financial, geographical, and other process barriers (waiting time, for example) impose the burden for such assessment on particular groups of persons. Thus, proposals to increase "cost sharing" by public program recipients, such as Mrs. Angst, the Medicare recipient discussed earlier, have a disproportionate effect on poorer recipients. Where it is felt that sociological and cultural barriers exist that prevent people from utilizing services, positive steps are needed to make certain that choices whether to seek care are informed ones.

Fourth, the fair equality of opportunity account remains silent on what to make of demands for strict equality with regard to certain features of the health care process. Certain features of the process through which health care services are delivered may have an effect on the satisfaction patients feel, even though there is no measurable effect on the quantity or quality of services delivered, judged from their impact on health status.

Where does all this leave Mrs. Bow and Mr. Arrow, our friends from an earlier discussion? The account suggests that Mrs. Bow, despite her poverty, be guaranteed whatever health care services are needed to ensure that her opportunity range is not diminished by disease or disability; Mr. Arrow, more comfortable financially, must be guaranteed the same thing. When the quality of care has an effect on its efficacy, then such quality must be equal as well. Here, medical services and food differ: medical services may have to be "more equal" in quality than cuisine.

RESOURCE ALLOCATION

The account of health care needs and their connection to fair equality of opportunity has several implications for resource allocation issues. First, I have already noted that there is an important distinction between the use of health care services to meet health care needs and their use to meet other wants and preferences. The tie of health care needs to opportunity makes the former special and important in a way not true of the latter. Moreover, there is a crude criterion—impact on normal opportunity range—for distinguishing the importance of different health care needs, though this fails to solve many difficult allocation questions.

Second, there has been much debate about whether the United

States' health care system overemphasizes acute therapeutic services as opposed to preventive and public health measures. Sometimes the argument focuses on the relative efficacy and cost of preventive, as opposed to acute, services. My account suggests there is also an important issue of distributive justice here. Suppose a system is heavily weighted toward acute intervention, yet it provides equal access to its services. Thus, anyone with severe respiratory ailments—black lung, brown lung, asbestosis, emphysema, and so on—is given adequate and comprehensive services as needed. Does the system meet the demands of equity? Not if they are determined by the approach of fair equality of opportunity. The point is that people are differentially at risk of contracting such diseases because of work and living conditions. Efficacy aside, preventive measures have distinct distributive implications from acute measures. The opportunity approach requires that we attend to both, through adequate funding and enforcement of public health and regulatory agencies.

Third, my account points to another allocational inequity. One important function of health care services, here personal medical services, is to restore handicapping dysfunctions (e.g., of vision, mobility, and so on). The medical goal is to cure the diseased organ or limb when possible. When a cure is impossible, we try to make function as normal as possible, through corrective lenses or prosthesis and rehabilitative therapy. But when restoration of function is beyond the ability of medicine per se, we begin to enter another area of services, nonmedical social support. Such support services provide the blind person with the closest he can get to the functional equivalent of vision—for example, he is taught how to navigate, provided with a seeing-eye dog, taught Braille, and so on.

From the point of view of their impact on opportunity, medical services and social support services that meet health care needs have the same rationale and are equally important. Yet for various reasons, probably having to do with the profitability and glamour of personal medical services and careers in them as compared with services for the handicapped, our society has taken only slow and halting steps to meet the health care needs of those with permanent disabilities. The problem is particularly acute for the frail and partially disabled elderly. These are matters of justice, not charity; we are not facing conditions of scarcity so severe that these steps to provide equality of opportunity must be forgone in favor of more pressing needs. I develop some of the implications of this point for the problem of long-term care for the frail elderly elsewhere.[35]

PROVIDER RESPONSIBILITY AND AUTONOMY

It is sometimes argued that the difficult access problems are ones deriving from geographical barriers and the maldistribution of physicians within specialties. In the United States, it is often argued that achieving more equitable distribution of health care providers would unduly constrain physician liberties. It is important to see that no fundamental liberties need be violated. Suppose that the basic tier of a health care system is redistributively financed through a national health insurance scheme that eliminates financial barriers, that no alternative insurance for the basic tier is allowed, and that there is central planning of resource allocation to guarantee that needs are met. To achieve a more equitable distribution of physicians, planners *license those eligible for reimbursement* in a given health planning region according to some reasonable formula involving physician-patient ratios.[36] Additional providers might practice in an area, but they would be without benefit of third-party payments for all services in the basic tier (or for other tiers if the national insurance scheme were more comprehensive). Most providers would follow the reimbursement dollar and practice where they are most needed.

Far from violating basic liberties, this scheme merely puts physicians in the same relation to market constraints on job availability that face most other workers and professionals. A college professor cannot simply decide there are people to be taught in Scarsdale or Chevy Chase or Shaker Heights; he must accept whatever jobs are available within universities, wherever they are. Of course, he is "free" to ignore the market, but then he may not be able to teach. Similarly, managers and many types of workers face the need to locate themselves where there is need for their skills. So the physician's sacrifice of liberty under the scheme (or variants of it, including a national health service) is merely the imposition of a burden already faced by much of the working population. Indeed, the scheme does not change in principle the forces that already motivate physicians; it merely shifts the locations in which it is profitable for some physicians to practice. The appearance that there is an enshrined liberty under attack is the legacy of an historical accident, one more visible in the United States than elsewhere, namely, that physicians have been more independent of institutional settings for the delivery of their skills than many other workers, and even than physicians in other countries.

A final implication of the account raises a different set of issues, namely how to reconcile the demands of justice with certain traditional views of a physician's obligation to his patients. The traditional view is that the physician's direct responsibility is to the well-being of his patients, that (with their consent) the physician is to do everything in his power to preserve patients' lives and well-being. One effect of leaving all resource allocation decisions in this way to the micro-level decisions of physicians and patients, especially when third-party payment schemes mean little or no rationing by price, is that cost-ineffective utilization results. In the current cost-conscious climate, there is pressure to make physicians see themselves as responsible for introducing economic considerations into their utilization decisions. But the issues raised here go beyond cost-effectiveness. The fair equality or opportunity account suggests that there are important resource allocation priorities that derive from considerations of justice. In a context of moderate scarcity, this suggests it is not possible for physicians to see as their ideal the *maximization* of the quality of care they deliver regardless of cost: pursuing that ideal upsets resource allocation priorities determined by the opportunity principle. Considerations of justice challenge the traditional (perhaps mythical) view that physicians can act as the unrestrained agents of their patients.

We need to modify the traditional view. The physician has the task of advising the patient about the best treatment package, the one with the greatest ratio of benefits to risks, available under the resource constraints imposed by considerations of justice. The physician remains in this way primarily the agent of the patient, though he operates under some social constraints. Still, the physician does not have to import into his own case-by-case decision making inferences from general social principles that, at another level, determine macro allocations. Such an arrangement need not jeopardize patient confidence in the physician. Moreover, the patient's entitlements to health care services are themselves constrained by considerations of justice. But the constraints are not ones the patient should see the physician as having imposed. It is not the physician who here implicitly puts a price on the patient's life.[37]

These remarks on applications are brief, and a fuller development of them is required if we are to assess the practical import of the fair equality of opportunity account. Nevertheless, the account suggests enough that is attractive at both the theoretical and practical level to warrant further development.

Notes

Acknowledgments: This chapter is a substantial revision of my "Health Care Needs and Distributive Justice," *Philosophy and Public Affairs* 10 (1981): 146–179, © 1981 Princeton University Press. I thank Princeton University Press for permission to use passages from the original. It also draws on other, more recent papers, as noted, all of which were funded by National Center for Health Services Grant Number HSO 3097, OASH.

1. See Allen Buchanan, "Justice: A Philosophical Review," in *Justice and Health Care*, ed. Earl Shelp (Dordrecht: Reidel, 1981), 3–22.

2. See my "Equity of Access to Health Care: Some Conceptual and Ethical Issues," *Milbank Memorial Fund Quarterly/Health and Society* 60 (1982): 59.

3. Indeed, major decreases in mortality and morbidity rates in the late nineteenth and early twentieth centuries were primarily the results of better nutrition and sanitation, but "scientific medicine" often gets the full credit.

4. Other industrialized countries introduced different forms of compulsory national health insurance schemes or even national health services.

5. See Karen Davis and Diane Rawland, "Uninsured and Underserved: Inequities in Health Care in the U.S.," the President's Commission for the Study of Ethical Problems in Medicine and Biomedical and Behavioral Research, *Securing Access to Health Care: The Ethical Implications of Differences in the Availability of Health Services,* Volume III. Appendices: Empirical, Legal, and Conceptual Studies (Washington, D.C.: U.S. Government Printing Office, 1983), 55–76.

6. I paraphrase Charles Fried, *Right and Wrong* (Cambridge, Mass.: Harvard University Press, 1978), 126ff. See my comments on Fried's proposal in "Rights to Health Care and Distributive Justice: Programmatic Worries," *Journal of Medicine and Philosophy* 4 (June 1979): 174–191. I ignore here an issue of paternalism that Fried may have wanted to pursue but that is better raised when fair shares are clearly large enough to purchase a reasonable insurance package. Should the premium purchase be compulsory?

7. Reasons why medical markets are not efficient are given in Arrow's classic paper, which traces its anomalies to the uncertainties in it. My analysis has a bearing on the further moral issue, whether health care ought to be marketed even in an ideal market. See Kenneth Arrow, "Uncertainty and the Welfare Economics of Medical Care," *American Economic Review* 53 (1963): 941–973.

8. See T. M. Scanlon, "Preference and Urgency," *Journal of Philosophy* 77 (1975): 655–669.

9. The difference might not be in the *extent* but in the *content* of the scale. An objective full-range satisfaction scale might be constructed so that some categories of key preferences are lexically primary to others; prefer-

ences not included on a truncated scale never enter the full-range scale except to break ties among those equally well-off on key preferences. Such a scale may avoid my worries, but it needs a rationale for its ranking. The objection raised here to full-range satisfaction measures applies, I believe, with equal force to happiness or enjoyment measures of the sort Richard Brandt defends in *A Theory of the Good and the Right* (Oxford: Clarendon Press, 1979), chap. 14.

10. See Scanlon, "Preference and Urgency," 660.

11. David Braybrooke, "Let Needs Diminish That Preferences May Prosper," in *Studies in Moral Philosophy*, American Philosophical Quarterly Monograph Series, No. I (Oxford, Eng.: Blackwell, 1968), 90 (my emphasis). Personal medical services do not count as course-of-life needs on the criterion that we need them all through our lives or at certain developmental stages, but they do count as course-of-life needs in that deficiency with respect to them may endanger normal functioning.

12. The account here draws on a fine series of articles by Chrisopher Boorse; see "On the Distinction Between Disease and Illness," *Philosophy & Public Affairs* 5 (Fall 1975): 49−68; "What a Theory of Mental Health Should Be," *Journal of the Theory of Social Behavior* 6, no. I: 61−84; "Health as a Theoretical Concept," *Philosophy of Science* 44 (1977): 542−573. See also Ruth Macklin, "Mental Health and Mental Illness: Some Problems of Definition and Concept Formation," *Philosophy of Science* 39 (September 1972): 341−362.

13. Boorse, "What a Theory of Mental Health Should Be," 77.

14. "Health is a state of complete physical, mental, and social well-being, and not merely the absence of disease or infirmity." From the preamble to the constitution of the World Health Organization. Adopted by the International Health Conference held in New York, 19 June−22 July 1946, and signed on July 22, 1946. *Official Record World Health Organization* 2, no. 100. See Daniel Callahan, "The WHO Definition of 'Health,'" *The Hastings Center Studies* I, no. 3 (1973): 77−88.

15. See H. Tristram Engelhardt, Jr., "The Disease of Masturbation: Values and the Concept of Disease," *Bulletin of the History of Medicine* 48 (Summer 1974): 234−248.

16. Boorse's critique of strongly normative views of disease is persuasive independent of some problematic features of his own account.

17. For example, we need an account of functional ascriptions in biology (see Boorse, "Wright on Functions," *Philosophical Review* 85 [January 1976]: 70−86). More specifically, we need to be able to distinguish genetic variations from disease, and we must specify the range of environments taken as "natural" for the purpose of revealing dysfunction. The latter is critical to the second feature of the biomedical model: for example, what range of social roles and environments is included in the natural range? If we allow too much of the social environment, then racially discriminatory environments might make being of the wrong race a disease; if we disallow

all socially created environments, then we seem not to be able to call dyslexia a disease (disability).

18. Anyone who doubts the appropriateness of treating some physiognomic deformities as serious diseases with strong claims on surgical resources should look at Frances C. MacGreggor's *After Plastic Surgery: Adaptation and Adjustment* (New York: Praeger, 1979). Even when there is no disease or deformity, there is nothing in the analysis I offer that precludes individuals or society from deciding to use health care technology to make physiognomy conform to some standard of beauty. But such uses of health technology will not be justifiable as the fulfillment of health care needs.

19. One issue here is to avoid "hijacking" by past preferences that themselves define the effective range. Of course, effective range may be important in micro allocation decisions.

20. Presumably, he must also claim that we improve satisfaction more by treating and preventing disease than by finding ways to encourage people to adjust to their conditions by reordering their preference curves.

21. I draw on John Rawls, "Social Unity and the Primary Social Goods," in *Utilitarianism and Beyond*, Amartya K. Sen and Bernard Williams (Cambridge: Cambridge University Press, 1982), 159–186.

22. Here again the utilitarian proponent of the satisfaction scale may issue a typical promissory note, assuring us that maximizing satisfaction overall requires institutional arrangements that act to minimize social hijacking.

23. The division presupposes, as Rawls points out in response to Scanlon, that people have the ability and know they have the responsibility to adjust their desires in view of their fair shares of primary social goods. See Scanlon, "Preference and Urgency," 665–666.

24. Satisfaction scales leave us no basis for not wanting to *be* whatever person, construed as a set of preferences, has higher satisfaction. To borrow Bernard Williams's term, they leave us with no basis for insisting on the *integrity* of persons. See Rawls, "Social Unity and the Primary Social Goods." The view that issues here turn in a fundamental way on the nature of persons is pursued in Derek Parfit, "Later Selves and Moral Principles," in *Philosophy and Personal Relations*, ed. Alan Montefiore (London: Routledge & Kegan Paul, 1973): 137–169; Rawls, "Independence of Moral Theory," *Proceedings and Addresses of the American Philosophical Association* 48 (1974–1975): 5–22: and my "Moral Theory and the Plasticity of Persons," *Monist* 62 (July 1979): 265–287.

25. See John Rawls, *A Theory of Justice* (Cambridge, Mass.: Harvard University Press, 1971), 302.

26. See Rawls, "Social Unity and the Primary Social Goods."

27. Some weighting problems will need to be faced in any case; see my "Rights to Health Care" for further discussion. Also see Kenneth Arrow, "Some Ordinalist Utilitarian Notes on Rawls' Theory of Justice," *Journal of Philosophy* 70 (1973): 245–263. Also see Joshua Cohen, "Studies in Politi-

cal Philosophy," Ph.D. diss. (Harvard University, 1978), Part III and Appendices.

28. See Ronald Greene, "Health Care and Justice in Contract Theory Perspective," in *Ethics & Health Policy*, ed. Robert Veatch and Roy Branson (Cambridge, Mass.: Ballinger, 1976), 111–126.

29. The primary social goods themselves remain general and abstract properties of social arrangements—basic liberties, opportunities, and certain all-purpose exchangeable means (income and wealth). We can still simplify matters in using the index by looking solely at income and wealth—assuming a background of equal basic liberties and fair equality of opportunity. Health care is not a primary social good—neither are food, clothing, shelter, or other basic needs. The presumption is that the latter will be adequately provided for from fair shares of income and wealth. The special importance and unequal distribution of health care needs, like educational needs, are acknowledged by their connection to other institutions that provide for fair equality of opportunity. But opportunity, not health care or education, is the primary social good.

30. Here I shift emphasis from Rawls when he remarks that health is a *natural* as opposed to a *social* primary good because its possession is less influenced by basic institutions. See Rawls, *A Theory of Justice*, 62. Moreover, it seems to follow that where health care is generally inefficacious—say, in earlier centuries—it loses its status as a special concern of justice and the "caring" it offers may more properly be viewed as a concern of charity.

31. Of course, the effects of family background cannot all be eliminated. See Rawls, *A Theory of Justice*, 74.

32. Rawls allows individual differences in talents and abilities to remain relevant to issues of job placement, as in their effects on productivity. So fair equality of opportunity does not mean that individual differences no longer confer advantages. Advantages are constrained by the difference principle. See my "Merit and Meritocracy," *Philosophy & Public Affairs* 7 (Spring 1978): 206–223.

33. See my "Am I My Parents' Keeper?" *Midwest Studies in Philosophy* 7 (1982): 517–540.

34. See my "Equity of Access," 73–75.

35. See my "Am I My Parents' Keeper?" 529–533.

36. See my "What Is the Obligation of the Medical Profession in the Distribution of Health Care?" *Social Science and Medicine* 15F (1981): 129–13°

37. See my "Cost-Effectiveness and Patient Welfare," in *Rights and Responsibilities in Modern Medicine: The Second Volume in a Series on Ethics, Humanism, and Medicine*, ed. Marc Basson (New York: Alan R Liss, 1981), 159–170.

Suggestions for Further Reading

Buchanan, Allen. "Justice: A Philosophical Review." In *Justice and Health Care*, ed. Earl Shelp. Dordrecht: Reidel, 1981.

Daniels, Norman. "Rights to Health Care and Distributive Justice: Programmatic Worries." *Journal of Medicine and Philosophy* 4 (June 1979): 174–191.

———. "Cost-Effectiveness and Patient Welfare." In *Rights and Responsibilities in Modern Medicine: The Second Volume in a Series on Ethics, Humanism, and Medicine*, Vol. 2, ed. Marc Basson. New York: Alan R. Liss, 1981, 159–170.

———. "What Is the Obligation of the Medical Profession in the Distribution of Health Care?" *Social Science and Medicine* 15F (1981): 129–133.

———. "Equity of Access to Health Care: Some Conceptual and Ethical Issues." *Milbank Memorial Fund Quarterly/Health and Society* 60 (1982): 51–81.

———. "Am I My Parents' Keeper?" *Midwest Studies in Philosophy* 7 (1982): 517–540.

Fried, Charles. *Right and Wrong*. Cambridge, Mass.: Harvard University Press, 1978.

President's Commission for the Study of Ethical Problems in Medicine and Biomedical and Behavioral Research, *Securing Access to Health Care: The Ethical Implications of Differences in the Availability of Health Services*. Vol. I Commission Report. Vol. II Appendices: Sociocultural and Philosophical Studies. Vol. III Appendices: Empirical, Legal, and Conceptual Studies. Washington, D.C.: Government Printing Office, 1983.

Rawls, John. *A Theory of Justice*. Cambridge, Mass.: Harvard University Press, 1971.

CHAPTER IX

Personal Responsibility for Illness

Daniel Wikler

Introduction

Much illness is avoidable. Ninety percent of those who die of lung cancer would not have contracted the disease if they had not smoked. Exercise, sensible diet, and compliance with treatment for high blood pressure would prevent countless episodes of cardiovascular disease. Use of seat belts and motorcycle helmets would reduce the devastating toll of vehicular accidents.

Increasing numbers of Americans make conscious efforts to prevent these illnesses, apparently with some success. Others try but fail. Still others do not try and regularly indulge in habits that they have been warned are potentially lethal.

The health care system currently does not make much of the differences between these groups. People are largely free to engage in any number of dangerous habits. No law penalizes those who smoke or fail to exercise, nor does the government move to make tobacco or cholesterol-rich foods unavailble. Those who take serious risks with their health are not charged more for their health insurance. And when a person becomes ill, his or her chances of obtaining health care, either at public expense or through his or her own resources, do not ordinarily depend on the degree of complicity in bringing on the illness. Medical care is sometimes given or denied according to ability to pay, or according to legal entitlement. In some cases of outright discrimination, care is denied because of race. But almost never are patients systematically rejected because of their role in the origin of their illness.

These benign attitudes and policies have begun to be questioned, at least among those who seek to influence the nation's health policies. During the past decade, various influential writers have sounded a theme of "personal responsibility for health" and from this have drawn recommendations for singling out for special treatment those who engage in unhealthy habits. Some of these proposals call for governmental action to prohibit or discourage the maintenance of the habits. Other proposals aim to require individuals with bad health habits to shoulder all of the indirect costs of the medical care required when illness strikes.

None of these proposals has been put into effect on a large scale. Health educators, the professional group most directly concerned with promoting healthy living habits, are generally inclined to use persuasion rather than coercion. Concern over the ethics of using coercion to promote health, then, is addressed not to existing practices but to a new kind of policy that some have urged on our society. We will be asking whether such coercion, in the form of prohibitions and penalties, would constitute a desirable reform of the current, no-fault, permissive system.

As might be expected, these proposals have been the subject of sharp controversy. Proponents have pointed to the possible gains in health that might result, to anticipated savings in the cost of health care, and to the greater fairness that they attribute to a system requiring those whose choices generate costs to shoulder the resulting burdens. Opponents have deemed the policies impractical and punitive and have questioned the motives of the proponents.

Because acceptance of the notion of personal responsibility for health could eventually cause our health care system and its ethical norms to be quite pervasively restructured, it is important to scrutinize these proposals for their logic and for their place in a larger vision of the ethics of health care. We will pursue this goal by means of a philosophical discussion of the aims and means involved in the so-called lifestyle proposals (the inexact term deriving from the notion that individuals must be made to alter their living habits, or lifestyle, or else be made to pay the price).

We must begin the search for an answer, however, with the standard philosopher's effort to clarify the questions. In the present case, this amounts to a requirement to place the controversy within its historical context, for the questions that interest us here are given not by philosophers but by players in the highly contested competition for influence and income that constitutes, in part, the health care system.

"Personal Responsibility": The Context of the Debate

The early 1970s were a turning point of sorts in political thinking about health care delivery in the United States. There had, until that time, been a steady expansion of federal provision of, or payment for, health services. The Medicare and Medicaid legislation of the previous decade had been landmarks in what seemed to be a broader drive toward universal health insurance, an item on the agenda of Democratic, and even some Republican, administrations for generations. The resistance of organized medicine, which had been an insurmountable roadblock for so long, finally seemed possible to overcome.

Yet, at about this time, the dream faded. New initiatives were less ambitious, proposing only such limited programs as protection from catastrophic health expenses, or coverage for small children, and even these were less than vigorously pursued. By the end of the decade, proposals for universal health insurance were effectively stricken from the political agenda.

The retreat from, or defeat of, the earlier goals of health policy was part of a general swing away from the Great Society welfare liberalism that marked domestic policy in the 1960s. This meant that less money was to be extracted from the taxpaying public to pay the cost of meeting the needs of the worst-off.

But there were also factors that were more specific to health care. The first of these, and perhaps the most important, was the beginning of a rapid inflation in health costs, a phenomenon that has continued unabated. The rise in prices made the provision of health care an extremely expensive proposition. This motivated the search for methods of containing costs, possibly including reducing the provision of health services. Although the long-term goal of cost-containment efforts was said to be a reduction in the rate of increase of overall national expenditures on health care, the immediate objective of governmental initiatives was a reduction of the government's health care budget, which meant a corresponding reduction in health care assistance for the elderly and the poor.

A second factor, especially important in academic circles, was a new wave of "therapeutic nihilism," or pessimism over the efficacy of medical care. Books and articles appeared that challenged the past, present, and even future claims of medicine to maintain and restore health. Attention was directed instead to other causes of illness, and the habits of individuals became a central focus. This theme jibed, though imperfectly, with a new public hostility toward technological medicine and a movement toward "healthy living," a "holistic medicine" that asked the individual to assume much of the responsibility of staying healthy.

Finally, this was an era of large-scale attempts to change individual habits that were thought to lead to cardiovascular illness and other maladies. A shift in habits of living did take place, and so did a noteworthy fall in the incidence of some of these illnesses. Here, then, seemed a great opportunity for improving the public's health.

"Responsibility for Health": Different Interpretations

Although this brief sketch cannot pretend to provide a full explanation of the interest in personal responsibility for health and illness that has arisen in the past decade, it can help us clarify the issues. We may very tentatively assign specific meanings to the notion of personal responsibility for health according to the uses to which the answers would be put.

One use for an assignment of responsibility to the individual would be to shift responsibility away from other candidates. It has been alleged, for example, that this may have been the goal of apologists for the medical profession, who may have sought to remove some of the opprobrium from the failures of medicine that the new therapeutic nihilists claimed to have documented. Talk of personal responsibility thus functioned, in the view of these skeptics, as a diversionary tactic.

Alternatively, the motive might have been to downplay the overall importance of health care, with a view toward undermining the claim that health care should be made available as a matter of right. A policy of cutbacks in entitlements to health care, and a refusal to extend access to care to all those lacking it, would stand a better chance of acceptance if health care were seen as ineffective and unimportant relative to factors under the control of the individual.

Were these charges to be accepted, what meaning should be attached to "personal responsibility"? At least one part of the notion in this context is that of *cause*: in many, perhaps most, cases the individual's own behavior is a more powerful determinant of health status than anything doctors do or fail to do. From this it would follow that criticism of the medical profession for lack of effectiveness almost always is misplaced. A similar tactic might be used by those who wish to direct public attention away from those who place or allow health hazards in the environment or the workplace. It is textile workers who choose to run the risk of developing brown lung, for example, and who must bear the costs if they do contract this disease, not those who own the textile mills.

In either case, we face a question of fact as well as ethics. The factual issue is, of course, what relative causal contribution to illness is made by the individual's own choices. The ethical issue concerns the extent to which the individual or some other party should be made to accept the burden of illness or the costs of preventing or remedying it. This involves a sense of responsibility that goes beyond causality, one that we will discuss shortly.

A second motive for insisting that responsibility for illness be assigned to the individual is to motivate people to take better care of themselves. The ascription of responsibility in this case is exhortatory; calling another responsible is merely a means of urging that person to act prudently. It is, in a sense, a reminder of an opportunity for health and of the potential for containment of health care costs. Alternatively, the assignment of responsibility may be a claim about the moral requirements of a certain social role, such as that of citizen or even of person. As such, the assignment does not make any causal claims (though obviously some causal contribution is assumed), nor does it necessarily assign any blame or call for any particular distribution of the burdens of illness. It is this sense of 'responsibility' that is found particularly in the movement for holistic medicine and self-help.

Finally, talk of responsibility for health care can be, and perhaps usually is, a means of assigning liability. If fault is found in the individual who becomes sick, such that the person can be largely blamed for being sick, then it seems right to insist that the individual bear some or all of the burdens of the sickness. Of course, the sick individual by definition shoulders the burden of the sickness itself. What is at issue is whether that person should be provided the health care he or she needs, especially if personal funds are lacking or if there is competition for the same health services by others who are not responsible, in the requried sense, for their illnesses. More generally, if individuals are responsible in this sense for their illnesses, then there is no general moral entitlement to health care, possessed equally and unqualifiedly by everyone, since the costs of illness would then be distributed wrongly. Thus the notion of personal responsibility, construed this way, is congenial to those who, for whatever reason, wish to deny that there is a general moral right to medical care.

There are other real or possible correspondences between meanings of "personal responsibility" and political programs. But we will not pause to identify them, nor, indeed, to fill in the sketch already given. That is the job of the political scientist. Our interest is in assessing the truth of the several claims about personal responsibility that have thus far emerged in our discussion.

Nonetheless, certain critics with an acute political sensitivity may fault us for doing so. The complaint would be that in taking the claims of personal responsibility seriously, we are treating them with more respect than they deserve. In the critics' view, these claims are in reality nothing more than rhetorical smokescreens. They argue that by making the effort to assess the claims we collaborate in turning the debate away from social responsibility for ensuring health to that of the individual. In doing so, we collaborate in hiding the environmental and social sources of illness, and in undermining the belief that, as much as is feasible, health care should be a matter of right. We thus join in the familiar ploy of "blaming the victim."

What sort of response can be made to this complaint, short of terminating the discussion prematurely? We may question the central claim, that is, that the introduction of the notion of personal responsibility for health has functioned almost entirely to distract attention from other sources of illness and from the failings of society and the health system. The claim requires documentation; it is, after all, an empirical one. It may be true, but it is not self-evident. Nor is it inconceivable that some of the proposed policy changes might be good ones, from the moral point of view, even though the motives of some of those who formulate them may be suspect. Finally, and most conclusively, we may question whether a discussion of the issues, such as this one, automatically represents a capitulation to one side of the debate. What prevents this is precisely the airing of concerns of the skeptics and the directive, here heartily endorsed, to take the charges seriously.

The Ethical Issue

The central ethical issue in the lifestyle debate has been the degree to which an individual's liberty may be restricted in order to keep him or her healthy. The issue thus involves two sorts of value judgments: first, that liberty is something that ought not be curtailed without good reason, and, second, that there exist valid reasons for restricting liberty in the interests of fostering health. The philosophical task is to amplify, and to assess the case for, each of these value judgments.

THE VALUE OF LIBERTY

The first of these issues—the value and importance of liberty—may seem at first not to demand much investigation. Nearly everyone in our society, which prides itself for its extensive civil liberty, holds that liberty is in general a good thing.

The standard reasons for this view are easily summarized. People usually know what is best for themselves and should be left to chart their own course. The act of choosing is an important educational experience, tending to make future choices better ones and developing desirable talents and other character traits. When one party, whether government or individual, denies another freedom of choice, it denies an equality of status within the relationship. Liberty is the mark of adulthood and, in free societies, of full citizenship. If property rights are those that confer powers to decide the use and disposition of that which is owned, liberty is essential for nothing less than ownership of one's own life.

These are some of the standard reasons for deeming liberty to be generally valuable. They do not form a full account or theory. But we will not pause to work one out, for we cannot hope to use it to arrive at a short answer to our inquiry concerning the right to risk one's health. There are two especially troublesome problems: first, the generality of these arguments for liberty; and, second, the difficulty of judging what does and what does not count as a curtailment of liberty.

Are all liberties valuable?

The fine properties of liberty that we have mentioned in its defense apply most straightforwardly to actions of a certain class: those performed by adult agents of good intelligence in possession of their faculties and of adequate information; made after due consideration of the relevant facts; free from coercion, compulsion, or uncontrolled impulses; in harmony with the agent's broad life goals; and with consequences affecting mainly the agent.

Actions that do not fit this description are much less likely to be intuitively thought protected by right. Actions that harm others are the most obvious sort of case. Actions of small children and wholly incompetent adults are also excepted, as are certain acts, such as refusing to make way for construction of a superhighway, that would impede social progress.

If these are legitimate exceptions to a general presumption in favor of liberty that is itself legitimate, it must be because the grounds for that general presumption do not apply in the exceptional case. A small child, for example, might not experience the sense of denigration involved in a restriction of his or her liberty in the same way that a competent adult would. Adults who are mentally incompetent may not in fact have a coherent notion of what is good for them, and their lives may be bettered if others make certain kinds of decisions on their behalf.

Our task in inquiring into the propriety of governmental coercion to promote health, then, is to determine whether the risk-laden actions in question (e.g., the habitual heavy smoker) are of the sort that deserve the protection afforded by the general presumption in favor of liberty. Of course, it may turn out that no definite answer can be arrived at simply by reflecting on general principles. In that case, we will have the further task of judging what governmental policy should be in the face of this intellectual uncertainty.

What counts as a curtailment of liberty?

Even if we are able to arrive at a firm judgment on what sorts of actions ought to be made free (i.e., which decisions are to be left to the judgment of individual agents), we will need a clear notion of what counts as liberty and what should be regarded as a curtailment.

Part of this problem is the definition of coercion, which is surprisingly difficult. An outright ban on tobacco products, for example, would certainly count as coercive. But what of a government-sponsored campaign to encourage the attitude that smoking is disgusting and rude? If successful, the campaign would create informal social sanctions against smoking. Would such a campaign be coercive?

Even less clear is the definition of manipulation. Advertisements that associate smoking with unattractive models, or that subtly push the message that abusers of alcohol are unfit parents or citizens, make their point by playing on concerns and fears that may be unconscious. Their primary goal is not to "educate" in the sense of providing information for viewers to use as their values and preferences dictate. It is difficult, even in theory, to determine which, if any, of these interventions abridges freedom. Yet this sort of judgment must be made if we are to arrive at a principled position regarding the lengths to which a government may go to promote health.

A further difficulty in defining the limits of liberty stems from the intellectual uncertainty in characterizing penalties. If I pick up an apple at a fruit stand, I must pay for it; but the payment requirement, if reasonable, does not aim to discourage me from obtaining the apple. In such cases, the requirement of payment coexists comfortably with liberty.

Because health promotion is more complicated, we have greater reason to be uncertain about the morality of governmental programs. Ordinarily, we would hold that coercion would be involved in a heavy tax on cigarettes or alcohol, such as those in Scandinavia that have attempted to make alcoholism a rich person's vice. A defender of the program, however, might respond that the tax merely recoups the losses to the state's treasury brought about through the costs of medical care and of lost earnings that can be attributed to alcohol and tobacco use. The tax, according to this defense, does *not* coerce; it merely requires the users of these drugs to pay their own way rather than to continue to have others subsidize their habit by paying part of the habit's true cost.

The effect of the tax may be a reduction in the use of the drugs, but that is not sufficient reason to call it coercive. A further example may clarify this point. Suppose a group of people decides to insure themselves through a mutual health insurance plan. What should the group decide about members who take unusual risks with their health? Supposing the members are indifferent to the habits of the members except as they affect insurance costs, the members have three alternatives. They can refuse to insure these choices, in which case no benefits will be paid if the illnesses are traceable to the individual's excesive risk-taking. Or they can charge higher premiums to those who are bound to take the risks. Finally, they can ignore the problem and spread the costs of the risk-taking among all members of the group.

Should any of these measures be regarded as coercive? Apparently not, as long as each person is free to accept or reject the various plans. The discouraging effect on risk-taking will merely be attributed to the workings of the insurance market. Indeed, the extra insurance cost to be attached to risk-taking under certain of these plans might even be seen as facilitating the habits rather than coercion against them. Those who wish to take risks are offered a method for paying their own way when they enroll in these plans, and this removes the interest that their neighbors might have in coaxing or coercing them to get rid of their habits. The truly committed smoker or drinker might welcome the chance to assume these costs if the alternative was prohibition.

What, then, is to count as a curtailment of liberty? What of a special tax on cigarettes, liquor, and hang gliders designed to pay the cost of the added health risks assumed by users of these products? Our intuitive argument suggests that such a tax would not count as coercive, even though it almost certainly would cause people to adopt healthier living habits. It is noteworthy that, assuming that the tax had no other policy goals, it would be considered a success if it covered all of the added health costs, even if it did not change behavior at all. This distinguishes such a tax from a similar tax measure that might be designed to discourage the habits. This latter tax would be considered successful if it promoted health, even if the administrative costs more than offset the added revenues and prevented the tax from paying any of the costs of health care necessitated by use of the hazardous products. Whether a given penalty, tax, or other state action ought to be seen as infringing on personal liberty, then, depends on various factors, possibly including legislative intent, in addition to the action's effect on personal behavior.

These considerations show a need to refine our ethical question. We began by asking whether an individual's liberty may justifiably be restricted in order to promote that person's health. We should now add to this the question of whether there are costs that should be imposed on persons who take risks with their health, even if the aim of imposing the costs is not to change behavior but to ensure that those who generate the costs be made to shoulder them. If this latter aim is not classified as infringing on liberty, then we should say that our interest is in the wider issue of assignment of costs of illness as well as in the limits of liberty. In the rest of this chapter, we will for convenience speak of "costs or penalties," ignoring this distinction; but the analytical difference should be kept in mind.

GROUNDS FOR CURTAILING LIBERTY

If liberty is ordinarily valuable, and ought to be respected, what reasons justify a governmental policy that restricts it? Who may properly be denied the right to make choices that risk his or her own health? Which choices, and under what circumstances?

We will consider three general reasons for coercive health promotion. We select these not because they have emerged as the most promising arguments in a debate among philosophers, but because of their prominence in the public pronouncements of figures in health policy debates. They are:

1. That fairness demands that those whose choices involve risks to health be made to suffer the consequences, including the costs of medical care, and that these not be imposed on others who take better care of themselves.
2. That some people need the government to impose healthy habits on them for their own good, and that this is a proper government function.
3. That the reform of lifestyles, coercive if necessary, is required to maintain the effectiveness and soundness of the health care system, and indirectly the nation's economy and defense.

We will outline these arguments in turn and attempt, in a concluding section, to determine the success of all of these arguments in justifying a new, more forceful, kind of governmental health promotion.

At Fault for Being Sick

The chief argument in favor of assigning responsibility for health and illness to the individual is that failure to do so is unfair to others. A person's illness has consequences for many people other than the one afflicted. Fellow citizens must do without the ill person's labor and the tax revenues that might have been forthcoming. Families and other dependents may have to find other sources of support or else suffer deprivation. And, most commonly, other people may have to pay some of the cost of medical care. It seems just and fitting, then, that if an individual decides to undertake a project or adopt a habit that he or she knows carries a significant risk of causing illness, then that individual ought not be free to disregard these unwanted effects on others. The costs incurred must be made a part of the individual's own cost-benefit calculation, which requires that they be charged to that individual alone.

Such is the intuitive argument. It is initially persuasive. It appeals to a commonly held principle, that of responsibility for the consequences of one's decisions, and this makes its conclusions seem just and fitting.

A single intuition, however, does not constitute a conclusive argument. A person's everyday moral code may consist of any number of rules and principles that spring individually to mind depending on the concerns of the moment. When a principle is recalled in a specific moment of moral judgment, it may mark one particular choice as just and fitting. In reality, however, that principle may conflict with others in the same person's collection, and these others might confer approval on one or more of the alternative choices. An important function of philosophical reflection on moral choices is making such conflict and complexity manifest. We are then in a position to make choices between the principles, or, better yet, to try to devise a comprehensive system of rules and principles (i.e., a moral theory, in which, ideally, such inconsistencies are eliminated).

In the case of health-related behavior, for example, proposals that call for some form of slighting of patients who are responsible for their plight seem to apply the principle of individual responsibility that we have spoken of here. But they simultaneously deny the principle of distribution of medical care according to medical need, and the notion of a societal obligation to provide a "welfare floor." Similarly, proposals for intervention by the state to prevent the unhealthy behavior would apparently violate rules of privacy, since some of the behavior that has adverse consequences for health, such as sexual conduct under certain circumstances, is of an intimate nature.

We will not attempt here to develop a general theory of ethics that would set priorities among these intuitive principles and sort out all apparent conflicts. Nevertheless, it will be useful to move temporarily to a more theoretical level, both in order to appreciate the source of the principle that people ought to be made to shoulder the burden of the health care costs they generate, and to see whether the influences made in invoking that principle withstand close scrutiny.

How, then, might we reflect on the intuition that a person who risks his or her health ought to pay for the costs of medical care that result? Or that his or her fellow citizens have no obligation to permit the risk-taking behavior in the first place?

To begin with, we might like a theory of responsibility for actions in general. Such a theory might tell us, for example, who should be deemed responsible for the health costs generated by the illness of a patient who did not comply with his physician's prescriptions. Is it the patient, who may "freely" have disregarded the doctor's sound advice? Or, as some conscientious physicians would insist, are the costs to be regarded as the doctor's fault on the grounds that a doctor who is doing his or her job well will acquire the skills and take the time necessary to guarantee patient compliance? And is a smoker's cancer the fault of the individual, or of a society in which smoking is a condition of admission into certain teenage social circles? There are multiple causes of any unhealthy behavior; in the absence of some larger theory or set of principles, the assignment of responsibility is left simply to custom or intuition.

A different sort of theory that would be of use in this context would be a theory of rights to health care, an account of what justice demands by way of public guarantees of access to health care by those who need it. One part of the complaint over self-imposed health needs is that the public purse may be tapped to pay the medical bills. In order to know whether this might be illegitimate, one must know what sort of entitlements exist as a baseline (i.e., before we take into account personal responsibility).

Libertarians, for example, deny that people have a claim on their neighbors when they are ill and in need, whatever the cause; personal responsibility for the illness and need, therefore, changes nothing.

Other authors have predicated a right to some health care services on a principle of equal opportunity, an element of the just society that illness can prevent and health care can restore. The emphasis on opportunity, rather than outcome, is perhaps congenial to the view that a person who chooses to continue unhealthy habits may legitimately be slighted by the health care system; for though they become as sick as anyone else with their disease, they once had the opportunity not to become so.

Finally, utilitarian theories may, in general, favor health care for all, as long as it is cost-efective, since the healthy person is a much better utility producer; but an assignment of responsibility to the individual for self-caused illness may have a useful deterrent effect. The utilitarian may argue for holding people responsible for illness they could avoid for the same reasons that he or she will want to hold people responsible for committing crimes they might not have committed.

We are able only to mention these large subjects here. But various issues are tied more closely to the "lifestyle" question to which we may turn our attention. These take the form of challenges to the view, or group of views, that find reason to assign responsibility to the individual for the costs of avoidable illnesses. These responses are that the financial burdens placed on others are not unfair; that the individual could not in fact have avoided the illness; and that the general rule under which responsibility would be assigned to the individual is unprincipled and arbitrary, and ultimately harmful to society.

ARE THE BURDENS UNFAIR?

Not every risk that, once chosen, eventuates in expense for others represents an unfair distribution of the burdens of the risk. The plainest example is once again a simple insurance scheme. A shipper may buy insurance to protect himself in case his ship sinks. Any decision to send his ship on a voyage entails a risk, and if the ship does in fact sink, the result will be a loss that must be borne by the insurance company's stockholders or by the future purchasers of marine insurance. The shipper takes risks in full knowledge of this, but need not feel ashamed of his actions. To be sure, some of the other policyholders may not like having to pay higher premiums because the policies were offered to all shippers regardless of their reputation for recklessness. Their ire, however, should be directed at the insurer for failing to place these high-risk clients into a special category that would be charged higher rates.

Similarly, an individual might, in theory, join up with other smokers, drinkers, and mountain climbers in order to protect herself against the possible financial burdens should illness or injury strike.

Perhaps we should think of medical care in general as a kind of insurance policy. It helps restore health, but, like health itself, its ultimate value lies in enabling us to do the things that we must be healthy in order to do. It would be possible for us to put health above all other goals in our lives, avoiding all risks. But such a life would be impoverished. We are better off crossing streets, mingling with others in public places, and bearing children, even though all of these involve health risks. Medical care helps lessen the risk and is valuable for that reason.

If we do think of medical care in this way (i.e., as a risk-limiting device that enables us to pursue non-health–related projects), the assumption of risk will carry positive rather than negative connotations. As long as each of us desires about the same amount of this insurance, none will have cause to complain.

Thus, actions involving risks with adverse consequences for others, even if deliberately and knowingly undertaken, need not involve unfairness. What must also be considered is the nature of any arrangements that might have been made to accommodate the risks in the interests of providing increased freedom of action. There will be cause for complaint about health risks only if some people insist that they do not want this insurance, preferring to avoid health risks by living healthy lifestyles. There are such people, of course, ranging from the average jogger to so-called health nuts. What is unlikely, however, is that there is anyone who places health as an *absolute* first priority, always choosing actions on the basis of their effects on health before anything else is taken into account. Those who, though devoted to healthy living, fall short of this extreme are still "guilty" of taking risks with their health and hence of being willing to impose the costs of voluntary health risks on others. The difference between them and those who smoke, drink, and fail to exercise becomes one of degree and not of kind. No simple principle of individual responsibility will suffice to justify a health promotion program that singles out, for example, those who engage in smoking or those who do not wear seat belts, who could in good faith reply, "Why me and not you?"

VOLUNTARINESS

Smokers and other risk-takers are not the only people who impose unusually burdensome health costs on others. People who suffer from cystic fibrosis or other genetic diseases will also use up more health care dollars than they are likely to contribute in premiums or in taxes. Why, then, are there demands to penalize the smokers but not the sufferers from genetic diseases? The answer is obvious: smokers choose to risk their health, but there is nothing (aside from wise choice of one's parents) that one can do to escape unhealthy genes.

Genetic disease, then, is unchosen and involuntary, and is thus classed, as far as we know, with a great many other diseases. If those who call for penalties on risk-takers are willing to support health care for these involuntary conditions, they are clearly letting much ride on the notion of free choice. The question then arises whether those who smoke, drink, or otherwise take grave chances with their health are making truly voluntary choices.

The notions of "free choice" and "voluntary" are classic problems for philosophy of action, ethics, and political philosophy and are understood in very different ways by different philosophers. In ordinary life, we usually think that we can tell free from unfree, voluntary from involuntary. No one, for example, *makes* a person ignore their seat belts, and that seems to show that that particular choice is a free one. But in fact our everyday notions are not nearly so clear. Clarence Darrow, the great trial lawyer, was able to convince juries that his clients' choices were neither free nor voluntary, even though the defendants made no claim that others had forced them to commit their crimes. Other juries, confronting similar data but lacking Darrow's analysis of the concepts involved, have been quite ready to convict.

In the case of tobacco and other drugs, voluntariness is put into question by the power of the substances to cause physical addiction. In theory, people are still free to seek professional help to kick their addiction and were free not to become addicted in the first place. But in fact no one can guarantee successful treatment of a tobacco or alcohol habit; and people usually start smoking while young and immature.

Habits such as failure to wear seat belts or motorcycle helmets cannot be traced to any physical addiction. But there is no shortage of further explanations of these kinds of behavior, invoking either social forces or else factors within the individual's psychology. If to understand the causes of another's behavior is tantamount to forgiving it, removing the ascription of fault, then these explanations undermine the simple certainty displayed above in distinguishing voluntary health risks from genetic and other involuntary health risks.

How, then, might we determine whether the chief behavioral risks to health are freely chosen? Again, pending further enlightenment from philosophical theory, we must despair of a firm answer. A person who regards society as the culprit responsible for an individual's self-destructive lifestyle is likely to be one who would hold society at least partly responsible for a deprived person's criminal offenses. The same is true for the pairing of opposite positions on these questions. But in each set of firmly held opinions, there is usually more ideology than philosophy.

ARBITRARINESS: A HIDDEN AGENDA?

If the justification for restricting the liberty of, or otherwise penalizing, those who adopt unhealthy habits is to reduce the extent to which costs are imposed on the wrong parties, we should generally expect such penalties to be applied whenever health care costs are generated. In fact, however, those who urge these penalties for fairness's sake have a small number of such practices on their agenda. Smoking always heads the list, and for good reason, given its lethality; sloth and gluttony are often added under more contemporary names. Lust is sometimes a candidate, because it can lead to sexually transmitted disease, but the list does not extend much further.

Yet the range of practices that involve health risks is huge. A woman who delays childbearing until she finishes graduate education runs a higher risk of cervical cancer. Any woman who bears a child must brave the hazards involved in that natural process. A person who enters a high-stress occupation, or lives in a polluted city, also endangers his or her health. Why are these choices, and many more, not also regarded as unfair in that they place on others the burden of paying for the medical care needed when the behavior engenders illness?

There are several likely answers. Public policy need not attack all problems at once and ought not be taken to task for starting somewhere. Smoking is a much more pervasive and lethal habit than some of the others. Detection is a practical problem with some habits, as would be attempts at prohibition. And some of the unhealthy habits, such as working in high-stress occupations are socially useful and therefore not to be discouraged even though the financial impact of the resulting health care costs are a drawback.

It is not at all clear, however, that these answers rebut the charges. The problems of detection and the like are narrow and technical and in any case do not apply to such decisions as having children. The philosophical question is whether such decisions should be regarded as imposing unfair burdens on others because of the health care costs that they generate, and this question may be raised before we determine the practicality of any government intervention to discourage them.

Intuitively, this question has a clear-cut answer regarding childbearing: barring an overpopulation crisis, and assuming a general entitlement to needed medical care, people should be free to decide to bear children without having to pay a penalty to cover the costs of medical care at birth; nor should childbearing be discouraged as a matter of state policy because of these costs, even when these are not offset by anticipated gains in productivity.

But what doctrine underlies this intuition? Do we have a rational basis for shielding childbearing decisions from penalties, but not smoking? Is there some class of decisions that generate health care costs for the rest of us that are somehow "private" and are to be left to the individual to decide? The childbearing example shows that there certainly *seems* to be such a class, but it does not suggest any way to define it. And in the absence of any reasoned criterion, we must suspect that the class is defined not on the basis of rational, and therefore defensible, principle, but by tradition, convention, and other factors.

There is nothing unusual about social policy being based on traditional mores. But a policy of coercive health promotion could not comfortably rest on such a foundation. Those who desire to continue in their chosen lifestyle will insist that their choices, even those that generate expenses, are "private" and ought also be shielded from penalty or other public intervention. And they will complain, with some reason, that those favoring state intervention may have hidden agendas. Perhaps sloth, gluttony, lust, and the others are opposed not because they impose costs of health care upon others—as we have noted, numerous everyday practices also do that—but because they are seen as *vices*. And this would suggest that the health promoters are less interested in assigning costs to those who incur them than in moral reform. Health-minded moralists of this sort have not been strangers to the American scene (though contemporary crusaders, unlike many of their forerunners, tend not to insist that health itself is a moral obligation). Moral crusades are not necessarily wrong, but they are quite different in character from the grounds for coercion with which we have been concerned here. Most important, they cannot be supported by reference to the intuitively appealing principles of allocation of costs with which the argument began.

Those who would press the argument from fairness, then, are obliged to seek a reasonable criterion for distinguishing habits that they wish to curb, such as smoking, from choices that the individual should be free to make without having to worry aobut indirect costs. One possibility is through some theory of privacy, according to which the protected actions have in common a connection with personal concerns that, for reasons to be specified in the theory, ought to be shielded from public authority. Another is the concept of a "risk pool," which permits each person to take risks with others' interests up to a certain limit, to be set by social choice constrained by the requirement that individuals be left with enough freedom from risks to retain substantial control over their own affairs.

However, neither of these approaches has been satisfactorily developed. The notion of privacy, in particular, remains contested, and theorists regularly call for abandonment of the attempt to make it precise; in any case, it is unlikely that a satisfactory theory of privacy would draw the distinction in the place desired by advocates of coercive health promotion (e.g., in such a way as to license curbs on promiscuous sexual behavior).

Even if there were no moral crusade lurking in the background, however, and in addition to its apparent arbitrariness, the appeal to fairness as a ground for coercive health promotion presents an unattractive aspect. Its doctrine seems to call for a kind of "feed the meter" society in which all of our actions, save those (arbitrarily?) protected as "private" are subject to being scrutinized for financial impact and to being discouraged by penalties or other state intervention. One consequence of such a policy would be that liberty would be available only to those with the means required to pay the penalties, and this would extend to a new domain the burden of poverty in a nominally free society.

These penalties might also be a further brake on creativity and experimentation in society, of which John Stuart Mill warned in *On Liberty*. Indeed, Mill argued that state intervention should not be used to protect society from "indirect" harms such as loss of revenue through an individual's being lazy; the state's role should be restricted, he thought, to enforcing specific obligations, such as a parent's duty to support a child. The health costs and lost productivity traceable to unhealthy lifestyles are "indirect" harms in the same sense.

Ought we, then, accept the argument from fairness for coercive health promotion? We have examined several grounds for doubt. The basic claim, that the costs generated by unhealthy habits are currently distributed unfairly, was shown to require a much subtler formulation than given at first. And the argument was shown to be founded on two theses that may defy rational demonstration—that lifestyle decisions are voluntary and that they are not "private".

The acceptance of the argument from fairness, then, seems to be a matter of ideology rather than moral philosophy. Of course, the same may be true of its rejection. Thus, our tentative conclusions do not necessarily tell against the fairness argument. They do, however, tend to undercut the claim of its proponents to offer a compelling argument for adopting a radically new kind of health policy.

Paternalism

Paternalism is a nasty-sounding word and is almost always used derogatorily. It is conceivable that some might offer a paternalistic justification for coercive health promotion? The answer is yes, if the program is not labeled as such. Health promotion aims at policies that are for the individual's own good; when they are coercive, they operate, by definition, without consent of those whose good they are intended to further. This fits the definition of paternalism that is, then, congenial to the subject.

A paternalistic rationale for coercive health promotion is simply one that sees sufficient justification for the policies in the health that they produce. To a paternalist, the moral criterion to be used in judging health promotion is *effectiveness*: whether a policy delivers the health benefits it promises. That the intervention was not requested by those affected, or may in fact have been resisted, is to be counted as relevant only insofar as the opposition impedes the program's political acceptability or in some way interferes with its administration. The paternalist's job, if he or she is in the field of health promotion, is to sell the policy to those in power, attempt to disarm the opposition of those in whose name the policy is to be enacted, and work to neutralize those who may have a stake in maintaining the harmful habits. Attempts to discourage smoking and to promote the use of seat belts, along with many other such campaigns, have proceeded along these lines.

Paternalists may assume that the moral propriety of their actions is practically guaranteed by the fact that their basic aim is to help people. But they are sure to be reminded of a fundamental moral objection—that because their interventions are intended to occur without the permission of those affected, liberty will be impermissibly restricted. Nor will it do simply to insist that the health benefits will be more valuable than the liberty would have been, for if liberty means anything it gives people the right to make such judgments for themselves.

JUSTIFYING PATERNALISM

A paternalistic rationale for health promotion must adopt a strategy for overcoming this objection. One possible way would be to deny that freedom is ordinarily a good thing, and that consequently there is no general presumption in its favor. We will not develop this suggestion here. A second sort of reply, hinted at earlier, is to deny that freedom is to be favored for all agents in all circumstances, and to show that coercive programs that discourage smoking, overeating, and other bad habits deny freedom just in those cases in which its value may be questioned.

That there must be some acceptance of paternalism in life is practically beyond dispute. The clearest case is that which the term directly suggests: parenthood. Small children simply cannot be entrusted with important decisions concerning their own welfare. Their decisions will often, perhaps usually, get them into trouble. There usually are other persons who will make decisions on their behalf that advance the children's interests. The frustration and indignity in lacking control over one's life will not be felt by young children, and in any case autonomy needs to be introduced in stages, a process that itself involves paternalism.

Do any of these conditions obtain in the case of adults? Clearly they do in extreme cases of mental disability. Few will argue with paternalism with respect to an adult who has been severely brain damaged. But the kinds of choices that advocates of coercive health promotion wish to guide are not generally those of mentally disabled people. They are, instead, decisions by people who sign contracts, invest their money without others' permission, vote, and otherwise assume the role of autonomous agents.

If these adults choose to eat cholesterol-rich foods, to become obese, to smoke, to drive without seatbelts, and to shun exercise, on what grounds may they be treated like children? Two kinds of paternalist arguments may be advanced. The weak approach holds that in certain respects the smoker and the others are after all like children, that they are not exercising effective control over their own affairs, and that control by others is therefore appropriate. The task here, of course, is to specify the respect in which the adults are not in control. The strong approach skips this step and asserts that the health benefits warrant intervention even in the case of fully autonomous adults.

WEAK PATERNALISM

As we mentioned in the previous section, those who engage in unhealthy practices may not be making choices that are wholly free and unconstrained. Tobacco and other drugs are physically addictive to some degree, and commercial and social forces apply pressures that are sometimes difficult to withstand.

In addition, much of the public is misinformed about health risks. Bogus advice on diet and other vital concerns is offered everywhere. Even when good information is provided, individuals may shield themselves from it in order to rationalize their continued indulgence in dangerous substances and unhealthy practices. Ill-informed choices fall short of the ideal of the autonomous, rational agent.

Finally, people are prone to the familiar human failings. We opt for short-term pleasure over long-term good, we self-decieve, we use hazy logic. Our actual behavior demonstrably falls short of perfect rationality, defined not as inhuman logic but as effectiveness in reaching the goals we set for ourselves.

These facts tend to support the paternalist's claim that the state might do better than the individual in guiding certain decisions that have a major impact on health. And they provide evidence for the paternalist's claim that the state would not be usurping decision-making power since the adults in question are not fully in control.

The weak paternalist case can be contested on two grounds: first, whether intervention would in fact benefit the individual and, second, whether the state may justifiably intervene even when it has good reason to believe that its actions will be of help.

The likelihood of benefit depends, of course, on the accuracy of the state's information linking habits of living to illness and on the effectiveness of its proposed interventions. Good data on illness prevention are difficult to come by, and the public has been treated in recent years to the spectacle of rival scientific committees and commissions clashing openly on the necessity of exercise, changes in diet, and stress reduction. Nor is behavior change an exact science — and penalties that do not change behavior provide a burden with no benefit.

In addition to these important practical difficulties is a philosophical problem of defining the individual's own good. In arguing that some adults need help in reaching their health goals, the weak paternalist implicitly assumes that if the individual were fully in control he or she would adopt healthy habits. Only on this assumption does the alleged lack of full control provide a justification for intervention given the weak paternalist's rationale. The individual in question, however, might dispute this. Even if he or she were influenced by advertising and used faulty logic, there is no guarantee that under ideal conditions the same choices would not be made. People do differ in their tastes. And since *everyone* at least occasionally sacrifices health and security for other goods, those who do this regularly cannot simply be deemed irrational. To insist that the individual should have different preferences is to slide off into strong paternalism.

Further, the individual who lacks information or is subject to compulsion or influence may yet retain a kind of "second order" autonomy, an ability to reflect upon, and act to change, his or her very lack of first-order control. Ignorant people may be told that they are ignorant, and if they are willing they may be instructed. People under the influence of advertising may be informed that they have been manipulated, and if this message is accepted the advertising may have less power. As long as second-order autonomy remains, the individual is ultimately in control.

A RIGHT TO BE FOOLISH?

The most fundamental objection to the weak paternalist case, however, is that people are morally entitled to be masters of their fate —even when they are not being perfectly rational, even when they are subject to influence and are not thinking very clearly. The liberty to which we have a right, it is said, includes the liberty to be foolish. Our welfare is simply not anyone else's business unless we make it so, and so attempts to force us to act rationally are illegitimate.

It is difficult to provide a full argument for this claim. But it forms part of the core of liberal social philosophy. We may accept it as generally correct, at least for argument's sake, without conceding to it the impropriety of all paternalistic health promotion. The most plausible reply to this assertion of fundamental right is the "social insurance" argument for weak paternalism: that rational agents who prize autonomy nevertheless will not favor social policies that preclude paternalism. The reason is simply that we have good reason to expect that we may on some occasion be short on rationality, because of temporary confusion, ignorance, or influence, and we want to ensure that we will be protected from ourselves. If it is the case that we all *would* want this protection, goes the argument, then it is not illegitimate to provide it when the occasion arises— even if no actual desire for the protection had been expressed.

To determine the sorts of intervention that are legitimate, according to this view, we should engage in thought-experiments that can reconstruct the sorts of *ex-ante* reasoning we expect rational individuals to conduct. When we do so, it is argued, we will find a significant role for the state in determining lifestyles. Tobacco habits, for example, are dangerous and hard to resist. We should welcome help from the state in strengthening our powers of self-discipline. Other lifestyle choices cannot be made wisely without thorough understanding of complex medical information, and the state does us a favor by relieving us of the task of staying current. We currently give to the state the job of determining which drugs we should be free to buy without prescription; the reasoning behind this paternalistic policy is sound and should be extended to other health choices.

Evaluation of this argument requires us to be aware of its presuppositions (premises assumed but not stated). For example, the argument requires us to believe that once the state has acquired the power to override our personal decisions in order to help us, it will not use this same power to exploit us. The social insurance argument also assumes that those who would intervene would do so competently, and that the overall cost to us of the intervention, in the form of blundering, administrative expense, and lost opportunities, will not outweigh the benefit. Those skeptical of government intervention in general will not accept this and hence will deny that rational individuals would want government protection even during spells of vulnerability.

If the social insurance argument is to make good on its promise of finding instances in which all rational individuals would be willing to cede liberty for protection, it must also assume that different individuals will attach the same importance, or lack of it, to retaining control for its own sake. Cultural and interpersonal differences make this supposition unlikely. And, most crucially, the argument assumes that we can move from the premise concerning what rational individuals "would want" to the conclusion concerning what we may currently do to nonrational individuals over their objections.

Each of these premises is subject to dispute. Still, the social insurance argument retains much appeal. If it is accepted in the abstract, the policymaker's task is to apply the general argument to specific kinds of interventions. It remains to be seen whether specific, determinate answers can be derived for such policy questions as coercive taxes on tobacco or higher health insurance premiums for nonjoggers.

STRONG PATERNALISM

Despite appearances, the weak paternalist in an important sense recognizes the legitimacy of a wide range of personal values and goals, none of which may be said to be more "correct" than the others. Although he wants to coerce people into adopting the health habits he considers to be benificial, the weak paternalist need not insist that his values are better than those whose behavior he wishes to influence. Weak paternalists, after all, want to intervene only when the individual's autonomy is in some way compromised or encumbered. The encumbrance prevents the individual from pursuing his good *as he would define it if unencumbered.* The individual needs assistance, according to the weak paternalist, in order to reach goals that are ultimately his own.

The strong paternalist, however, has no hesitation to set himself up as a higher arbiter of values. It does not matter to the strong paternalist whether the individual is fully autonomous or fully in control. Nor would it make a difference if the individual were effectively pursuing the goals of an ordinary life, answering to values developed in ordinary ways within our culture. The strong paternalist believes that there are choices that would be better for the individual than the ones he now makes, where "better" is defined by an objective ideal rather than by reference to the individual's subjective preferences.

If a person likes to smoke, and does not mind trading off his security from illness for the pleasures of tobacco, he is, in the view of the strong paternalist, *mistaken*. He would be objectively better off with security than he is with the pleasure. Since the state knows this, it will do the individual a favor by forcing a different pattern of choices, and, in the view of the strong paternalist, this is a legitimate role for the government.

The ideal to which the individual should be made to conform, it should be noted, need not be a moral one. The strong paternalist claims that the individual will be best off if healthy, not that there is a duty to be healthy or that illness would be immoral. Thus the strong paternalist, though he insists on steering others in the direction of abstract ideals, need not be caricatured as a moral crusader.

IS STRONG PATERNALISM PLAUSIBLE?

Open advocates of strong paternalism are relatively rare among political theorists in this country. We have raised tolerance and pluralism to the status of supreme virtues. Few are willing to say in public that they know better than others what is good for them, when those others are fully informed, free, and rational.

There are good reasons to be hesitant to make such claims, even apart from the fact that they are perceived as offensive. No one has been able to show that he has a special pipeline to the truth regarding morality or lifestyle. If there is an objectively ideal way to lead one's life, much evidence suggests that the path remains inaccessible to reason. And no one has been appointed Keeper of the Truth. Even if someone were sure that he knew what was best for everyone, that person would need some sort of legitimacy before he could impose that vision on the rest of us. Few of us are willing to grant such authority.

However, when it is not identified as such, strong paternalism is treated more favorably. Public officials may consider it a part of their duty to provide "moral leadership," using the strength of the state to impose certain goals and values on the population for their own good. And not all advocates of coercive health promotion are likely to forswear this aim.

Cannot a reasonable case be made for strong paternalism? It should start by challenging the antipaternalist's respect for received values. If certain people in our society seem to favor minor pleasures of the moment over greater longevity, and to blithely pass up the opportunity of greater vigor and the opportunities it provides, why should these preferences be honored? We should not accord automatic respect for another's values simply because they are "his own." Not all preferences and values originate in the rational deliberations of a reflective agent. Many, if not most, are simply taken over unthinkingly, from the individual's psychological milieu. If these are the values that a person has picked up from his surroundings, claims the strong paternalist, surely it is not unreasonable to suggest that the person has been ill-served.

Indeed, even John Stuart Mill, the apostle of liberal antipaternalism, did not shy from asserting that some preferences are better than others. He who has experienced both high and low pleasures, according to Mill, is in a position to know that the higher pleasures are more valuable. The unfortunate person who has enjoyed only the lower pleasures is not. If the person of greater experience states flatly that people would be better off enjoying the higher pleasures (assuming the capacity to do so), he is not being capricious, arbitrary, or arrogant.

Thus, according to the strong paternalist, it is entirely reasonable to hold that individuals are not the final authorities on what is best for them. Others may know better, either because they are acquainted with a better condition and recognize it as such, or because they have arrived at the ideal through careful reflection.

Nevertheless, the problem of legitimacy remains. We cannot have every person who thinks he has the key to human betterment imposing his ideals on others, even if some of these reformers happen to be correct. The task for the strong paternalist interested in requiring others to be healthy is to formulate a principle of government that would selectively empower the wise paternalists.

We are led, then, to the basic issue: on what basis can health authorities claim to know what is best for people? Why should their priorities be regarded as wiser or better than those of the people they want to reform?

The bold paternalist will not shrink from an answer at this point. He will cast modesty aside and argue directly for the value of health. In this effort, the strong paternalist will not be alone: liberals who argue for a right to health care, for example, have proceeded from the premise that health is objectively good and important, and not merely subjectively desired.

We will skip over the details of the argument for health's objective value and importance. Instead, we will ask a different question: Does the propriety of strong paternalist intervention in private choice for health's sake depend only on the success of that argument? For if it does, the strong paternalist position is more plausible than usually acknowledged. Many are ready to endorse the claim that health is objectively good for people.

At this point, then, the contest is most clearly defined. The advocate of coercive health promotion advances the claim that health is good for people whether they know it or not. The antipaternalist accepts this claim, at least for the sake of argument, but denies that it licenses the state to intervene in personal choice.

The winning argument in this debate has not been found. But one approach to it is the general strategy with which we began our discussion of paternalism, which involves a determination of whether the general reasons for favoring liberty apply to unhealthy lifestyles.

The problem of denigration, of being placed in an inferior status, is even graver in the case of strong paternalism than in weak, for there is not even the excuse that the individual's autonomy had been encumbered in some way. People deprived of control over health-related habits do lose out on an opportunity to learn; it is a primary subject for the exercise of self-discipline.

But the key questions are whether the individual left to his own devices will hurt himself, and whether others are likely to make better choices. These are, in part, the same empirical questions about the effectiveness and benevolence of government operations that we encountered in discussing weak paternalism. They raise, however, a more fundamental issue. Clearly, if we regard welfare as subjectively defined by the fully autonomous, rational individual, strong paternalism cannot make a person better off. This is ruled out by definition. The case for strong paternalism, then, rests in large part on a rejection of one of the key elements of liberal political philosophy. This conclusion does not automatically deny the strong paternalist case, but it ties it to a political stance with implications broader than the lifestyle question. Whether this stance should be adopted depends, of course, on issues beyond the scope of this chapter.

We have not, then, drawn firm conclusions on the paternalist arguments for coercive health promotion. But perhaps we have managed to identify the questions to which the paternalist must respond if his policies are to survive critical scrutiny. It is an interesting exercise to examine proposals for coercive health promotion with an interest in evaluating the success of their paternalist arguments. It is unfortunate for health policy that paternalism, labeled as such, is so much a taboo that the task of its forthright defense is rarely joined.

Social Benefits of Coercive Health Promotion

Thus far we have identified two reasons for requiring people to take better care of themselves: to benefit the person whose behavior is guided and to ensure that others are not unfairly saddled with the expense of avoidable illness. The beneficiaries of these two programs, then, include those who have unhealthy lifestyles and everyone else, respectively. That takes in the entire population.

There is, however, a sense in which concern for the entire population constitutes a third rationale for coercive health promotion. The goal here is to produce a range of social benefits, goods either for society as a whole or for a broad range of individuals not clearly identifiable beforehand. This rational is only marginally paternalistic, since most of the beneficiaries will not have been coerced into adopting new lifestyles. It is not quite the fairness argument, either, though, because there is no suggestion of fault. The argument proceeds instead from the premise that there exists an opportunity for the realization of various goods by altering lifestyles. The goods themselves are to justify the intervention.

The benefits could be of many sorts. For example, a healthier population makes a better work force, and a better resource pool for future military needs. These benefits might serve as enough excuse for government regulation of personal lifestyle; certainly they justify coercive programs in a wide varitey of non-health–related contexts. The principal hope for coercive health promotion, however, has become the possibility of major reductions in health care spending. This concern has been prompted by the rapid inflation of health care costs. This inflation had been especially burdensome to the federal budget because the government's health care delivery programs have been constructed on an entitlement basis, using funds from a pool not fixed in advance.

Because of the concern for the health budget, and for spending on health care generally, new interest has been shown in behaviorial solutions. If it is true that lifestyle is a major contributor to illness, it is reasoned, then it makes much more sense to change lifestyles than it does to spend ever-increasing billions of dollars to repair the damage. This sort of argument quickly translates into the language of obligation: taking care of oneself is necessary if one's country is not to run out of funds needed for health care (or defense, or other needs); good citizenship, then, calls for jogging and teetotaling. And if there exists a civic obligation, and there are people who are failing to meet it, perhaps it would be proper for the government to enforce it.

CAN EXPECTED SOCIAL BENEFITS JUSTIFY
COERCION OF LIFESTYLES?

The cost of these social benefits is liberty: freedom to smoke, to drink, to drive without seat belts fastened, worrying only about the impact of illness on oneself. The social benefits argument for coercive health promotion presents the claim that we, as a nation, can no longer afford this liberty. How may such a claim be evaluated?

The first move by those who wish to be free to take risks might be at the level of absolute principle: that smoking and other elements of the unhealthy lifestyle are to be decided by the individual as a matter of right, that the government tramples on basic principles of liberty in conducting such programs. But this is unlikely to be a sound approach. The government restricts liberty in ways both great and trivial in most of its daily workings. Unless one adopts a libertarian position, in which case the critique of government action would be vastly more sweeping and radical than opposition to coercive health promotion, this kind of argument needs to endow unhealthy habits with some special kind of status. There is no "right to smoke" unless smoking is somehow shown to be essentially private or otherwise privileged, and, as we saw earlier, that is unlikely.

If no absolute principle protects smoking and other unhealthy practices from state intervention, there remain important reasons to question the social benefits argument. The argument is, as we have said, currently made in reference to the need for containment of health care costs. As such, it presents an image of crisis. Only with such an alarm can it be plausible to insist that we are suddenly unable to afford unhealthy behavior.

But this is only half a truth. There does indeed seem to be a sort of crisis in financing health care, if only because costs have diverged so sharply from willingness to pay. But this does not in itself show that the state ought to enforce a duty of self-protection. There are numerous other sources for savings, both within the federal budget and in the economy generally. What is missing from the social benefits rationale for coercive health promotion is a comparative evaluation of liberty in lifestyle as opposed to these other sources. Without such an evaluation it is not at all obvious why we should address the budget problem by restricting liberty rather than, say, increasing income or sales taxes. That lifestyle and health care financing are similar in being elements of the health care picture is insufficient reason to insist that funding problems in the latter be remedied by raising money from the former. And once this inference is undermined, the suggestion of crisis loses its force: it simply is not true that we must choose between the freedom to choose our own lifestyles and the financial integrity of the health care system. There are many other alternatives, and, once more, we are left with the task of determining whether "lifestyle" deserves some measure of protection from state intervention as long as reasonable alternative sources of budgetary savings remain.

The most pressing difficulty with the social benefits argument, however, is that coercive health promotion might not produce any appreciable savings. One of the arguments that helped launch the National Health Service in the United Kingdom was the promise that, by reducing the need for health care, and thus the need for funds to pay it, the program would pay for itself. This benefit was never realized. It is conceivable that an intensive, strong-handed program of health promotion would reduce illness and health care costs, but this is nothing to count on. Numerous forces promise to counter any such trend. Use of doctors, for example, is determined by many factors other than objective need. And, according to the "target income" hypothesis, physicians with little to do tend to treat more in order to increase their income.

Conclusions

Should proposals for coercive health promotion be taken seriously? Should people who show little interest in taking care of themselves be made to shape up? Must medical considerations be placed first in choosing habits and activities, regardless of individual preferences?

The primary objection to coercive health promotion, and presumably the reason such programs have not been put in force, is that individual liberty would be compromised. In a society that prides itself on the degree of liberty (in the sense of freedom from state intervention) it provides, this is always a powerful argument.

But the argument should not be won simply by declaring choice of lifestyles inviolate. There is no argument in sight that would demonstrate a fundamental human right to smoke or drink, a right that would be violated by any law or Constitutional provision that permitted the state to intervene for a legitimate purpose.

In practice, the state regularly restricts liberty to engage in various activities, for paternalistic reasons and many others. True, there are some activities that are not subject to regulation by the state. These are primarily civil liberties, such as free speech and the secret ballot. Certain other actions have been extended the same protection under other doctrines, such as the alleged Constitutional right of privacy that has been held to protect the right of abortion. It is noteworthy, though, that for each of these actions some further principle seems to be required; it is not enough merely to insist on a general right of liberty.

Thus, we should be skeptical of arguments that attempt to resolve the debate over coercive health promotion by invoking absolutes. The issue is not one of fundamental right, but instead one in which a range of solutions might be fully just, the choice among which should be left to political processes. The arguments we have surveyed here do not, then, settle the issue before the fact, but might serve as considerations for those empowered to make policy.

Which of the arguments for compromising individual choice of lifestyles ought to be given serious consideration by policymakers? If our discussion is correct, the argument from fairness, moving from allegation of culpability for health care costs to proposals for restriction of liberty, involves a high degree of arbitrariness; and, given this, the selection of targets seems to reflect an ideological bias. And of the three rationales that we considered, it comes closest to the kind of victim-blaming exercise that critics of the lifestyle debate have complained of.

The social benefits argument involves a degree of the same sort of arbitrariness in identifying lifestyle change as the source of budgetary savings and is premised on promises of efficacy that may be difficult to fulfill. Further, its conjunction with concern over cost containment is a warning signal that the emphasis on lifestyle may serve as a diversion from the unfinished task of ensuring universal access to needed health care. The social benefits argument would be more apealing if it were premised on the need to reduce the strain on health care resources in order to make room for those not yet included.

An openly paternalistic program of health promotion also has the potential of serving the needs of ideology. It too calls attention to the individual as the source of his or her own health problems, which is only a partial truth, and the health promotion might be offered as a substitute for needed access to curative and preventive medical services. It has the advantage, however, of being motivated by direct concern for the individuals affected; and, in its weak version, it can ask to be welcomed by rational individuals wary of their own powers of self-discipline and protection.

The debate over the ethics of coercive health promotion, then, may turn on the ability of its proponents to argue for an explicit and justifiable paternalism.

Suggestions for Further Reading

Two government documents that set out the case for changing lifestyles to promote health care are *Healthy People* (Surgeon General's Report on Health Promotion and Disease Prevention, [Washington, D.C.: U.S. Government Printing Office, 1979]) and *A New Perspective on the Health of Canadians: A Working Document* (Lalonde, Mark, "A New Perspective in the Health of Canadians" [Ottawa: Report of the Government of Canada, 1974]).

The charge that risk-takers unfairly burden the public was made by John Knowles in his influential essay "The Responsibility of the Individual," in *Doing Better and Feeling Worse*, ed. J. H. Knowles (New York: W.W. Norton, 1977). An interesting series of papers by Robert Crawford dissects the ideological underpinnings of Knowles's followers: "Individual Responsibility and Health Politics in the 1970s," in *Health Care in America: Essays in Social History*, ed. Susan Reverby and David Rosner (Philadelphia: Temple University Press, 1979), 247–268; "You are Dangerous to Your Health:

The Ideology and Politics of Victim Blaming," *International Journal of Health Services* 7 (1977): 663–680; and "Healthism and the Medicalization of the Everyday Life," *International Journal of Health Services* 10 (1980): 365–388.

Philosophical treatments of the issue include Gerald Dworkin, "Voluntary Health Risks and Public Policy," *Hastings Center Report* 11 (October 1981): 26–31; Robert Veatch, "Voluntary Risks to Health," *Journal of the American Medical Association* 243 (January 4, 1980): 50–55; Daniel Wikler, "Persuasion and Coercion for Health: The Government's Role in Changing Lifestyles," *The Milbank Memorial Fund Quarterly: Health and Society* 56 (1978): 303–338; and Daniel Wikler, "Holistic Medicine: Concepts of Personal Responsibility for Health," in *Examining Holistic Medicine*, ed. Douglas Stalker and Clark Glymour (Buffalo, N.Y.: Prometheus Press, 1985).

CHAPTER X

Concepts of Health

Christopher Boorse

Introduction: Controversies About Health

A need for clear definitions of health and disease arises in the analysis of a variety of legal and public policy issues. Even more commonly, debates over the scope and limits of health occur within health professions themselves. In either context, controversy may be of two types. One type is a general controversy over the limits of health—for example, whether mental health is genuinely health, or whether there can be positive health beyond freedom from disease. The second type is a specific dispute over the classification of individual conditions such as pregnancy, drug addiction, homosexuality, or psychopathy as medical disorders. In this chapter, I examine some examples of each type of controversy and sketch an analytical framework for their resolution.

Within the law, abortion provides an example of a general dispute about the scope of health. Laws (including the Supreme Court decision in *Roe v. Wade*, 410 U.S. 113 (1973)) that allow abortion for the sake of the pregnant woman's health raise the issue: what counts as maternal health? Is mental as well as physical health included—and if so, must the risk justifying abortion be a serious mental illness, or merely some degree of psychological pain? The U.S. Supreme Court, in *U.S. v. Vuitch*, 402 U.S. 62 (1971), rejected a lower court's opinion that health is an unconstitutionally vague concept; it ruled that the "modern understanding" of health includes "psychological as well as physical well-being" and can be equated with "soundness" of body and mind. In *Doe v. Bolton*, 410 U.S. 179 (1973), the Court went on to say that a physician's medical judgment regarding abortion "may be exercised in the light of all factors—physical, emotional, psychological, familial, and the woman's age—relevant to

359

the well-being of the patient," on the grounds that "[a]ll these factors may relate to health." Thus the Court seems to adopt a broad definition of health, one encompassing emotional well-being[1] and strongly reminiscent of the World Health Organization's famous definition: "Health is a state of complete physical, mental, and social well-being and not merely the absence of disease or infirmity."[2]

Somewhat analogous controversies over mental health occur within medicine, although some form of psychiatry has been a feature of Western medicine since Hippocrates. Recent critics of psychiatry, notably Thomas Szasz,[3] claim that the concept of mental health makes no sense and serves as a cover for psychiatric oppression of dissident minorities. Szasz argues that a genuine medical disorder must involve physiological abnormality. At apparently the opposite pole are contemporary "holistic" physicians, who view mental and spiritual factors as causally relevant to all diseases. Holistic medicine also criticizes traditional medicine for its neglect of positive health transcending mere freedom from disease. Among psychologists and other nonmedical therapists, a large and growing literature attacks the "medical model" of mental illness, though writers seldom agree on what the medical model is. Finally, surveys[4] of criteria of mental health used by clinicians show a wide diversity of ideals of the healthy personality; nor do theorists agree on whether such theories should be rooted in empirical data, social value judgments, or the theorist's own values.

The disease status of many specific conditions has also sparked intense debate. Within the law, notable examples include alcoholism and heroin addiction: the Supreme Court in *Robinson v. California*, 370 U.S. 660 (1962), held that heroin addiction was a disease and its punishment therefore unconstitutional under the cruel and unusual punishment clause. Four dissenting justices took the same view of alcoholism in *Powell v. Texas*, 392 U.S. 514 (1968).[5] Criminal trials involving the insanity defense[6] always require categorizing the defendant's mental condition as a "mental disease" (or "mental defect"), since all four major legal definitions of insanity use this term. But experts disagree whether such psychiatric diagnoses as psychopathy, explosive personality, or post-traumatic stress syndrome should qualify as mental diseases for the insanity defense. Further legal debate over the concept of health occurs in a series of cases dealing with the curious question whether pregnancy is a disease for purposes of employer disability benefits. The Supreme Court majority in *General Electric v. Gilbert*, 97 S.Ct. 401 (1976), came close to endorsing the district court's finding that pregnancy is not a disease, citing as grounds that pregnancy is often a voluntary and desired condition.

Within the health professions, by far the most vigorous recent dispute about whether a specific condition is a disease was the 1973 American Psychiatric Association (APA) controversy over homosexuality.[7] At issue was whether the APA should continue to list homosexuality in its official *Diagnostic and Statistical Manual (DSM)* of mental disorders. Gay activists and liberal psychiatrists argued that homosexuality is a healthy, normal variant of sexual development, and homosexuals constitute merely one more persecuted minority. Conservative psychiatrists continued to view homosexuality as a sign of severe psychological immaturity and conflict. After heated internal debate, including the highly unusual step of a referendum to all members, the APA ultimately deleted homosexuality from the new edition (*DSM-III*)[8] and replaced it with "ego-dystonic homosexuality," a condition consisting not in homosexuality but in conflict over it. Other traditional perversions such as voyeurism and sadomasochism remained in the nomenclature regardless of their adherents' attitude. The APA debate was criticized widely for politicizing an ostensibly scientific issue. But it also resulted in some interesting attempts, which we shall discuss below, to define "mental disorder" in objective terms.[9]

Clearly, the issues mentioned above are similar in that their resolution requires some analysis of health and disease. One cannot sensibly discuss whether pregnancy, homosexuality, alcoholism, or psychopathy is a disease without knowing what a disease is. Nor can one decide whether mental health is health, or whether it includes complete emotional well-being, without an analysis of health. I will now try to provide such a general analysis,[10] and in the process try to suggest answers to at least the following questions:

1. Are health judgments value judgments? If so, what kind of values do they express, and should they be a patient's, a clinician's, or a society's? Can we expect health to vary with an observer's ethics, politics, and social philosophy?
2. Are health judgments scientific judgments? Can physical health and disease be biologically defined? What is the relation between medicine and biology?
3. How do the concepts of health, disease, disorder, illness, normality, and pathology interconnect?

4. Is a mind the kind of thing that can literally be healthy or unhealthy? Is behavior? If the idea of mental health makes sense, by what process should ideals of mental health be derived?
5. To what extent does a definition of health determine the scope of clinical professions? Is medicine concerned only with health? What are the implications of an analysis of health for the ethics of medicine and psychotherapy?

Health Concepts in Medicine

Traditional medicine deals with a vast range of conditions that are departures from ideal health and employs a rich variety of terminology to describe them. Physicians speak of defects, disorders, abnormalities, anomalies, injuries, lesions, illnesses, and handicaps. Patients are described as deteriorating, stabilizing, improving, or recovering; their condition is guarded or serious or critical. Underlying this diversity, however, is a basic theoretical conception of health as freedom from the whole range of medically abnormal conditions—or, as it is often described, freedom *from disease*. This description is accurate, however, only on an extremely broad usage of the word *disease*. Such usage occurs mainly in the headings of reference works such as the AMA's *Standard Nomenclature of Diseases and Operations*.[11] This book breaks down the range of medical conditions into the following categories:

0. *Diseases due to genetic and prenatal influence.* E.g., cleft palate, webbed fingers, undescended testis, patent ductus arteriosus, Down's syndrome, agammaglobulinemia, color blindness, congenital absence or duplication of any body part.
1. *Diseases or infections due to a lower plant or animal parasite.* E.g., plague, cholera, malaria, tuberculosis, syphilis, vaccinia, chickenpox, common cold, carbuncles, warts.
2. *Diseases or infections due to a higher plant or animal parasite.* E.g., scabies, ringworm, athlete's foot, flea or lice infestation, tapeworm, trichinosis, histoplasmosis.
3. *Diseases due to intoxication.* E.g., arsenic, cyanide, lead, mercury, alcohol, opium poisoning; drug reactions; allergic reactions including hives, eczema, hay fever; insect stings.
4. *Diseases due to trauma or physical agent.* E.g., abrasions, bruises, scars; stab wounds, gunshot wounds, animal bites;

bone fractures and dislocations; sprains and strains; burns, frostbite, radiation injury; asphyxiation, electrocution.

50. *Diseases secondary to circulatory disturbance.* E.g. coronary occlusion; portal hypertension; gangrene.

55. *Diseases secondary to disturbance of innervation or of psychic control.* E.g., muscular paralysis or spasm; seasickness; abnormalities of sensation; neurogenic impotence.

6. *Diseases due to or consisting of static mechanical abnormality.* E.g., foreign body in stomach; dental malocclusion; thrombus or embolus; gallstones; varicose veins; diverticulosis; myopia, astigmatism, glaucoma.

7. *Diseases due to disorder of metabolism, growth, or nutrition.* E.g., malnutrition and obesity; vitamin deficiency diseases including pellagra, rickets, scurvy, pernicious anemia; pituitary giantism, adrenal virilism; inborn errors of metabolism including phenylketonuria; acne, vitiligo; benign hypertrophy of prostate; senile osteoporosis.

8. *New growths.* All tumors, benign and malignant, including carcinomas, sarcomas, adenomas, lipomas, myomas; leukemias and lymphomas.

9. *Diseases due to unknown or uncertain cause with the structural reaction manifest.* E.g. atherosclerosis, liver cirrhosis; muscular dystrophy; gastrointestinal ulcers; rheumatic heart disease; psoriasis, hereditary baldness; Dupuytren's contracture.

x. *Diseases due to unknown or uncertain cause with the functional reaction alone manifest.* E.g., epilepsy, narcolepsy, migraine; essential hypertension; paroxysmal tachycardia; functional impotence or dysmenorrhea; loss of sense of smell; proctalgia fugax.

As a rule, the term 'disease' is used more narrowly, in such a way that many conditions listed would not be called diseases. In narrower senses of 'disease'[12] many writers contrast diseases with static defects, such as a scar or missing limb; with injuries, such as a gunshot wound or broken bone; with "functional" disorders such as migraine or spastic colon; or with miscellaneous other kinds of disorders including poisoning, environmental traumas such as heat stroke, and unusual susceptibilities such as allergies. Narrower uages of 'disease' are seldom clear or consistent in medical writings: Acosta's disease and caisson disease are environmental effects, the disease hemosiderosis is chronic iron poisoning, and even classic infectious diseases like diphtheria resemble injuries and poisonings in various ways. For our purposes, narrower ideas of disease are important only in that under any of them, health in medicine is *not* the absence of disease—since medicine regards all the conditions above as inconsistent with perfect health.

The term 'disease' has a further well-established connotation of specificity. Medical science divides the field of unhealthy conditions into individual diseases, the units of theory and diagnosis. A well-defined "disease entity" is characterized in terms of its *etiology*, or precipitating causes; its *pathogenesis*, or process of development; its *pathophysiology*, or derangement of normal physiologic mechanisms; its *pathology*, or lesions to tissues and fluids; its *clinical features*, including *signs*, *symptoms*, and *course*; and its appropriate *therapy*. Rarely are all these features fully specific—that is, unique and invariant for the disease in question. On the contrary, usually one feature defines the disease and the rest vary. As Kendell notes, this means that medical disease classifications rest on highly heterogeneous bases:

> Each of these waves of technology has added new diseases, and from each stage some have survived. A few, like senile pruritus and proctalgia fugax, are still individual symptoms. Others, like migraine and most psychiatric diseases, are clinical syndromes—Sydenham's constellation of symptoms. Mitral stenosis and hydronephrosis are based on morbid anatomy, and tumours of all kinds on histopathology. Tuberculosis and syphilis are based on bacteriology and the concept of the etiological agent, porphyria on biochemistry, myasthenia gravis on physiological dysfunction, Down's syndrome on chromosomal architecture, and so on.[13]

Disease categories also evolve with the growth of scientific knowledge. A vague clinical entity, consumption, becomes a more precise pathologic entity, tuberculosis, on discovery of the characteristic tubercle lesion, and an even more precise bacteriologic entity on identification of *Mycobacterium tuberculosis*. Old diseases subdivide into new ones; what was pneumonia or rheumatism to the eighteenth-century physician would be many distinct diseases today.

Fortunately, we can abstract from all problems of disease classification and definition by using a more general term; *pathological*. All the conditions in the *Nomenclature* are correctly described as pathological,[14] or medically abnormal, however classified or subdivided. I suggest that the distinction between normal and pathological conditions is the basic theoretical concept of Western medicine. A bodily state or process is disease, disorder, injury, lesion, defect, sickness, or illness only if it is abnormal in the sense of pathological; in other words, these are all specific kinds of pathological conditions.[15] What makes a condition pathological I will try to define in the next two sections. The term applies primarily to parts or processes rather than whole organisms; although liver function or kidney structure or color perception may be pathological, one does not speak of pathological people. Nevertheless, if one defines a medically ideal (and nonexistent) human being as one completely free of all pathological phenomena at every level of physiological function, one might draw up the following rough taxonomy of *grades of health* (see Figure 10–1).

The figure is meant to suggest the following points. First, death, the complete cessation of organic functions, is the most extreme form of pathology. Second, pathological conditions may exist but be clinically undiagnosable, such as minor liver cirrhosis, tiny pancreatic cysts, transient cardiac arrhythmias, and early atherosclerosis. Patients with such undectectable abnormalities are *theoretically abnormal* but *diagnostically normal*. Third, diagnostic abnormalities, in turn, may need no treatment, as is the case with some benign tumors, small skin lesions, or gallstones in the elderly. Such patients are theoretically and diagnostically abnormal but *therapeutically normal*. Finally, a patient is *sick* or *ill* when pathological processes rise to a systemic level that produces global incapacitation of the whole organism. Athlete's foot, myopia, intestinal polyps, and bursitis are pathological (and disease processes), but they are not ill-

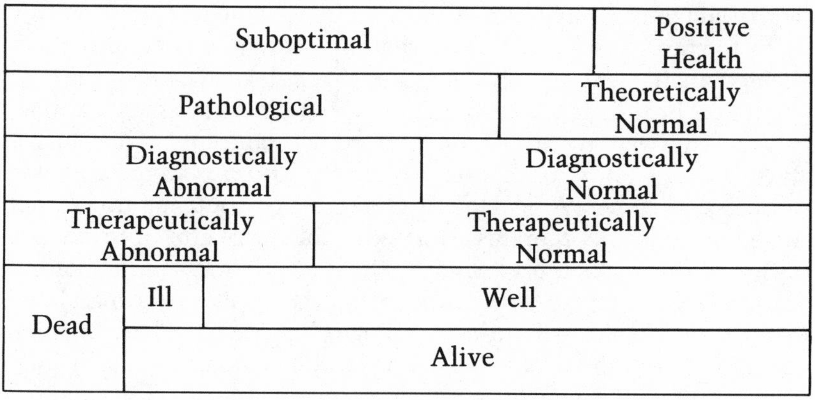

Suboptimal		Positive Health
Pathological		Theoretically Normal
Diagnostically Abnormal		Diagnostically Normal
Therapeutically Abnormal		Therapeutically Normal
Dead	Ill	Well
	Alive	

FIGURE 10.1. Grades of Health

ness because they involve no systemic incapacitation.[16] Finally, the figure allows for the debatable possibility of "positive health," or superhealth beyond the already utopian goal of complete normality.

Defining Health and Disease: The Context of Debate

Our main task now is to analyze the normal-pathological distinction in traditional medicine. A correct analysis, or reportive definition, must conform to medical usage—that is, it must fit the stock of recognized pathological conditions. Definitions that are wider or narrower than his stock are incorrect. For example, traditional medicine never describes pregnancy, menstruation, male or female fertility, penile foreskins, or Oriental ancestry as pathological, or as diseases. Thus, when one psychiatry textbook defines a disease as "any condition associated with discomfort, pain, disability, death, or an increased liability to these states, regarded by physicians and the public as properly the responsibility of the medical profession"[17] the example of pregnancy, which meets all the conditions but is not a disease, refutes the definition. In this section, we will survey some popular approaches to defining health and disease and criticize them according to this basic ground rule. Although most authors take their target concept to be "disease" rather than "pathological condition," similar criticisms usually apply in each case.

One important general dimension of definitions of health is *value-ladenness* or *value-freedom*. Most definitions of disease make health judgments, at least in part, value judgments. Such writers seem to start from the intuition that diseases are *bad* conditions of the organism—physiological evils, or psychological evils in the case of mental health. On this normativist view, health and disease belong to the welfare-harm family of ethical concepts. The normativist writer's job is to distinguish medical from nonmedical evils —unless like the World Health Organization (but not traditional medicine) one incorporates every kind of well-being into health. Other writers, notably Szasz,[18] Kass,[19] Klein,[20] and Boorse,[21] seem to begin instead with an intuition that places health and disease in the life-death family of biological concepts. These writers' accounts of health are naturalistic or value-free, making health judgments empirical, scientific claims resting on biological facts about a species.

A rare illustration of the two (almost) pure types of view, norma-tivist and naturalist, occurs in the following interchange between Sedgwick and Kass. Sedgwick writes:

> Outside the significances that man voluntarily attaches to cer-tain conditions, *there are no illnesses or diseases in nature*. . . . Are there not infectious and contagious bacilli? Are there not definite and objective lesions in the cellular structures of the human body? Are there not fractures of bones, the fatal rup-tures of tissues, the malignant multiplications of tumorous growths? . . . Yet these, as natural events, do not—prior to the human social meanings we attach to them—constitute ill-nesses, sicknesses, or diseases. The fracture of a septuagenari-an's femur has, within the world of nature, no more signifi-cance than the snapping of an autumn leaf from its twig. . . . Out of his anthropocentric self-interest, man has chosen to consider as "illnesses" or "diseases" those natural circum-stances which precipitate the death (or the failure to function according to certain values) of a limited number of biological species: man himself, his pets and other cherished livestock, and the plant-varieties he cultivates for gain or pleasure. . . . Children and cattle may fall ill, have diseases, and seem as sick; but who has ever imagined that spiders and lizards can be sick or diseased?[22]

On Sedgwick's view, diseases are not discovered in nature. One discovers new natural phenomena, but to classify these phenomena as diseases is a nonscientific imposition of human values.[23] Kass replies, however, that the disease status of some phenomena is as much a biological fact as the phenomena themselves:[24]

> [H]ealth, although certainly a good, is not therefore a good whose goodness exists merely by convention or by human de-cree. Health, illness, and unhealth all may exist even if not dis-covered or attributed. That human beings don't *worry* about the health of lizards and spiders implies nothing about whether lizards and spiders *are* healthy, and any experienced student of spiders and lizards can discover—and not merely invent—ab-normal structures and functionings of those animals. Human indifference is merely that. Deer can be healthy or full of can-cer, a partially eaten butterfly escaping from a blue jay is not healthy but defective, and even the corn used to nourish para-sites becomes abnormal corn, to the parasite-grower's de-light.[25]

Most normativist writers (including Sedgwick by his reference to death) employ factual as well as evaluative concepts in their definitions. One very common type of definition I will call a "3-D" definition: it analyzes diseases as conditions causally associated with certain specified evils, such as death, disability, discomfort, or deformity. Examples of "3-D" definitions are the Goodwin-Guze formulation above and the following version by Engelhardt:

> [A]ny physiological or psychological processes or states not under the immediate control of a person which (1) preclude the goals chosen as integral to the general life of humans (inability to engage in the range of physical activity held integral to human life); (2) cause pain (if that pain is not integral to a process leading to goals held integral to human life); (3) preclude a physical form that other humans would hold to be normal (not deformed)—will count as diseases.[26]

Clearly, a "3-D" definition is value-laden insofar as any of the "D" concepts is value-laden. In Engelhardt's definition, both the disability and the discomfort clauses require value judgments about what is "integral" to human life, while the deformity clause refers to social values concerning appearance.

3-D definitions seem to face two main difficulties. First, by their focus on gross, clinically evident effects—death, discomfort, disability, deformity—they tend to exclude many types of minor, local, or compensated pathology. Consider a small internal benign tumor, mild liver cirrhosis, an intestinal diverticulum, or a tiny wart or scar on the skin. These conditions are pathological, but they may have no gross effects on a person's quality of life at all. The 3-D theorist must reply that such conditions nonetheless raise the risk of gross effects. It is true that diverticula can become infected; so, however, can normal tissue, such as the appendix. It is quite incredible that every scar, no matter how tiny and invisibly located, poses an appreciable risk to life and happiness.

Furthermore, the gross performance of one person with well-compensated pathology may be superior to that of a second normal person. A large, mildly cirrhotic liver may outperform a small normal one; a champion athlete with a muscle disease may beat a normal nonathlete in every event. To these last two examples one may reply that the first person's gross output would be even better if the large liver or muscles were free of disease. But small hearts and muscles would likewise perform better if large. The second problem for the 3-D theorist is thus to explain how to distinguish disease from the low end of a normal range of variation. If this point and the previous one are addressed in detail, I expect the 3-D approach to converge on the definition in the next section in terms of statistical normality of part-function.

An additional difficulty for normativist definitions is the phenomenon of desirable pathology. At least in some circumstances, a disease state may be preferable to normality: it is advantageous to have cowpox in a smallpox epidemic, rubella prior to pregnancy, myopia or flat feet during a military draft, or oviduct blockage if one wishes no more children. A normativist may reply that at least the typical cases of any disease are undesirable. Perhaps diseases are *prima facie* undesirable, and desirable only under unusual circumstances. But it is certainly not obvious that infertility is only rarely a blessing. A normativist must also deal with the fact that some normal conditions are far worse than some pathological conditions. For example, short stature, low intelligence, and moderate ugliness are by most standards greater handicaps than athlete's foot or myopia— even if the latter last a lifetime.

I conclude this section by mentioning some other recurrent ideas in definitions of disease and their characteristic difficulties. Since the antonym of "pathological" is "normal," many writers define diseases as *statistically abnormal*. But statistical abnormality is not sufficient for pathology, since unusual intelligence or strength or aerobic capacity is medically abnormal. It is also statistically normal to have some pathology; everyone has skin lesions, and tooth decay is nearly universal. Many writers appeal to the *treatment* of a condition *by physicians* to explain why it is a disease. But physicians treat many normal conditions, as when they deliver babies, prescribe contraceptives, circumcise males, or do cosmetic surgery. Conversely, many diseases such as muscular dystrophy or paraplegia are untreatable, so that treatment by physicians is neither necessary nor sufficient for a condition to be pathological. Biological concepts often used in definitions of disease include *homeostasis, defense mechanisms*, and *adaptation*. Homeostasis fails as a general account of health because many life functions (e.g. locomotion, vision, or reproduction) are not homeostatic. Defense mechanisms like inflammation and the immune response occur in many pathological states, but not all; consider blindness or deafness. Finally, a definition of health as adaptation must cope with the fact that an individual with compensated or minor pathology may be better adapted to his environment than another person with none, who falls near the low end of the normal range of variation.

A Statistical-Functional
Definition of Normality

It is a virtual truism of medicine that health is *normal function*, and what is pathological is *abnormal function*. I believe this truism, suitably analyzed, is the only correct definition of the normal-pathological distinction in medicine. The relevant concept of a function belongs primarily to biology, not medicine. Ordinary medicine borrows its theories of part-function from physiology, a subfield of biology. Normality of function, in turn, is a statistical concept based on what is typical of a species (or subclass thereof). On this analysis the normal-pathological distinction is a naturalistic one: the essence of the pathological is *statistically species-subnormal part-function*, or more carefully:

> A condition of a part or process in an organism is *pathological* when the ability of the part or process to perform one or more of its species-typical biological functions falls below some central range of the statistical distribution for that ability in corresponding parts or processes in members of an appropriate reference class of the species.[27]

Figure 10.2 may be helpful:

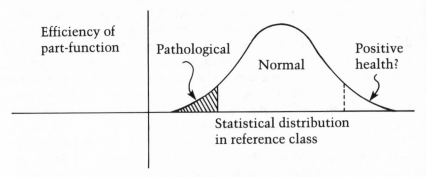

FIGURE 10.2. Pathological Condition

Three points will clarify this figure. First, the reference class for normality is only a fraction of a species, because medical normality is relative to sex and age (and possibly to race). For example, normal males must have prostate glands though most humans (females) do not; normal babies cannot walk even though most humans can. The best reference class for explaining medical judgments of normality may be an age group of a sex of a species. Second, the lower limit of normal functional ability—the line between normal and pathological—is arbitrary. Although statisticians often use of 95 percent central range, no reason for such a choice applies here. The concept of a pathological state has vague boundaries—though the vast majority of disease processes involve functional deficits by any reasonable standard. Third, this definition uses "function" in a biological sense, which means there is no such thing as excess of function. The function of the oxyntic cells of the stomach wall is to secrete acid to aid digestion. But excess stomach acid is ultimately even more dysfunctional than deficiency. The right-hand tail of a function's distribution is maximal physiological efficiency—not maximal quantities of stomach acid or insulin or leukocytes, any of which are, on the contrary, pathological.

To analyze the idea of biological function on which this definition rests is beyond the scope of this chapter. The problem is widely discussed by philosophers of biology.[28] Clearly, one cannot be content with Galen's definition of the function of an organ as "what it does best." Organs like the liver or hypothalamus have countless functions; furthermore, the heart makes heart sounds (a nonfunction) about as well as it circulates the blood. Most recent writers[29] hold some version of the following view: the functions of an organ are its species-typical causal contributions to the organism's survival and reproduction. Other writers, notably Larry Wright,[30] argue that the functions of an organ are those effects that, via evolutionary theory, explain its existence. Given Darwinian evolution, the two analyses usually agree on particular cases. My thesis is that whatever the correct analysis of biological function statements, *physiology determines pathology*. A pathological state, in ordinary medicine, is a state in which one or more physiological part-functions are performed at a species-subnormal level of efficiency.

This definition of medical normality in terms of statistically typical biological part-function avoids the difficulties of other approaches.[31] Local part-dysfunctions need not have any gross effects on disability or deformity or distress. A small skin lesion or intestinal polyp is pathological because it involves local dysfunction or nonfunction of parts (i.e. cells and tisues). But such local pathology often leaves the gross abilities of the organism unscathed. Liver cells, to be normal, must perform a host of metabolic functions because that is what liver cells collectively contribute to survival and reproduction. But a large number of liver cells can be pathological without clinically detectable effects or appreciable risk of such effects. Finally, pathology is occasionally desirable just because biological functions are occasionally undesirable. Reproduction, for example, is a quintessential biological function; but there is no reason why everyone should want to reproduce at every opportunity. A woman who has her tubes tied after five children deliberately acquires a pathological condition in the interests of values she prefers to normality.

This naturalistic account of health as biological normality is value-free, or as value-free as biology itself.[32] Some writers suggest that the science of biology is value-laden in that it presupposes a commitment to the value of life. But biologists who study fungi or cicadas or sharks need not assume that the life of such organisms is beneficial to anyone. Biology is, by definition, the science of life; that is what distinguishes its subject matter from that of physics and chemistry. But to define life and death, or to study the functional subprocesses on which they depend, requires no value judgments. My claim is that the same is true of health. The distinction between health and disease, like the distinction between life and death, is a fact of biological science.

In a similar vein, Engelhardt[33] has criticized the above approach for its implicit value commitment to the biological goal of species survival, which conflicts with medicine's concern for individual patients. First, however, it is incorrect that biological functions aim at species survival: the units of selection are the genes of individuals, and therefore biological functions work to preserve the individual and his close kin. Secondly, the definition above incorporates no value judgments; it only states what health (i.e. medical normality) *is*, namely biologically normal part-function. The normal-pathological distinction is a reasonable foundation for medical practice because biological normality is almost always in the interests of the patient. Where this presumption fails, however—as with continuous fertility—other values take precedence over health. Although the value of health is usually important, it is also limited, a theme to which I shall return in the final section.

Mind, Brain, and the "Medical Model"

Let us now ask whether there is such a thing as mental health, or mental disease or mental illness. The status of psychiatry as a medical speciality seems to presuppose an affirmative answer. In the last century, indeed, psychiatry has expanded its scope enormously. Although some of what we now call psychoses have ranked as medical disorders since Hippocrates, contemporary psychiatric classifications go beyond psychoses to far more subtle (and controversial) disorders of feeling, personality, and behavior.

The vast scope of contemporary psychiatry is evident in the APA's *Diagnostic and Statistical Manual* or any textbook of abnormal psychology. For the most part, *DSM-II*[34] could be rearranged into the following general categories:[35] *psychoses*, both organic (due to drugs, poisons, traumas, tumors, infections, etc.) and functional (schizophrenia, paranoia, and affective psychoses such as mania and depression); *neuroses*, such as hysterical, phobic, obsessive-compulsive; *personality disorders*, including neurotic and psychotic personalities (hysterical, paranoid, schizoid), sexual deviations (homosexuality, sadomasochism, pedophilia), drug dependencies (alcoholism, heroin addiction), and antisocial personality (psychopathy); *psychosomatic disorders* such as migraine, eczema, asthma; *behavior disorders of childhood and adolescence* (enuresis, hyperkinesis); *speech and learning disorders* (aphasia, dyslexia); *mental retardation*; and *transient situational disturbances*. For purposes of such a list, clearly, "mental disorder" and "physical disorder" are not incompatible terms. The DSM classification seeks to include all disorders with any significant psychological component, whether that component is etiology (psychosomatic diseases), primary pathology (schizophrenia), or clinical signs (alcoholic psychosis).[36]

As psychiatry has expanded its scope, it has also encountered widespread criticism that the new conditions do not fit the "medical model" of health and disease. Critics of the medical model, however, give very diverse descriptions of it. Sometimes such critics attack theoretical assumptions: that mental disorders are qualitatively different from normality, that there are disease entities in psychopathology with specific etiologies, or that mental disorders are brain diseases. Other critics attack views about therapy: e.g., that only physicians are qualified to treat mental disorders, or that such treatment ought to be by traditional "medical" methods such as drugs rather than psychotherapy, or that treatment should be of single patients rather than families or social environments. Still other critics focus on social or legal consequences of viewing a condition as medical: that the patient deserves the Parsonian "sick role,"[37] may be involuntarily hospitalized, or merits coverage by medical insurance. All these theses, however, are distinct and

374 · CHRISTOPHER BOORSE

mostly independent of one another. To take only one example, the fact that a condition is pathological does not mean that only M.D.s can treat it; dentists, optometrists, podiatrists, and nurses all treat genuine diseases. Many attacks on the "medical model" distort or oversimplify ordinary medicine, as with the thesis that pathology must be discontinuous with normality.

I will consider only one essential requirement for "medicalizing" mental conditions: that they concern mental *health* (i.e., psychological normality and pathology). In a famous series of essays and books, Szasz[38] argued that the concept of mental health is a dangerous metaphor that makes no literal sense. One of his arguments was that whereas the norms of physical health are objective and factual, the norms of "mental health" are essentially value-laden:

> The concept of illness, whether bodily or mental, implies *deviation from some clearly defined norm.* In the case of physical illness, the norm is the structural and functional integrity of the human body. Thus, although the desirability of physical health, as such, is an ethical value, what health *is* can be stated in anatomical and physiological terms. What is the norm deviation from which is regarded as mental illness? . . . It is a norm that must be stated in terms of *psychosocial, ethical,* and *legal* concepts.[39]

Szasz cites chronic hostility, vengefulness, divorce, and murder as traits or acts that one can brand "mental illness" only by selecting ethical or legal ideals of "health"—that is, by making value judgments about desirable human behavior.

I agree with Szasz that defining physical health and disease is a factual enterprise, and therefore anything properly called "mental health" must be similarly identifiable without appeal to values. What Szasz does not show to my satisfaction is that psychological normality *cannot* be so defined. Why cannot psychology (like physiology) discover "the structural and functional integrity" of the human mind? Szasz is right that American psychiatry has, in fact, too often illegitimately used social value judgments as a criterion of disease. For example, *DSM-II's* category 000-x60 (sociopathic personality disturbance) was for individuals "ill primarily in terms of society and of conformity with the prevailing cultural milieu"; one of its subcategories covers professional criminals of the Mafia type. But such use of social values was roundly criticized, and largely repudiated, in the APA homosexuality debates. Szasz's general arguments that values are inseparable from psychological normality are to my mind unconvincing.[40]

Another argument against the concept of mental health, suggested by Szasz and elaborated by Sarbin,[41] takes the form of a dilemma. Either "mental diseases" are brain diseases, in which case they should be defined and diagnosed in neurophysiological terms; or they are diseases of an immaterial soul, in which case they are not medical diseases at all. However, such arguments against "mentalistic" vocabulary are no stronger in psychiatry than in psychology at large. Nearly all psychologists, like psychiatrists, believe that mental processes (both normal and pathological) occur in the brain. But a brain process may be best described and explained in mentalistic rather than neurophysiological terms. Terms such as 'drive,' 'affect,' 'motive,' 'belief,' and the like are familiar in psychological theories. Though they no doubt ultimately refer to brain processes, they are not currently definable in neurophysiological language and may never be conveniently so definable. It may be unrealistic to expect neurologists ever to be able to tell by a brain autopsy whether a dead person admired Charlemagne or knew that Berg wrote *Lulu*. Perhaps a computer analogy is helpful: functional defects in computers are often best described in program rather than electronic terms. If mental disorders are like software diseases, they may forever remain best described in psychological vocabulary.[42]

The preceding point can be strengthened by noting that many organic conditions are classified as diseases only by psychological criteria. Some physical causes, of course, kill brain cells—for example, CNS syphilis, lead poisoning, or Alzheimer's disease—and by that physiological criterion are pathological. But in other cases, a physical condition is pathological only because of its psychological effects. Cortisone overdose can produce mania, and LSD can induce a schizophrenialike psychosis; some recent investigators claim to correlate depression with neurotransmitter deficiency or homosexuality with low plasma testosterone. In all these examples, a biochemical *abnormality* is identified but no evident biochemical *dysfunction*. If neurotransmitter deficiency is pathological, that is because it leads to depression and depression is a psychological dysfunction; similarly for testosterone and homosexuality. Physiological abnormalities in themselves, as with low cholesterol or low blood pressure, may be signs of superior health. In practice, therefore, organic psychiatry itself leans heavily on a concept of normal psychological function—that is, a concept of mental health.

Mental Health: Psychoanalysis
and Anthropology

Our analysis implies that the concept of mental health makes sense on one condition: that human psychology be divisible into part-processes with biological functions. Mental health and mental disorders exist if and only if there are counterparts to anatomy and physiology for the mind. This does not mean that psychology, to support a concept of mental health, must *be* physiology. Contrary to much usage in mental health literature, "biological" does not mean "physicochemical"; biology is not the same as chemistry and physics. Biology is the study of inherited functional structures of organisms produced by evolution. As such it embraces, as Darwin clearly realized, species-typical psychology as much as species-typical physiology. What a psychological theory must do to support a concept of mental health is to take physiology as a *model* (i.e., to make a serious effort to anatomize the mind and assign its part-processes functions).

Some psychological theories give the mind too little structure to justify talk of health and illness; that is clearly true of radical behaviorism and perhaps also of "self-realization" theorists such as Maslow and Rogers. The best example of a personality theory with specific mental part-functions is psychoanalytic theory[43] developed by Sigmund Freud and his followers from about 1890 onward. Current psychoanalysis divides the mind into three substructures—the id, ego, and superego—and assigns fixed functions to each. The id, an unconscious system of primitive sexual and aggressive drives, serves as a reservoir of motivational energy. The superego, a punitive agency arising in the Oedipal phase by internalization of parental values, confines behavior within socially acceptable bounds by means of feelings of guilt and shame. The ego serves many integrative and self-preservative functions, including perception, reasoning, and reality testing; its prime job is to coordinate drive gratification in the least destructive channels. Such activities are correctly called biological functions, and psychoanalysts view all forms of psychopathology as involving dysfunction in these three subagencies or their relations. A relatively mild weakness in the ego's ability to resolve conflicts among the demands of id, superego, and reality may result in symptom neurosis, character neurosis, or perversion. A massive ego defect constitutes a psychosis, which may involve a break with reality manifested in hallucinations or delusions.[44]

One advantage of a deep personality theory like psychoanalysis is the light it sheds on the second most puzzling question (besides mind-body perplexities) about mental health: the paradoxes of cultural variation. The American anthropologist Ruth Benedict, in her classic book *Patterns of Culture*,[45] propounded the thesis that the abnormal personality types of some culture are the normals of another, and therefore normality is a cultural construct:

> One of the most striking facts that emerge from a study of widely varying cultures is the ease with which our abnormals function in other cultures. It does not matter what kind of "abnormality" we choose for illustration, those which indicate extreme instability, or those which are more in the nature of character traits like sadism or delusions of grandeur or of persecution, there are well-described cultures in which these abnormals function at ease and with honor, and apparently without danger or difficulty to the society.[46]

Benedict illustrated this thesis with many examples. Mystical experience, the ability to enter trance states and have supernatural visions, is aberrant in Western culture but highly valued in most others, forming the basis for the shaman or "witch doctor" role. Homosexuality has been tolerated or rewarded in cultures as diverse as American Indian societies and classical Greece. Benedict also cites cultures in which the predominant, or "modal," personality type seems to be a form of psychopathology in Western psychiatry. The Kwakiutl, a Northwest Pacific Indian society, organized their social life around the potlatch, a wildly grandiose ceremonial of wealth aimed at cruelly humiliating one's rivals. Benedict describes the personality of a Kwakiutl chief as megalomaniac and paranoid. Even more paranoid were the Dobu of Melanesia, a culture in which everyone viewed everyone else, even family members, as out to poison him and steal his crop of yams by black magic.

Benedict's view, inspired by such examples, was that each culture selects a certain range of "normality" from a continuum of human personality types and condemns the rest as deviant:

> Every society, beginning with some slight inclination in one direction or another, carries its preference farther and farther, integrating itself more and more completely upon its chosen basis, and discarding those types of behavior that are uncongenial. Most of those organizations of personality that seem to us most incontrovertibly abnormal have been used by different civiliza-

CHRISTOPHER BOORSE

tions in the very foundations of their institutional life. Conversely the most valued traits of our normal individuals have been looked on in differently organized cultures as aberrant. Normality, in short, within a very wide range, is culturally defined.[47]

To evaluate this thesis of the cultural definition of normality, one must distinguish cultural variation from cultural relativism. Cultural *variation* in judgments of normality is a fact, even in the realm of ordinary medicine. Many conditions considered pathological by Western medicine have been viewed as normal by other cultures. The Greeks saw epilepsy as a divine gift; the Navajo reportedly viewed congenital hip dislocation as normal; one African tribe takes dyschromic spirochetosis (a skin diease) to be so normal that its absence is a disease making one unsuitable for marriage. Culture *relativism* is the further thesis that no culture's views about normality are objectively right or wrong. This thesis our analysis forces us to reject. If—and it is a large assumption—a given culture judges normality by the biological concept of pathology in Western medicine, the culture can be just as mistaken about what is normal as about any other biological fact, such as the origin of babies or the migration of butterflies. Any culture can be wrong about biological function and dysfunction—including Western psychiatry when it relies on social values to define abnormality.

A depth psychology like psychoanalysis suggests two fundamental points regarding Benedict's cross-cultural data. First, one must distinguish among behavior, personality, and deep psychodynamics. A form of behavior (homosexual acts) or even surface personality trait (paranoia) may have different psychodynamic significance in different cultures. For example, a Plains Indian shaman who sees visions of, say, tree spirits is likely to have a much healthier personality and psychodynamics than a New York investment analyst who has the same vision. The latter is schizophrenic or organically psychotic; the former, not necessarily. It may not be, in fact, "our abnormals" who function in other societies with prestige and distinction.[48] Psychoanalysts agree with Benedict that the "definite fixed symptoms" of Western descriptive psychiatry may change their diagnostic significance across cultures. But it may be possible to state universal criteria of normality at a deeper level of psychological theory. In nontechnical terms, psychoanalytic universals of health might include freedom from crippling anxiety, deep and stable love relations, full and unconflicted development of one's abilities, and the capacity for orgasmic sexual release.

A second psychoanalytic thesis about normality and culture is that normality cannot be equated with social acceptance. Deviance is not psychopathology and is often a poor indicator of it. As Benedict suggests herself near the end of her essay, universal criteria of normality will locate the abnormals of each culture not only among its outcasts but also in its most prestigious members. In Western society, these "abnormals of extreme fulfillment of the cultural type" might, to the psychoanalyst, include compulsively ambitious politicians and business executives, fanatical intelligence agents, and religious extremists such as fundamentalist preachers, priests, and nuns. Such individuals find their personal psychopathology rewarded by their culture with a special, even prestigious, niche, as did Greek epileptics or (depending on one's diagnosis of shamans) Indian shamans. But it is crucial to the psychoanalytic view that social prestige—resulting as it does from the adventitious cultural choices Benedict describes—is no index of normality defined in functional psychological terms.

Mental Health: Atheoretic Psychiatry

Mainstream psychiatry, especially in America, has been deeply influenced by psychoanalysis. But psychiatry before and after Freud also described and classified mental disorders apart from any deep theory of psychological part-function. As one might predict from the history of medicine and our analysis of health, this atheoretic approach—currently enjoying a resurgence illustrated by the new DSM-III classification—faces serious difficulties.

As the current canon of psychopathology emerged under Kraepelin toward the end of the nineteenth century, it rested mainly on two criteria of abnormality: social values and faculty psychology. By faculty psychology I mean the commonsense division of mental functioning into "faculties" such as sensation, perception, memory, reason, belief, imagination, and will. Such a theory though primitive, may be enough to identify catastrophic psychiatric disorders (e.g., psychoses) as pathological. The delusions, hallucinations, and bizarre abnormalities of reasoning and speech in schizophrenia leave little doubt that species-typical human psychological functions are grossly impaired. However, the faculty approach is less helpful with less severe impairments. Should one recognize a faculty of conscience, for example, or of heterosexuality or religious faith, in order to brand as abnormal psychopathy, homosexuality, and atheism? Lacking a clear methodology for determining normal psychological faculties, nineteenth-century psychiatry in practice used social disfavor to classify perversions, addictions, and antisocial behavior as pathological.

Since the 1973 homosexuality controversy, American psychiatry has tended to disavow social value judgments as a test of normality. But its attempts to justify the DSM classification on atheoretic, nonevaluative grounds raise many of the classic difficulties of faculty psychology. One of the most sophisticated such attempts at defining mental disorder appears in an article by Spitzer (chair of the APA nomenclature committee) and Endicott:

> A medical disorder is a relatively distinct condition resulting from an organismic dysfunction which in its fully developed or extreme form is directly and intrinsically associated with distress, disability, or certain other types of disadvantage. The disadvantage may be of a physical, perceptual, sexual, or interpersonal nature. Implicitly there is a call to action on the part of the person who has the condition, the medical or its allied professions, and society.
>
> A mental disorder is a medical disorder whose manifestations are primarily signs or symptoms of a psychological (behavioral) nature, or if physical, can be understood only using psychological concepts.[49]

This "3-D" definition of medical disorder is based on distress, disability, and disadvantage. Spitzer and Endicott defined 'disability' as "some impairment in a wide range of activities," hoping by the term 'wide' to avoid psychiatric value judgments about which activities are "basic" or "essential." Still, their examples of broad-range impairment include antisocial personality—which they concede covers a large proportion of criminals—mania, and alcoholism. Most controversial, the authors recognize, is their category of "disadvantage." Their psychiatric examples of kinds of disadvantage include "atypical and inflexible impulse-driven behavior which often has painful consequences" (sadism, kleptomania, compulsive gambling) and "impairment in the ability to experience sexual pleasure in an interpersonal context" (anorgasmia, fetishism).

Spitzer and Endicott realize that their somewhat heterogeneous list (pp. 20–21) of forms of disadvantage, like traditional lists of faculties, invites criticism as ad hoc—that is, designed solely to produce a certain psychiatric classification, in this case roughly *DSM-II* without homosexuality. Why must normal sexuality be "interpersonal," so that homosexuals but not fetishists or bestialists can be normal? Among traditional interpersonal perverts, sadomasochists, transvestites, exhibitionists, and pedophiles are abnormal by the clause on atypical inflexible sexual behavior. But by this clause, the authors let a social reaction to a condition (the "painful consequences") determine its normality. Spitzer and Endicott allow for normal homosexuality because, although many social environments penalize homosexuals, more tolerant cultures or subcultures make their condition painless. By contrast, the authors believe no society can tolerate the other perversions or kleptomania or crime with equanimity. But this judgment is open to question, and so is the notion that social reaction should determine normality or pathology at all.

Nevertheless, it is instructive to compare the Spitzer-Endicott definition with the one that ultimately appeared in *DSM-III* (though *DSM-III* denies that it is intended as a definition):

A mental disorder is conceptualized as a clinically significant behavioral or psychologic syndrome or pattern that occurs in an individual and that typically is associated with either a painful symptom (distress) or impairment in one or more important areas of functioning (disability). In addition, there is an inference that there is a behavioral, psychologic, or biologic dysfunction, and that the disturbance is not only in the relationship between the individual and society. When the disturbance is limited to a conflict between an individual and society, this may represent social deviance, which may or may not be commendable, but is not by itself a mental disorder.[50]

Here Spitzer and Endicott's distinction between disability and disadvantage has disappeared. Further, the idea of dysfunction has been demoted from a "cause" to an "inference," on our analysis a change for the worse. The definition does not indicate when a dysfunction may be "inferred"; nor does it explain what a "behavioral dysfunction" might be. The remarks on pure social deviance mean, perhaps, that one society's evaluation of a condition is never enough to make it pathological. On this reading, the deviance clause explains why the manual does not consider Soviet political dissidents or "egosyntonic" American homosexuals as abnormal. But as written it leaves mysterious *DSM-III*'s treatment of other perversions, psychopathy, and organized crime. In the end, the DSM-III definition buries problems and distinctions elucidated by Spitzer and his colleagues, relying on an unanalyzed category of "disability" that leaves most of the problems of faculty psychology untouched.[51]

The history of medicine shows that an atheoretic, purely clinical approach to identifying diseases is of limited value. Gifted clinical observers like Hippocrates or Sydenham succeeded in recognizing well-marked syndromes, such as gout or typhoid fever. As a global strategy of classification, pure clinical description risks producing sterile compendia of symptoms like the encyclopedic nosology of Boissier de Sauvages, with its scores of kinds of "fluxes" (bodily discharges). Psychiatry faces a special difficulty in recognizing what is or is not a symptom. Without a deep theory of psychological part-function, how is one to decide whether exclusive homosexuality is abnormal, or exclusive heterosexuality, or both, or neither? Ordinary medicine also has had uncertainties over the normality of gross signs; some nineteenth-century physicians, for example, found it normal for menstruating women to cough blood. In psychiatry, however, controversy over the normality of specific behaviors seems more the rule than the exception.

Current disease classifications, now grounded in a century of scientific physiology and pathology, reveal a converse danger in the clinical approach: it favors acute symptomatic disorders over more serious chronic ones. Clinicians may recognize gout as a disease but not hypothyroidism; measles, but not systemic lupus. There are interesting psychiatric parallels. A pure clinician may view a phobia or compulsion (symptom neurosis) as abnormal, perhaps calling it a "volitional disability." Less clinically apparent is the graver chronic "defeat of will" (character neurosis) that paralyzes a person from vigorous pursuit of his ambitions and goals. A noted surgeon who suffers hysterical paralysis or a severe phobia seems, to the clinical eye, to have a disorder. But a psychoanalyst may see the surgeon as far healthier than a symptom-free accountant who surrendered dreams of medical school out of neurotic conflict. The accountant's "symptoms" are his whole life and character. For various reasons, then, it may be questioned whether atheoretic psychiatry can succeed in proving much more than the psychoses to be genuine mental disorders.

Health, Medicine, and Society

I conclude with some remarks on the relation between health, medicine, and social values. Clearly, almost all traditional medical therapy aims at promoting health. Medical treatment in this *core sense*[52] is the removal, mitigation, or prevention of pathology. An example of removal is a total cure of an infectious disease; examples of mitigation (substitution of mild for severe pathology) include most other medical treatments and all surgery. The justification for medical therapy in the core sense is that normal biological functional ability is almost always desirable. Of course, a patient's choice between two forms of pathology (or levels of risk) may depend on the patient's personal values; for that very reason, however, such decisions seem not distinctively medical ones. It is the overwhelming presumption of the value of biological normality that creates the sense of objectivity and moral urgency in traditional medicine.[53]

Contemporary medicine now also includes various *peripheral* forms of treatment: procedures requiring medical expertise and therefore performed by physicians, but not aimed at health promotion. Current examples include cosmetic surgery, vasectomy, and circumcision. Undoubtedly future surgical and pharmacologic technology will present physicians with a vast range of techniques for assisting patients in optional self-modification. Unlike traditional physicians of a generation ago, I would not argue that health promotion is medicine's only legitimate business. Contraceptive prescriptions are now accepted practice; and history is far from kind to the Victorian editor of Lancet who opposed obstetrical anesthesia because pain in childbirth is normal. Still, one must keep the two kinds of medical treatment conceptually distinct. Peripheral medical treatment is medical only in that physicians do it; moreover, the decision to do it usually lacks the objectivity and moral urgency of the medicine of health promotion.

Unfortunately, core and peripheral medicine are thoroughly confused in many contemporary writings on abortion. If our analysis of health in traditional medicine is correct, the typical elective abortion is not a medical treatment in any core sense. It is no more medical than a nose job; indeed, it is less medical insofar as it involves killing a human organism. Typical elective abortions are not medical procedures because a fetus is not pathology and unhappiness is not ill health—even ill mental health. The World Health Organization's expansive definition of health, which the Supreme Court seems to endorse, is both an incorrect analysis and a powerful vehicle for what Szasz calls "bootlegging humanistic [better, liberal] values through psychiatry."[54] Similar remarks apply to infant "euthanasia" motivated by concern for parents rather than the baby. A decision or procedure is not medical in any interesting sense simply because doctors are the agents. Physicians might well make the most expert executioners, as they are now the safest abortionists; but that hardly would make capital punishment therapy.

To turn from ordinary medicine to psychotherapy, our discussion implies that insofar as psychotherapy aims at mental health, its standards of success should be based on a substantive theory of psychological part-functions. A concept of "mental health" based purely on the therapist's own values, or even the patient's own values, is not an ideal of mental *health*. Even psychoanalytic writers sometimes miss this point, as when Hartmann suggests that "individual conceptions of health differ widely among analysts themselves, varying with the aims which each has set himself on the basis of his views concerning human development, and also of course with his philosophy, political sympathies, etc."[55]

A genuine ideal of mental health should vary no more with a therapist's social philosophy or politics than an ideal of physical health in ordinary medicine. Liberal and radical psychotherapists are especially prone to this confusion. Arnold Lazarus, describing the goals of "behavior therapy," wrote a virtual feminist manifesto:

In behavior therapy we aim to teach women how to be assertive and truly emancipated from an oppressive regime of domestic drudgery; how to be successful while never hiding their intellectual prowess and never denigrating their own achievements; how to be genuinely uninhibited, fully recognizing their rights and gently but persuasively showing many of their exploited sisters how to modify a wide range of proscribed roles.[56]

Whether or not these ideals are admirable, the quotation clearly presents a specific political program as an ideal of health. That is precisely what should not occur, on our analysis. At bottom, there is much similarity between feminist therapists calling feminist ideals mental health and Soviet psychiatrists diagnosing political dissidence as "sluggish schizophrenia": in both cases, the vocabulary of medicine is being abused to mask political ends.

As for the extraprofessional social issues discussed earlier, our analysis of health suggests a modest generalization. Rarely are medical judgments of the presence or even severity of pathology the whole of a social issue; occasionally they are not the issue at all. In the second category is the dispute over pregnancy benefits, as the Supreme Court realized in *General Electric* and *Geduldig v. Aiello* (417 U.S. 484, 1974). Pregnancy is certainly not a disease; nonetheless, arguably it should be covered for the same reasons diseases are covered, especially since neither benefit plan in the two cases covered all diseases and only diseases. By contrast, an issue in which pathology is relevant but not the whole story is the insanity defense. All major tests of criminal insanity use the concept of "mental disease."[57] All but the *Durham* rule, however, add conditions beyond mere (causal) psychopathology; the *Durham* rule itself would have been abandond far more rapidly had it been literally applied. Criminal insanity is not just mental disorder, but mental disorder *that ought to excuse* criminal conduct. Which mental disorders ought to excuse conduct is inescapably a moral, not a psychiatric question; this remains true even if the further legal requirements chosen correlate roughly, as the *M'Naghten* knowledge test may, with severity of disease.

Homosexuality, finally, is an issue with respect to which our analysis separates several questions that are often confused. We can agree with the new psychiatric view in *DSM-III* that mere social condemnation is not enough to make a condition pathological. Whether homosexuality is pathological depends on whether it involves a biological mental dysfunction. On general biological principles, the exclusive homosexual (but not the bisexual) looks pathological by virtue of his or her reproductive failure. Some recent biologists suggest models (e.g., kin selection) by which evolution could favor genes for homosexuality in the population. Unless some such model is vindicated, exclusive homosexuality seems likely to be a form of mental pathology, as psychoanalysts have always maintained.

Nevertheless, to judge homosexuality pathological settles the issue of its inclusion in *DSM* only if *DSM* is intended as a list of all pathological conditions. Many writers, including Spitzer himself[58] view the nomenclature instead as a list of *serious* abnormalities justifying a "call to action" on the part of society, patients, and the medical profession—roughly, what we called "therapeutic abnormalities" earlier. To judge homosexuality as biologically abnormal says nothing about its severity; it might be a minor form of pathology, like a wart or red-green color blindness, and one as consistent with happiness as any other abnormality (e.g., oviduct blockage) producing infertility. Freud's own position was that homosexuality, though abnormal, was not an illness.[59] On no interpretation of *DSM*, in any case, is it easy to justify including homosexuality or other perversions while excluding celibacy. Perverts have some sex life, which is more than one can say for the total celibate.

The most crucial point is that judgments of pathology (whether of presence or degree) are not equivalent to social or legal judgments. A psychiatric nomenclature is not a hunting license for social and legal discrimination. For any disease category, some discriminations will be justified and others will not. Each issue requires a social policy judgment grounded in rational ethical and legal debate. For example, if homosexuality were shown both pathological and contagious to young children, that might justify disqualifying homosexuals from teaching elementary school. It would not justify disqualifying homosexuals from holding government jobs, renting apartments, or enjoying basic civil rights and liberties. A different array of justified discriminations would apply to psychotics, another to psychopaths, another to agoraphobes, and so on. Such questions are indeed "political"[60] in the best sense (i.e., they concern morality and law). But just for that reason they are not psychiatric issues. It has been a central thesis of this essay that medicine is not morals, nor morals medicine; the same goes for psychiatry and politics. Even more surely, attempts to resolve all professional and social issues with a simple sick-well dichotomy are bound to fail.

Notes

1. In the abortion context, the broad definition means that an abortion is arguably necessary to the mental health of any woman who strongly wants one. In California in 1968, 92 percent of all abortions were medically justified on mental health grounds. See Lynn D. Wardle and Mary Anne Q. Wood, *A Lawyer Looks at Abortion* (Provo, Utah: Brigham Young University Press, 1982), 35.

2. Caplan, Arthur L.; Engelhardt, H. Tristram, Jr.; and McCartney, James J., eds., *Concepts of Health and Disease: Interdisciplinary Perspectives.* (Reading, Mass.: Addison-Wesley, 1981), 83.

3. Szasz, Thomas S., "The Myth of Mental Illness," *American Psychologist* 15(1960):113–118; *The Manufacture of Madness* (New York: Harper and Row, 1970); *The Myth of Mental Illness.* Rev. ed. (New York: Harper and Row, 1974); *Ideology and Insanity* (Garden City, N.Y.: Anchor, 1970); *Schizophrenia: The Sacred Symbol of Psychiatry* (New York: Basic Books, 1976).

4. Jahoda, Marie, *Current Concepts of Positive Mental Health* (New York: Basic Books, 1958); Offer, Daniel, and Sabshin, Melvin, *Normality* (New York: Basic Books, 1974).

5. Four justices in the *Powell* plurality read *Robison* to bar conviction only for a disease itself (addiction, alcoholism), not for its symptomatic acts (public drunkenness). This disease-symptoms distinction was rejected by Justice White as well as by the four dissenters, making an apparent majority for the thesis that *Robinson* bars conviction at least for acts "irresistibly compelled" by disease

6. LaFave, Wayne R., and Scott, Austin W., Jr., *Handbook on Criminal*

Law (St. Paul, Minn.: West Publishing, 1972); Moore, Michael S., *Law and Psychiatry: Rethinking the Relationship* (Cambridge: Cambridge University Press, 1984).

7. Bayer, Ronald, *Homosexuality and American Psychiatry* (New York: Basic Books, 1981).

8. American Psychiatric Association, *Diagnostic and Statistical Manual of Mental Disorders*, 3d ed. *(DSM-III)* (Washington, D.C., 1980).

9. Besides the examples in the text, psychiatric diagnoses arousing considerable controversy include premenstrual syndrome, hyperactivity in children, senile dementia, and depression. Some feminists also have attacked all psychiatric theories of female psychology as oppressive to women.

10. My discussion, however, is limited to ideas of health in traditional Western medicine. Contemporary scientific medicine is the most sophisticated available theory of health and disease. Although it is also of interest to study lay ideas, or non-Western ideas, or innovative medical ideas, evaluating their significance requires an understanding of traditional medical views. The analysis below is restricted by this assumption.

11. American Medical Association, *Standard Nomenclature of Diseases and Operations*, ed. Richard J. Plunkett and Aladine C. Hayden, 4th ed. (New York: Blakiston, 1952).

12. Culver, Charles M., and Gert, Bernard, *Philosophy in Medicine: Conceptual and Ethical Issues in Medicine and Psychiatry* (New York: Oxford University Press, 1982), 65–66.

13. Kendell, R. E., "The Concept of Disease and Its Implications for Psychiatry," *British Journal of Psychiatry* 127 (1975): 307.

14. The term *pathological* is wider than pathology (e.g., concrete lesions to tissues or fluids). It also covers functional disorders (*Nomenclature* category x) with no known pathology. But for stylistic convenience, I will hereafter often use "normality and pathology" instead of "the normal and the pathological." A more leisurely discussion also would distinguish *pathologic* (constituting disease) from *pathogenic* (causing disease) and *pathodictic* (indicating disease).

15. Culver and Gert note the need for a "genus" term covering all these medical conditions and propose "malady." But "pathological" is already in established medical usage in this role. See *Philosophy in Medicine.*

16. This definition of illness assumes that one cannot be physically sick or ill without some pathophysiology. It also implies that one can feel sick without being sick and be sick without feeling it. The definition is a marked revision of my earlier discussion of illness, making illness virtually as value-free as disease. See my "On the Distinction Between Disease and Illness," *Philosophy & Public Affairs* 5 (1975): 49–68.

The distinctions in the figure, though useful, are at best a gesture in the direction of a theory of *health comparisons*, which are fundamental in therapy and in many extraprofessional issues. Space prevents discussion of this important topic.

17. Goodwin, Donald W., and Guze, Samuel B., *Psychiatric Diagnosis*, 2d.ed. (New York: Oxford University Press, 1979) 68.

18. Szasz, "The Myth of Mental Illness," 113–118.

19. Kass, Leon, "Regarding the End of Medicine and the Pursuit of Health," *The Public Interest* 40(1975):11–42.

20. Klein, "A Proposed Definition," 64.

21. Boorse, Christopher, "On the Distinction Between Disease and Illness."

22. Sedgwick, Peter, "Illness—Mental and Otherwise," *Hastings Center Studies* 1(1973):30–31.

23. A pure normativist view implies that a radical shift in values can produce a radical shift—even a reversal—in what count as health and disease. Suppose we believed (like some medieval Christians) that life is bad, death good, and suffering beneficial. On a pure normativist view, what we now see as disease would be health, and health disease. On a naturalistic view, the otherworldly Christian, in devaluing life, devalues health automatically—and is still dying of disease.

24. Kass is not, however, best described as a "naturalist" in that he seems to reject the fact-value distinction. He describes health as "a natural standard or norm," "an activity of the living body in accordance with its specific excellences." I cannot grasp the Aristotelian notion of a "natural norm." Kass also believes in positive health beyond the absence of disease. See Leon Kass, "Regarding the End of Medicine and the Pursuit of Health," *The Public Interest* 40(1975):11–42.

25. Kass, "Regarding the End," 13–14.

26. Engelhardt, H. Tristram, Jr., "Human Well-Being and Medicine: Some Basic Value Judgments in the Biomedical Sciences," in *Science, Ethics and Medicine*, ed. Engelhardt and Daniel Callahan (Hastings-on-Hudson, N.Y.: Hastings Center, 1976), 136.

27. This definition omits some details necessary to avoid medical counterexamples. Such refinements might include clauses on qualitative structural abnormalities (see my "Health as a Theoretical Concept," *Philosophy of Science* 44(1977):565–566); distinct sustaining cause (Culver and Gert, *Philosophy in Medicine*, 72–74); and normal limitations of one function by another. A similar approach to the definition in the text can be found in Donald F. Klein, "A Proposed Definition of Mental Illness," in *Critical Issues in Psychiatric Diagnosis*, ed. Robert L. Spitzer and Donald F. Klein (New York: Raven Press, 1978), 41–71.

28. Sober, Elliott, ed., *Conceptual Issues in Evolutionary Biology* (Cambridge, Mass.: MIT Press, 1984).

29. Ruse, Michael, "Functional Statements in Biology," *Philosophy of Science* 38(1971):87–95.

30. Wright, Larry, "Functions," *Philosophical Review* 82(1973):139–168.

31. A word about universal diseases: the definition in the text makes universal disease impossible. In the case of aging or atherosclerosis, this result is not far from traditional medical views. What is pathological is *premature*

aging or atherosclerosis. The same view is less plausible for tooth decay; for some remarks on this problem see my "Health as a Theoretical Concept," 566.

32. I suspect, however, that adding a disvalue clause to the definition in the text—making conditions pathological when they meet the definition *and* are prima facie undesirable—would leave most controversies untouched. The crucial element of most disputes is the matter of conformity to species design.

33. Engelhardt, H. Tristram, Jr., "Ideology and Etiology," *Journal of Medicine and Philosophy* 1 (1976): 264.

34. American Psychiatric Association, *Diagnostic and Statistical Manual: Mental Disorders*, 2nd ed. (*DSM-II*) (Washington, D.C., 1965).

35. *DSM-III* both deletes some of these categories (neuroses) and adds to others (tobacco dependency), as well as introducing a multiaxial diagnostic scheme too complex to discuss here. An extended comparison of *DSM-II* and *DSM-III* is included in *DSM-III*.

36. If one must distinguish between mental and physical disorders, the most useful criterion is probably mental causation, in the sense of psychological etiology or primary pathology. Often, however, the distinction causes much unnecessary confusion.

37. Talcott Parsons ("Definitions of Health and Illness in the Light of American Values and Social Structure," in *Patients, Physicians, and Illness*, ed. E. G. Jaco [New York: Free Press, 1979]), 120–144, describes the sick role as including two exemptions and two duties: (1) the patient is not responsible for his or her illness; (2) the patient is exempt from normal social responsibilities; (3) the patient is obliged to want to get well and also (4) the patient is obliged to seek competent assistance in doing so.

38. Szasz, "The Myth of Mental Illness;" *The Manufacture of Madness, The Myth of Mental Illness, Ideology and Insanity, Schizophrenia: The Sacred Symbol of Psychiatry*.

39. Szasz, "The Myth of Mental Illness," 114.

40. For example, Thomas Szasz (ibid.) argues that a patient who believes he is Napoleon can be called delusional only by "a covert comparison" of his ideas with those of the psychiatrist or society. But whether the patient is or is not Napoleon is a fact, not a value judgment. If the patient had a delusion about his blood pressure, any ordinary physician would feel free to disagree. So the example seems to mark no difference between medicine and psychiatry.

41. Sarbin, Theodore, "The Scientific Status of the Mental Illness Metaphor," *Changing Perspectives in Mental Illness*, ed. Stanley C. Plog and Robert B. Edgerton (New York: Holt, Rinehart and Winston, 1969).

42. Similarly—contrary to many psychiatrists and jurists over the past century—metaphysical materialism provides no support for psychiatric organicism. Organicism amounts to the view that mental disorders are the result of brain pathology of the *same kinds* found in other organs—infections, toxins, tumors, metabolic abnormalities. As the computer analogy sug-

gests, though the brain is an organ, it may suffer unique kinds of pathology not seen in other organs, kinds best described in psychological vocabulary.

43. Brenner, Charles, *An Elementary Textbook of Psychoanalysis*, 2d. ed. (Garden City, N.Y.: Anchor, 1973); Waelder, Robert, *Basic Theory of Psychoanalysis* (New York: International Universities Press, 1960).

44. Two notable disanalogies between psychoanalytic and medical normality may be the folloing. First, psychoanalysis uses an ideal conception of normality in terms of which no one is fully normal; it is not clear that medical normality is, as Freud says of the normal mind, an "ideal fiction." Second, developmental arrest is central to psychoanalytic psychopathology, but far from central in ordinary medicine.

45. Benedict, Ruth, *Patterns of Culture* (Boston: Houghton Mifflin, 1934).

46. Benedict, Ruth, "Anthropology and the Abnormal," *Journal of General Psychology* 10(1934):59–82. Reprinted in Rabkin, Leslie Y., and Carr, John E., eds., *Sourcebook in Abnormal Psychology* (Boston: Houghton Mifflin, 1967), 10.

47. Ibid, 15–16.

48. Wegrocki, Henry J. "A Critique of Cultural and Statistical Concepts of Abnormality," *Journal of Abnormal and Social Psychology* 34 (1939): 166–178.

49. Spitzer, Robert L., and Endicott, Jean, "Medical and Mental Disorder: Proposed Definition and Criteria." In Spitzer and Klein, *Critical Issues*, 18.

50. American Psychiatric Association, *DSM-III*, 363.

51. My discussion of the two definitions above is indebted to Michael S. Moore, *Law and Psychiatry: Rethinking the Relationship* (Cambridge: Cambridge University Press, 1984), and Culver and Gert, *Philosophy in Medicine*.

52. Boorse, "On the Distinction Between Disease and Illness."

53. Beyond this, social tradition licenses physicians virtually to put patients' health above all other considerations. Thus doctors may treat a dictator's heart disease, or a pickpocket's arthritis, without being accomplices to their crimes or even incurring moral criticism.

54. Szasz, *Ideology and Insanity*, 87–97.

55. Caplan, Engelhardt, and McCartney, *Concepts of Health and Disease*, 364.

56. Lazarus, Arnold, "Women in Behavior Therapy," in *Women in Therapy*, ed. Violet Franks and Vasanti Burtle (New York: Brunner-Mazel, 1974), 226.

57. LaFave and Scott, *Handbook on Criminal Law* ; Moore, *Law and Psychiatry*.

58. Spitzer and Endicott, "Medical and Mental Disorder," 17.

59. Bayer, *Homosexuality*, 27.

60. Ibid., 5.

Suggestions for Further Reading

A voluminous literature exists on each of the controversies of section I. For a survey of abortion law, see Lynn D. Wardle and Mary Anne Q. Wood, *A Lawyer Looks at Abortion* (Provo, Ut.: Brigham Young University Press, 1982).

A useful discussion of empirical research and legal doctrines about addiction is parts III and IV of Herbert Fingarette and Ann Fingarette Hasse, *Mental Disabilities and Criminal Responsibility* (Berkeley: University of California Press, 1979).

On the insanity defense, a survey of basic law is chapter 4 of Wayne R. LaFave and Austin W. Scott, Jr., *Handbook on Criminal Law* (St. Paul, Minn.: West Publishing, 1972). More extended and sophisticated discussions include Abraham Goldstein, *The Insanity Defense* (New Haven: Yale University Press, 1967); Herbert Fingarette, *The Meaning of Criminal Insanity* (Berkeley: University of California Press, 1972); Fingarette and Hase, *Mental Disabilities*; and Michael S. Moore, *Law and Psychiatry: Rethinking the Relationship* (New York: Cambridge, 1984). An interesting survey of mental illness and murder is Donald J. Lunde, *Murder and Madness* (New York: Norton, 1979).

The history of the APA homosexuality controversy is recounted at length in Ronald Bayer, *Homosexuality and American Psychiatry* (New York: Basic Books, 1981), and further documented in Bayer and Robert L. Spitzer, "Edited Correspondence on the Status of Homosexuality in DSM-III," *Journal of the History of the Behavioral Sciences* 18(1982):32–52. Philosophical introductions to empirical and ethical theories about homosexuality include Michael Ruse, *Homosexuality: A Philosophical Perspective* (Berkeley: University of California, forthcoming), and the chapter by Joseph Margolis in Tom Regan and Donald VanDeVeer, *And Justice for All* (Totowa, N.J.: Rowman and Allanheld, 1982).

The diversity of existing clinical criteria of mental health is explored in Marie Jahoda, *Current Concepts of Positive Mental Health* (New York: Basic Books, 1958), and in Daniel Offer and Melvin Sabshin, *Normality* (New York: Basic Books, 1974).

The contemporary assault on psychiatry by Szasz and others is illustrated by Thomas S. Szasz, "The myth of mental illness," *American Psychologist* 15(1960):113–18; *The Manufacture of Madness* (New York: Harper and Row, 1970); *The Myth of Mental Illness*, rev. ed. (New York: Harper and Row, 1974); *Ideology and Insanity* (Garden City, N.Y.: Anchor, 1970); and *Schizophrenia: The Sacred Symbol of Psychiatry* (New York: Basic, 1976). An introductory anthology on Szasz's work is Richard E. Vatz and Lee S. Weinberg, *Thomas Szasz: Primary Values and Major Contentions* (Buffalo: Prometheus, 1983). On anti-psychiatry see also Peter Sedgwick, *Psycho Politics* (New York: Harper, 1982).

On the scope of the medical concept of disease, see Edward T. Thompson and Adaline C. Hayden, eds., *Standard Nomenclature of Diseases and Operations*, 5th ed. (New York: McGraw-Hill, 1961), or any basic textbook of medicine such as Paul B. Beeson and Walsh McDermott, eds., *Textbook of Medicine*, 14th ed. (Philadelphia: Saunders, 1975) or *Harrison's Principles of Internal Medicine* 8th ed. (New York: McGraw-Hill, 1977). Historical materials on the development of medical concepts of disease include Knud Faber, *Nosography* (New York: Hoeber, 1930) and the essays by Cohen, Veith, King, Temkin, and Kendell in Arthur L. Caplan, H. Tristram Engelhardt, Jr., and James J. McCartney, eds., *Concepts of Health and Disease: Interdisciplinary Perspectives*. (Reading, Mass.: Addison-Wesley, 1981).

A useful factual summary of the history of medicine is Charles Singer and E. Ashworth Underwood, *A Short History of Medicine* (New York: Oxford, 1962). See also the essays collected in Owsei Temkin, *The Double Face of Janus* (Baltimore: Johns Hopkins University Press, 1977). Aspects of ancient medicine are discussed in Ludwig Edelstein, *Ancient Medicine*, ed. and trans. Owsei and C. Lilian Temkin (Baltimore: Johns Hopkins University Press, 1967) and the classical roots of modern psychiatry in Bennett Simon, *Mind and Madness in Ancient Greece* (Ithaca, N.Y.: Cornell University Press, 1978).

The contemporary psychiatric classification is presented in American Psychiatric Association, *Diagnostic and Statistical Manual of Mental Disorders*, 3d. ed. (Washington, D.C.: 1980), and analyzed in depth in Alfred M. Freedman, Harold I. Kaufman, and Benjamin J. Sadock, eds., *Comprehensive Textbook of Psychiatry*, 2d.ed. (Baltimore: Williams and Wilkins, 1975) and almost any current textbook of abnormal psychology. The appendix to Karl Menninger, *The Vital Balance* (New York: Viking, 1963) is an invaluable historical compendium of psychiatric classifications.

On the history of psychiatry in general see Franz Alexander and Sheldon T. Selesnick, *The History of Psychiatry* (New York: Harper, 1966); Henri Ellenberger, *The Discovery of the Unconscious* (New York: Basic Books, 1970); and Gregory Zilboorg and George W. Henry, *A History of Medical Psychology* (New York: Norton, 1941). Particularly helpful on late nineteenth-century concepts of "moral insanity" is Henry Werlinder, *Psychopathy: A History of the Concepts* (Stockholm: Almqvist and Wiksell, 1978).

Some basic sources on contemporary psychoanalysis are Charles Brenner, *An Elementary Textbook of Psychoanalysis*, 2d ed. (Garden City, N.Y.: Anchor, 1973); Robert Waelder, *Basic Theory of Psychoanalysis* (New York: International Universities Press, 1960); Philip Holzman, *Psychoanalysis and Psychopathology* (New York: McGraw-Hill, 1969); and the article by Meissner, Mack, and Semrad in *Comprehensive Textbook of Psychiatry* (above).

On the anthropological issue of culture and normality, see Ruth Benedict, *Patterns of Culture* (Boston: Houghton Mifflin, 1934), and "Anthropology and the Abnormal," *Journal of General Psychology* 10(1934):59–82, reprinted in Leslie Y. Rabkin and John E. Carr, eds., *Sourcebook in Abnormal*

Psychology (Boston: Houghton Mifflin, 1967), for the classic statement of cultural relativism. A critique of Benedict still worth reading is Henry J. Wegrocki, "A critique of cultural and statistical concepts of abnormality," *Journal of Abnormal and Social Psychology* 34(1939):166–78. More recent sources include Anthony F.C. Wallace, *Culture and Personality* (New York: Random House, 1970), Robert A. LeVine, *Culture, Behavior, and Personality* (Chicago: Aldine, 1973), and Warner Muensterberger, ed., *Man and His Culture*, (London: Rapp and Whiting, 1969), specifically on cross-cultural psychoanalysis. Jane Murphy "The recognition of psychosis in non-Western societies," in *Critical Issues in Psychiatric Diagnosis*, ed. Robert L. Spitzer and Donald F. Klein [New York: Raven Press, 1978], 1–13) is one of several recent writers to question whether primitive concepts of psychosis differ very greatly from those of Western psychiatry.

On the basic topic of this essay, the problem of defining health and disease, the best single source is Caplan, Engelhardt, and McCartney, *Concepts of Health and Disease* (above). Most of the essays in this volume deal with the concept of health. An important essay recently translated is Georges Canguilhem, *The Normal and the Pathological* (1966), trans. Carolyn R. Fawcett (Dordrecht: Reidel, 1978). Among many other works on this topic, the interested reader may consult Charles M. Culver and Bernard Gert, *Philosophy in Medicine: Conceptual and Ethical Issues in Medicine and Psychiatry* (New York: Oxford University Press, 1982), chapters 4 and 5; Robert Brown, "Physical Health and Mental Illness," *Philosophy and Public Affairs* 7(Fall 1977):17–38; Daniel Callahan, "The WHO definition of health," *Hastings Center Studies* 1(1973):77–87; H. Tristram Engelhardt, Jr., "Human Well-Being and Medicine: Some Basic Value Judgments in the Biomedical Sciences," in Engelhardt and Daniel Callahan, eds., *Science, Ethics and Medicine* (Hastings-on-Hudson, N.Y.: Hastings Center, 1976); R. E. Kendell, "The Concept of Disease and its Implications for Psychiatry," *British Journal of Psychiatry* 127(1975):305–315; Donald F. Klein, "A Proposed Definition of Mental Illness," in Spitzer and Klein, *Critical Issues*, 41–71; Joseph Margolis, "The Concept of Disease," *Journal of Medicine and Philosphy* 1(1976):238–255; and the articles by Robert Spitzer and his coworkers: Robert L. Spitzer and Jean Endicott, "Medical and Mental Disorder: Proposed Definition and Criteria," in Spitzer and Klein, *Critical Issues*, 15–40, and Spitzer and Janet Williams, "The Definition and Diagnosis of Mental Disorder," in W. R. Gove, ed., *Deviance and Mental Illness* (Beverly Hills, Ca.: Sage, 1982).

One of the fuller discussions of the relation of health to medical practice is still Leon Kass, "Regarding the End of Medicine and the Pursuit of Health," *The Public Interest* 40(1975):11–42, reprinted in Caplan, Engelhardt, and McCartney, *Concepts of Health and Disease.*

CHAPTER XI

Ethical Autonomy in Nursing

Martin Benjamin and Joy Curtis

Introduction

Nurses frequently find themselves in situations that raise questions of allowing to die, informed consent, experimentation on human subjects, treating incompetents, abortion, and so on. But before a nurse begins to address these and related questions in health care ethics, she must have a clear, defensible understanding of the extent to which she is entitled or required to have and act upon a position *of her own* on these matters. In other words, she must determine the degree to which she is, in her role as a nurse, morally autonomous or self-determining.

Traditionally, nurses have been discouraged from developing and acting on their own ethical judgments. Although the institutions of nursing and medicine developed separately until the late eighteenth century, the increasing importance of the hospital in health care brought nursing under the dual command of physicians and hospital administrators.[1] Thus in 1903 the *Journal of the American Medical Association* complained that the nurse is "often conceited and too unconscious of the due subordination she owes to the medical profession of which she is a sort of useful parasite." Three years later, the same journal editorialized that "Every attempt at initiative on the part of nurses . . . should be reproved by physicians."[2] Leaders of the nursing profession later echoed this conception of nursing. In 1917, for example, Sarah Dock, who is said to have been "a considerable influence on nursing in her time," wrote in the *American Journal of Nursing*:

In my estimation obedience is the first law and the very corner-stone of good nursing. And here is the first stumbling block for the beginner. No matter how gifted she may be, she will never become a reliable nurse until she can obey without question. The first and most helpful criticism I ever received from a doctor was when he told me that I was supposed to be simply an intelligent machine for the purpose of carrying out his orders.[3]

Certainly if the conception of nursing expressed in these passages is correct, a nurse might have an interest in health care ethics as a citizen or a patient, but she would have no special interest or responsibility as a nurse. For as a "sort of useful parasite" to the physician, as "simply an intelligent machine for the purpose of carrying out his orders," she would, in her role as a nurse, lack the self-direction presupposed by the notions of moral deliberation, decision, and responsibility.

The most basic ethical question for nursing, therefore, is whether nurses should think and act for themselves on matters involving ethical questions in health care, and, if so, to what extent. To say that this is the most basic ethical question for nursing is to say that a nurse's response to other questions in health care ethics depends on her response to it. Under the traditional conception of nursing, for example, a nurse's only ethical obligations, in her capacity as a nurse, are to follow the orders of physicians and the regulations of the hospital. She has no ethical concern, bound up with her professional responsibilities, with the problems of allowing to die, informed consent, experimentation on human subjects, treating incompetents, abortion, and so on. Only if we can show that nurses are, as nurses, morally responsible for some of the consequences of their particular actions can we show that nurses have a professional interest in health care ethics. And we can show this only if we can show that nurses, as nurses, possess some degree of ethical autonomy or moral self-direction.

In what follows we will argue that nurses should, as nurses, be permitted and encouraged to think and act for themselves on matters involving health care ethics. We acknowledge, however, that being ethically autonomous currently is problematic and sometimes personally hazardous in nursing. This is because the traditional conception of nursing, though out of favor with many nurses and nursing leaders, remains deeply embedded in the health care system and in the eye of the public.[4] Therefore, nurses who aspire to moral autonomy will all too often be at odds with the hospital or agency (that employs them), the physician and other nurses (with whom they work), and the patient (for whom they provide care). Although we believe that the system is gradually becoming more accommodating to the ethically autonomous nurse, various instances will occur in which individual nurses will find the price of ethical autonomy extremely high. Thus we will suggest that ethical autonomy requires attention not only to particular cases as they arise but also to those aspects of the health care system that make the exercise of autonomy in these cases especially problematic. Finally, we will identify certain difficult questions that remain to be explored by morally autonomous nurses.

Ethical Autonomy

CASE I: THE RECALCITRANT PATIENT

Mr. Wilson is a seventy-two-year-old patient in an extended care facility, where he is receiving physical therapy following a recent stroke. Although he has made definite gains in strength and mobility, his left arm and leg are partially paralyzed. He is, however, very irritated at his slow recovery and does not want to continue the daily physical therapy, which he finds difficult and monotonous. Lupe Garcia, his primary nurse, believes that, as in similar cases, exercise during the next few weeks will lessen Wilson's long-term disability, and she has tried to persuade him to continue exercising. His therapist and physician have also explained to him the benefits of continuing his therapy, but Wilson is adamant and refuses further cooperation.[5]

A matter of ethics
Whatever Lupe Garcia decides to do in this case, her problem is in large part an ethical one. At issue are questions of informed consent, paternalism, deception, and a possible conflict between the value of patient autonomy, on the one hand, and maximal therapy benefit, on the other. If, for example, Lupe believes that patient autonomy and informed consent are more important than maximal therapeutic benefit, she may, after assuring herself that Wilson knows what he is doing and is capable of weighing the alternatives, again explain the likely consequences of both continuing and discontinuing therapy. She can then offer to help Wilson determine, clarify, and examine his values to ensure that his decision is based on them. If after

this, he still elects to discontinue the physical therapy, and if she acts in accord with her values, she will respect his decision.

If, however, Lupe believes that maximizing therapeutic benefit is more important than patient autonomy and informed consent, she may try to override his expressed wishes on paternalistic grounds. If she justifies paternalistic intervention by claiming that maximizing therapeutic benefit is more important than patient autonomy or informed consent, she will be embracing what is usually labeled *strong* paternalism. Strong paternalism involves doing what is ostensibly for the patient's own good or welfare regardless of the patient's capacity to consent. If, however, she bases an intervention on a judgment that Wilson is mentally incapable of making an autonomous decision on this matter because of the effects of his stroke, his medication, or other factors that have severely restricted his capacity for autonomous choice, she will be relying on what is sometimes called *weak* paternalism. Weak paternalism involves acting to benefit a person or limit harm when, because of mental impairment, the person is substantially unable to make the decision for him- or herself. The distinction between strong and weak paternalism is important because each appeals to quite different lines of justification; and, as a rule, strong paternalism is more difficult to justify than weak paternalism.

Finally, if Lupe does decide to be paternalistic in this case, whether it be strong paternalism or weak, she must determine whether to be coercive or deceptive. For instance, it is likely that if she becomes rather stern and scolds and chastises Wilson, he will grudgingly relent and begin exercising again. But she will have to scold and chastise him almost daily to obtain his continued participation over the ensuing few weeks. Nevertheless, it is equally likely that Wilson will resume his physical therapy if she tells him that unless he continues to exercise for three more weeks he will regress and be unlikely to walk again. This, however, she knows to be untrue. Wilson will be able to walk whether he continues with the therapy or not; the point of the therapy is simply to reduce his ultimate level of disability. Although Lupe may agree that lying is generally wrong, she may nonetheless think that deceiving Wilson in this way will be much less painful for both of them than scolding and chastising.

Ethical autonomy: the elements

In working her way through the ethical considerations involved in this case, Lupe Garcia has the opportunity to exercise ethical autonomy. That is, she can within limits exercise independent thought and judgment about what she ought to do and then act accordingly.[6] As a result, she will be morally responsible for what she does and for the foreseeable consequences.

To say that an action is ethically autonomous is roughly to say that it is free and the result of rational deliberation involving values and principles that are based on moral reflection. Free action, rational deliberation, and moral reflection are the elements of ethical autonomy.[7]

Free action. To say that an action is free, in the sense that concerns us here, is to say that it is not the result of threats, exploitation, or deliberately inculcated false belief. "Your money or your life" is a threat, and when you hand over your money to save your life there is a sense in which you do not do so freely. Similarly, if your options are severely limited because of circumstances beyond your control, and an unscrupulous employer will pay you only subsistence wages because he can get away with it, your working for him is not entirely a free action if the only alternative is going without food and shelter. This is exploitation. In both this and the previous example, you act under duress. Finally, if as a result of being deceived you believe that you have only one alternative when you actually have three, your freedom is also limited. In short, then, an action is not wholly free, in the sense that concerns us here, when it is attributed to coercion (threats, exploitation) or manipulation.

Rational deliberation. An autonomous action is one that is performed after the knowable alternatives and their foreseeable consequences have been evaluated. Rational deliberation on the part of physicians, nurses, hospital administrators, and so on requires not only biomedical, social, and scientific knowledge but also knowledge of the values and ethical considerations underlying various alternative courses of actions. It also requires conceptual clarity and the capacity to identify, construct, and evaluate the arguments for and against various alternatives (see the introduction to this volume). Finally, just as coercion and manipulation limit free action, so too do various forms of mental disability or psychopathology limit rational deliberation. The former, we might say, undermine autonomy from without while the latter do so from within.

Moral reflection. Insofar as a free action involves rational choice, it is ethically autonomous only if the choice involves ethical values or principles and the person performing the action not only has reflected critically upon the values or principles underlying the final decision but also has endorsed or adopted them as his or her own. Of course, our upbringing, religion, and culture all equip us with a set of values and principles long before we are able to reflect on them critically. If we are morally autonomous, however, we will examine these prereflective values and principles, determine the extent to which they are independently justifiable and consistent, and compare their overall adequacy with other values and principles. In so doing, as S. I. Benn, a contemporary Australian philosopher, expresses it:

> [W]e discover our principles changing as we discover reasons for setting old ones aside as empty that once we thought serious and weighty. The critical junctures in our lives occur when we discover that a principle or attitude that we had taken to be constitutive of our characters, as making certain kinds of action "unthinkable," has been eroded by our acceptance alongside it of others that now seem basic. We discover experientially what considerations really matter to us, or what amounts to the same thing, who we really are. Such discoveries are possible only to the extent that we are autonomous.[8]

As a result of our moral reflection, then, we embrace, at least provisionally, certain values and principles as our own. And the free actions that result from rational deliberation in accord with these values and principles are, in the strongest sense, ethically autonomous. Whatever their moral quality, we are responsible for them and the foreseeable consequenes of acting on them.[9]

Ethical autonomy: an illustration

We can now show how Lupe Garcia can be ethically autonomous in deciding how to respond to Mr. Wilson's refusing further physical therapy.

First, as a primary nurse, Lupe is responsible for the total twenty-four-hour nursing care of Wilson. She interviews him on admission, makes a nursing diagnosis, issues orders, and coordinates his activities with his physicians, family, and other health care workers. Another staff nurse, termed an associate, cares for Wilson when Lupe is off duty, though the associate may phone Lupe to seek a change in nursing orders.[10] Thus, as primary nurse, Lupe is free to decide how best to respond to Wilson's refusal. Whatever she decides to do, however, she will inform others involved in his care—his physician, his physical therapist, and her associates—of what she has done and why.

Second, we assume that Lupe has had a long-standing interest and some background in health care ethics. She recognizes her various options outlined earlier and the values and principles underlying them. She then begins to examine the arguments for and against different courses of action. She also tries to determine with as much certainty as possible certain empirical and conceptual factors. What is the likelihood and degree of impairment that Wilson will suffer if he does not continue the therapy? To what extent is his wish to stop physical therapy a product of temporary depression or a mental impairment related to his stroke or medication? What is the difference between strong paternalism and simply imposing one's values on someone else? In critically analyzing various arguments and in becoming as clear as possible about relevant empirical and conceptual considerations, Lupe is engaging in what we have called rational deliberation.

Finally, we assume that Lupe has given careful consideration to the values and principles involved in questions of informed consent, patient autonomy, paternalism, maximal therapeutic benefits, deception, and so on. She believes, as a result of past and ongoing moral reflection, that certain values and principles, though not beyond question, are more well grounded than others; and she uses these values and principles in making her decisions.

Whatever she decides to do in this case, Lupe's action as described will be ethically autonomous; it will be free and based on rational deliberation and moral reflection. This, however, is not to say that her decision will necessarily be morally correct. As we will show later, it is possible for two people to be ethically autonomous and yet disagree because of empirical uncertainty and moral complexity. And even Lupe, if she appreciates the complexity of health care ethics, must admit that it is possible that she has overlooked some important factor, failed to draw a relevant distinction, reasoned badly, and so on. Nonetheless, as an ethically autonomous decision her choice is one for which she is morally responsible; and if this doesn't guarantee that it is the best decision, it does ensure that she is, and ought to be respected as, a morally responsible person.

The value of ethical autonomy

But, one might ask, what is the value of a person being ethically autonomous? What can be said in its behalf? There are two main lines of argument for ethical autonomy. The first claims that ethical autonomy is valuable in and of itself; and the second bases the value of ethical autonomy on its consequences. The first type of argument we will label an *intrinsic* argument because of its emphasis on the intrinsic value of ethical autonomy. We will label the second type of argument an *extrinsic* argument because it holds that the value of ethical autonomy is based on factors extrinsic to the act itself.[11]

Intrinsic arguments generally are regarded as providing the more basic or fundamental justification of ethical autonomy. According to one argument, being able to think and act for ouselves on ethical and other matters is what gives our lives unity and identity while providing the basis for personal dignity and self-esteem. Without a certain degree of autonomy we would not be able to lead our lives. For to lead a life, as opposed simply to having a succession of experiences, presupposes shaping it according to certain goals, principles, and ideals. And we can do this only if we are able to determine these goals, principles, and ideals and act in accord with them. Furthermore, our dignity and self-esteem derive in part from our accepting responsibility for what we do. If we are responsible for what we do, we can then take credit for those actions that make the world (or, more modestly, our immediate community) a better place. And we can claim responsibility for such changes only if they are the result of free actions based on rational deliberation and values and principles that we have adopted or endorsed after moral reflection. Ethical autonomy, then, provides the foundation for moral responsibility; and being morally responsible for certain states of affairs is part of what it means to be, and be respected as, a person.

In addition, utilitarians and others who base the value of actions on their consequences often provide extrinsic arguments for ethical autonomy. For example, although an action's being autonomous is no guarantee of its being morally correct, there is good reason to believe that free actions based on rational deliberation and moral reflection are more likely to be right than actions determined in other ways. This is especially true when people of various religious, cultural, and national backgrounds must arrive at ethical decisions on matters of great complexity in a rapidly changing world; for we will not be able to resolve ethical disagreements if each of us relies on an uncritical acceptance of received moral views. We are much more likely to arrive at well-grounded, widely shared decisions that are sensitive to the complexities of the issues if we discuss them with others and make them on the basis of rational deliberation and moral reflection. A second extrinsic argument for the value of ethical autonomy turns on the consequences of people's being held morally responsible for what they do. For to the extent that we are regarded as morally responsible for our actions, we are less likely to participate or acquiesce in actions that are, by practically any standard, morally wrong. The rise of Nazism and the mass suicide at Jonestown on November 18, 1978, are two particularly dramatic examples of what can happen when large numbers of people surrender their ethical autonomy.

The ethically autonomous nurse

We can now show that ethical autonomy in nursing can be supported on both intrinsic and extrinsic grounds. First, nurses are persons with goals, principles, and ideals. Self-esteem, personal integrity, and being respected as persons are no less important to nurses than to anyone else. Therefore, being regarded as a "sort of useful parasite" to the physician or as "simply an intelligent machine for the purpose of carrying out his orders" is demeaning and incompatible with what a nurse is—a self-determining person. The intrinsic value of thinking and acting for oneself on ethical matters is so important that we might even say that any occupational role that seems to require the surrender of ethical autonomy ought to be abolished. Thus, if the role of the traditional nurse requires the surrender of ethical autonomy, this role must give way to a conception of nursing that provides more room for the exercise of ethical autonomy.

There is, however, an objection to this line of argument that must be addressed. In a contemporary defense of the traditional conception of nursing, the philosopher Lisa H. Newton of Fairfield University argues that one can be an autonomous person without being an autonomous nurse.[12] There is an important difference, she maintains, between "an autonomous person—one who, over the course of adult life, is self-determining in all major choices and a significant number of minor ones, and hence can be said to have chosen, and to be responsible for, his own life—and an autonomous *role*—a role so structured that its occupant is self-determining in all major and most minor role-related choices."[13] Newton uses this distinction to argue that "an autonomous person can certainly take on a subordinate role [such as that of the traditional nurse] without losing his personal autonomy."[14] Thus, just as an actress can retain her autonomy as a person while submitting to the directives of the playwright and the director, so, too, Newton maintains, a traditional nurse can retain her overall autonomy as a person while submitting to the directives of the physician and hospital bureaucracy.

Two difficulties with this argument are apparent. First, Newton assumes that in occupying a subordinate role one's exercise of autonomy in others areas of life is unaffected. But a recent article by Adina Schwartz, formerly a philosopher at Yale, and currently pursuing legal studies, suggests that the character of nonautonomous work spills over into people's personal lives, making them less autonomous generally.[15] She cites various studies by social scientists showing that occupations that explicitly limit independent thought and judgment hinder those who hold them "from developing the intellectual abilities that they must have if they are rationally to frame, adjust, and pursue their own plans during the rest of the time."[16] Although the evidence marshaled by Schwartz is not conclusive, it is strong enough to show that Newton's assumption that a person's occupational role and his or her life as a whole can be neatly compartmentalized with regard to autonomy is far from self-evident.

Second, and more important, even if Newton's assumption were true, significant differences between nursing and most other occupational roles seriously weaken her argument. A nurse is constantly placed in situations in which patients, family members, physicians, nursing supervisors, hospital administrators, employing agencies, and so on claim and presuppose her personal fidelity on matters of importance. But often she cannot be faithful to one party without breaking faith with another.

Consider, for example, what a hospital nurse should do when a mentally competent patient with whom she has built a close and trusting relationship asks for information about his condition, but the physician does not wish him to have this information. Suppose, too, that the physician expects and trusts the nurse to put the patient's questions off or, failing this, to lie to him throughout her eight-hour shift. Furthermore, suppose that the nurse has strong grounds for believing that the patient both has a right to the information and will not be harmed by it. A nurse who remains subordinate to the physician in this situation compromises her own integrity as well as the integrity of her relationship with the patient. In pretending to maintain a close and trusting interpersonal relationship with the patient while withholding the information, the nurse betrays the patient and her relationship with him. And in doing something that she herself believes is, at bottom, duplicitous and unjustified, she betrays herself.[17]

An actress has no comparable loss of integrity if she plays Saint Joan on one day and Lady Macbeth on another. For we all know that actresses, as actresses, are always only playing roles. But a nurse is trusted by patients and physicians because each party assumes that she is not simply playing a role. Nurses are presumed by both patients and physicians to be personally honest, open, and loyal to each party. And in cases in which both sets of expectations cannot be met, when the nurse is quite literally caught in the middle, she typically cannot maintain a sense of herself as a whole person unless the physician is prepared to recognize her ethical autonomy. This is not, however, to say that the physician must always agree with whatever the nurse believes to be ethically correct. Rather, it is to say that physicians and nurses must respect one another as autonomous moral agents. And this means, among other things, addressing each other's ethical concerns, mutually deliberating and reflecting about various courses of action, and in some cases agreeing with or accommodating the other's ethical views. Thus although there may be, as Newton suggests, subordinate roles that are compatible with personal autonomy, nursing is not one of them.

We turn now to the extrinsic value of nursing autonomy. First, nurses who carefully think for themselves about ethical and other matters are more likely to be sensitive to the complex personal, emotional, and physical needs of their patients. They will, in short, be able to provide more effective nursing care for their patients. Moreover, they are more likely to be responsive to unanticipated changes in the patient's condition and to represent the patient's vital interests when these seem to be threatened by medical oversight or bureaucratic indifference. Thus, nursing autonomy should result in better patient care.

A second extrinsic consideration, while also focusing on benefits to patients, is related to the intrinsic value of ethical autonomy. Hospital nurses in the United States display a well-documented problem of "burnout."[18] After a few years, many conscientious, sensitive, and highly skilled nurses feel "burned out" by the stresses and strains of their work and leave nursing. As a result, the costs of hospital care go up while the quality goes down. One commonly identified cause of nursing burnout is the difficulty many nurses have in maintaining personal integrity in their work.[19] Therefore, providing more room for ethical autonomy may contribute to reducing burnout among nurses and, as a result, lower the costs and raise the quality of hospital care.

We have shown that ethical autonomy in nursing has both intrinsic and extrinsic value. Yet because the traditional conception of nursing is still deeply embedded in the health care system, exercising autonomy is often problematic and sometimes personally hazardous. Therefore, we now turn to some of the questions and complexities that confront the would-be autonomous nurse. In so doing, we will deepen and refine our account of ethical autonomy in nursing.

Between Patient and Physician

CASE 2: "IS IT RIGHT?"

Ann Fiske enjoyed the first seven months on a medical unit, her first nursing position. But since being assigned as primary nurse to James Bering, a seventy-one-year-old retired widower suffering from a rapidly growing, highly malignant sarcoma of the peritoneum, Ann is finding her job unsettling. Bering's days and nights are filled with intractable pain, and despite her care and that of others, he suffers greatly from insomnia and discomfort. Further, his various medications often cloud his mind. During the past two days, Bering has talked briefly with Ann of his approaching death.

Today, after Bering's attending physician, Dr. Rhodes, checked him and spoke at length with Bering's two children, he increased Bering's morphine dosage and frequency. As he handed the chart to Ann, he said, "I want you to begin this now." Ann understood that although it would provide additional control for his pain, the increased morphine dosage would further depress Bering's already depressed respirations and, as a side effect, increase the likelihood that he would soon die. Although the likelihood of an earlier death for Bering was not in itself troubling to Ann, she doubted whether Bering had explicitly consented to this course of action.

Since Ann knew that Dr. Rhodes was a highly respected physician with years of experience, she hesitated a moment before asking him whether Bering had given his consent. But when she did, Dr. Rhodes quietly explained that he had not discussed the issue with Bering because to do so would be needless cruelty. Nor, he said, would he saddle the relatives with "the burden of making this decision." In fact, he added, "I never ask families to make decisions that would leave them feeling guilty." Then he said, rather firmly, "I've made hundreds of these difficult decisions—sometimes it's a little less potassium, sometimes too much oxygen, sometimes morphine—and you, if you're a good nurse, should know better than to say anything.

If you're not going to be a good nurse, I'd better call your supervisor."[20]

Recognizing both that Dr. Rhodes expected all nurses to follow his orders unquestioningly and that he was one of the nursing supervisor's favorite physicians, Ann thought that if she balked at his orders, she would face problems not only with him but also with the nursing supervisor. Ann did not want to make trouble for herself, but she was concerned about Bering. She asked herself, "Is it right for us to administer treatment that may hasten his death without his permission?"

Ethical disagreement

The conflict of values in this case centers on the choice between simply administering the additional morphine, which will not only reduce pain but perhaps also hasten death, and trying to determine whether, when informed of the consequences, Bering (or—if he is not competent—his family) wants the increased morphine. Underlying the first alternative are the values of reducing pain, suffering, and guilt; underlying the second are the values of self-determination and informed consent.

Inasmuch as this issue turns on a conflict of values, when Ann questioned Dr. Rhodes's decision, she in no way challenged his specialized medical knowledge and expertise. Nothing in Dr. Rhodes's training certified him as an expert on ethical matters, if indeed there are any experts of this sort. And in asking for his reasons and even subjecting them to critical examination, Ann is not venturing into matters beyond her competence.

If Ann discusses the matter further with Dr. Rhodes, it will be to her advantage if her position is based on rational deliberation and moral reflection rather than intuition or "gut feeling." Dr. Rhodes has already given reasons for preferring his course of action. Ann, if she is to maintain her position, must be able to provide stronger reasons for obtaining informed consent before proceeding.

The main consideration to which Ann could appeal is the respect that is owed to Bering as a person. Bering has a right to accept or refuse various forms of medical treatment. This right is based on the right to self-determination, which is itself based on the respect that is owed persons as autonomous beings. As far as we can tell, Bering has not chosen to die sooner rather than later. He knows that death is immiment, but he has not consented that it be hastened. To administer the additional morphine, however, is likely to hasten his death. Therefore, to provide medical treatment that will, as a side effect, be likely to hasten Bering's death without his explicit informed consent is to deny his freedom and dignity as an autonomous being, a person.

On the surface, this argument for Ann's position is at least as strong as Dr. Rhodes's argument for administering the morphine without further discussion with the patient or his family. If Ann is to be thorough in her deliberations, however, she must be able to anticipate and respond to the objections Dr. Rhodes might make against her reasoning. First, he might emphasize that although the principle of informed consent is fine in theory, it is often inapplicable in practice. Self-determination and informed consent presuppose that the patient (or if not the patient, the patient's family) is capable of rational deliberation in situations like this one. But this, according to Dr. Rhodes, is not often the case and is certainly not the case with Bering or his family. Bering, Dr. Rhodes might claim, is not mentally competent to make this decision himself, and his family would be plagued by guilt if it were to be thrust upon them.

The question of patient autonomy is a complex conceptual-empirical matter.[21] If Ann is to neutralize this objection, she must be able to show that either Bering or his family can understand and decide on this matter or at least that Dr. Rhodes has not yet determined that they cannot do so; and since patient autonomy must be presumed, the burden is on Dr. Rhodes to show why they lack this capability.

A second possible objection to Ann's line of reasoning is that increasing the morphine will maximize happiness. Appealing to the principle of utility, Dr. Rhodes could point out that not only would Bering's suffering be diminished, but also his family would be spared the agonies of decision making as well as of witnessing Bering's pain and distress. Furthermore, since obtaining informed consent would take valuable time, Dr. Rhodes and Ann would have more time to provide the sort of medical and nursing care for which they have been prepared.

As is often the case, however, these utilitarian considerations may be neutralized by others. In the long run, for example, it is likely that if the practice of hastening the deaths of suffering persons without their explicit consent were to become more widely practiced and more widely known, it would result in a loss of trust throughout the health care system. Any suffering person with a terminal illness might wonder whether this or that treatment would hasten his or her death. And such loss of trust might create anxiety and a fear of medicine that actually would reduce the net balance of happiness.

Thus, as matters stand, Ann's doubts appear to be well grounded. The question remains, however, of whether ethical autonomy requires that she go further than simply discussing the matter with Dr. Rhodes.

The question of free action

Let us suppose that Dr. Rhodes either refuses to discuss the matter with Ann any further or that after discussing it he stands by his initial decision. Let us also assume that he has rather cavalierly decided that Bering and his family are in no condition to decide the matter themselves. However, Ann has good reason to believe that at least one of them is perfectly capable of doing so. If, then, Ann were to give the injections at this point, she would be acting contrary not only to what she regards as Bering's rights but also to her own deeply held moral convictions. She would be compromising her intregity as a person. What, then, should she do?

There is an adage in ethics that "ought implies can," which relates to Ann's dilemma. It is usually taken to mean that if we say that someone morally *ought* to do something, it must be true that he or she *can* do it. If a person cannot do something, it makes no sense or is morally unjust to say that he or she morally should do it. Thus, if a person cannot swim, we cannot say that he ought to have gone into deep water to rescue a drowning swimmer. And if a physician is prevented at gunpoint by a terrorist from treating a wounded hostage, we cannot say that she ought nevertheless to have treated him. Thus, in determining what Ann ought to do in the case before us, we must try to clarify what she *can* do.

Deciding what she can do, however, is no easy matter, for unlike Lupe Garcia in the earlier case, Ann's freedom of action is in doubt. On the one hand, perhaps Ann is being coerced into following Dr. Rhodes's orders. If, for example, she resists giving the injection, Dr. Rhodes may find various ways to make things difficult for her. He may also report her to her nursing supervisor, who may have considerable power over her. Because she is relatively new in the unit and this is her first position, Ann may fear losing her job. Perhaps she has heard about the case of Jolene Tuma, a nurse in Idaho who in 1977 lost her nursing license for giving information to a patient about alternative cancer treatments.[22] The charge against Jolene

Tuma was that she interfered with the doctor-patient relationship. If there were no other hospital in town and Ann were the sole support of her ailing mother, the risk of losing her job would indeed be serious. Thus, in light of these de facto conditions, we might conclude that Ann is not entirely free to act in accord with her ethical views.

On the other hand, perhaps Ann finds herself in more favorable circumstances. Experienced and with a strong record, she believes that being harassed by Dr. Rhodes or being reprimanded or disciplined by her nursing supervisor is a small price to pay for protecting Bering's rights and for acting in accord with her deepest ethical convictions. Suppose, too, that she is not committed to living in the area where she is currently employed or that she could readily find another nursing position if things became too unpleasant. If this were Ann's situation, we might conclude that she is not being coerced into following Dr. Rhodes's orders. As a result, she is free to act in accord with her considered moral views, and therefore she ought to do so.

The main question, then, is this: Is Ann free to act in accord with the results of her rational deliberation and moral reflection or is she coerced into giving the injections? If we conclude that she is not free to act in accord with the results of her rational deliberation and moral reflection, then she is neither fully autonomous nor fully responsible for giving the injection. If, however, we conclude that, despite the circumstances, she is free to act in accord with her considered ethical judgments, then she is both autonomous and responsible for what she does.

We have no simple solution to the problem of free action in nursing. On the one hand, we admire nurses who risk punitive responses from physicians and others for the sake of patients' rights and their own moral integrity. We think that such nurses generally should be commended and supported. On the other hand, we recognize that many nurses find themselves in situations in which it will be extremely difficult to withstand the threat of punitive responses. Moreover, we do not believe that nurses should have to be heroines or make large personal sacrifices to do what they have good reason to believe is morally right or to preserve their moral integrity. We will, therefore, later suggest some systematic changes that may reduce the incidence and severity of such predicaments. In the following case, we will explore an additional clinical situation in which the nurse's ethical autonomy is a critical factor.

CASE 3: "MEDICAL MISTAKE"

Linda Kane, a nurse with eight years' experience in maternity nursing, worked in a postpartum unit on the three-to-eleven shift. One evening about 8:00 P.M., her patient, Jane Jones, a thirty-two-year-old woman with three previous births, began to bleed heavily. Jane had had a precipitous delivery of twins about 5:00 P.M. and Linda knew that Jane was a prime candidate for postpartum hemorrhage. Linda assessed Jane's condition, called the resident (a physician undergoing specialized clinical training) on duty, and then returned to the patient to clean her and change the linens. When the resident came to check Jane, he decided that she was not hemorrhaging. Approximately forty-five minutes later when Jane again began to bleed heavily, Linda once more phoned the resident. This time, however, he declined to return to the unit and told Linda, "Don't call me again." Linda, believing that Jane had an immediate problem, decided to call Jane's physician and detailed her assessment to him. Thereupon, he called the resident, who later returned to the floor in a rage against Linda. The resident did, however, write orders for medication and for the nurses to "carefully monitor the patient's vital signs," which, of course, Linda had already been doing throughout the evening as a part of her ongoing assessment. The next evening Linda saw on the chart that Jane Jones had received blood transfusions that morning.[23]

Conflicting obligations
    Unlike Ann Fiske's disagreement with Dr. Rhodes, which turned principally on differing ethical views, Linda Kane, in questioning and ultimately going over the head of the resident, is challenging his knowledge and expertise as a physician. Although Dr. Rhodes can make little claim to ethical expertise, the resident has a strong claim, in virtue of his training and certification, as an expert on medical matters. Thus, on the face of it, Linda is much more susceptible than Ann to charges that she is not qualified or competent to question the physician.
    Yet our prereflective response may be to say that she was justified in doing what she did and to commend her actions. Indeed, it is situations of this sort that help provide extrinsic grounds for the value of ethical autonomy in nursing. But, in moving beyond an intuitive response, what considerations or principles can we cite to support our conclusion?

First, we must note that given the rapid growth and complexity of medical knowledge and technology, certain nurses, through in-service education, college or university courses, independent study or experience, and the like, may know more about some aspect of a particular treatment or machine or condition than do the physicians with whom they work. For example, an experienced and knowledgeable nurse working full-time in an intensive care unit may know more about certain treatments in that unit than a physician working there only briefly during his educational program. In addition, some nurses, who in certain cases spend more time with patients than do physicians, often know considerably more about those patients' strengths, weaknesses, desires, and needs than do some physicians, who may see patients only during short visits. In the case before us, then, it is likely that Linda Kane's eight years' experience in maternity nursing, together with her close monitoring of the patient, explains her having a greater understanding of the patient's condition than the resident. Thus, although physicians generally will know more about medical matters than nurses, at times a nurse will know more about a specific matter.

What is a nurse to do when efforts to correct what she has good grounds to believe is a medical mistake require that she disregard a physician's directives? On the face of it, the nurse seems to have conflicting obligations. On the one hand, she has an obligation to restore and further the health of the patient. On the other hand, she has an obligation to comply with the medical directives of physicians. And in this case Linda cannot do both.

But are these obligations equally basic or stringent? Moral reflection, we believe, reveals that they are not. For as a health care provider a nurse's primary obligations are, in the end, to patients and not to physicians. The reason a nurse works with a physician and generally complies with his or her medical directives is to help provide the patient with the best possible health care. In other words, the nurse's prima facie obligation to comply with the medical directives of the physician is derived from her more basic obligation to the patient. In most cases, then, in following a physician's medical directives a nurse will be partially fulfilling her obligations to the patient. But whenever a nurse has good grounds for believing that a particular medical directive will be more harmful to a patient, her prima facie obligation to the physician is overridden. Thus, we may justify our prereflective positive response to what Linda Kane did by arguing that her obligation to her patient overrode her obligation to follow the directives of the physician.

The spectrum of urgency

But it is sometimes argued that despite occasional medical mistakes, nurses must always follow a physician's directives. For, the argument goes, hospitals, like most large, complex bureaucratic institutions, require that employees perform assigned tasks, follow chains of authority and established protocols, and refrain from taking initiative. As Newton puts it:

> These requirements are common to all bureaucracies, but dramatically increase in urgency when the tasks are supposed to be protective of life itself and where the subject matter is inherently unpedictable and emergency prone. Since there is often no time to re-examine the usefulness of a procedure in a particular case, and since the stakes are too high to permit a gamble, the institution's effectiveness, not to mention its legal position, may depend on unquestioning adherence to procedure.[24]

If, then, the hospital and physicians are to fulfill their purpose, which is to save life and promote health, the inevitably tense and urgent atmosphere in which this is to be accomplished demands that "all participating activities and agents [including nurses] must be completely subordinate to the medical judgments of physicians."[25]

Underlying this argument is the assumption that relationships between nurses and physicians in the hospital are invariably characterized by high stakes and breathless urgency. But, as we have pointed out elsewhere,[26] decision points in the hospital are located on a wide "spectrum of urgency"—that is, on a continuum of cases in which the available time to make decisions varies considerably. The spectrum begins at one end with problems that may be solved at a leisurely pace, allowing time for reflection, collection of further data, debate, and discussion, and ends at the other end with urgent questions that demand quick solutions and immediate actions. The low-urgency end of the spectrum includes such situations as those in which a physician and a nurse disagree about the extent to which hospitalized children of various ages should be informed of the nature of their illnesses or injuries. In such a situation, the physician and nurse can take time to study and discuss all aspects of the situation. The high-urgency end of the spectrum includes emergency situations in which a physician and nurse disagree about an order for actions that must be carried out immediately. For example, a nurse and a physician may be inclined to allocate care differently for three accident victims admitted simultaneously to the emergency room.

In cases in which a nurse is inclined to question a hospital's policy or a physicians's order, she may use the spectrum of urgency to decide what to do. If the case falls on the low end of the spectrum and she believes that her misgiving or suggested alternative is well grounded, considerations of bureaucratic efficiency or medical crisis carry no weight at all and she should express her misgiving or make her suggestions. If, however, the case falls at the other end of the spectrum, the argument for the nurse's following the policy or order without question is much stronger. A rule-utilitarian argument in this case supports the nurse's compliance even if she judges that the particular policy or order is not, all things considered, the best. That is, always following such policies or orders in situations of great urgency is likely to have the best overall consequences. Even here, however, there are two important qualifications. First, if a nurse disagrees with a physician's orders but complies with them under emergency conditions, she should, after the crisis has passed, carefully express her misgivings in order to determine how best to deal with similar cases in the future. And second, if a physician's order is clearly outside the bounds of acceptable medical practice, a nurse should not obey it even in an emergency.[27]

Authority and collaboration

The problems encountered by Ann Fiske and Linda Kane stem in part from the authoritarian nature of the traditional relationship between physicians and nurses. But as our discussion of the spectrum of urgency suggests, an authoritarian conception of the physician-nurse relationship is best replaced in many contexts by a collaborative conception. In collaborating to meet the health-related needs of patients while respecting their rights, physicians and nurses share knowledge, discuss differences, and work together with mutual respect.[28]

This is not to deny, however, that authoritarian structures sometimes are needed and morally justifiable. In our discussion of the spectrum of urgency, we indicated that emergency situations often require such structures. In addition, as John Ladd, a philosopher at Brown University, has suggested, specialized contexts such as the operating room are highly suited to the exercise and recognition of medical authority:

> In an operating room, the authority of the surgeon might be likened to the authority of the conductor of an orchestra: the surgeon is the chief performer and the one who "orchestrates" the proceeding. Let us grant that the aim of the procedure is to save

the patient's life, i.e., a morally worthy goal. But here, as with the orchestra, we are dealing with a precisely defined, limited enterprise involving goals that we may assume are shared by all the parties involved, or, to be more nearly accurate, we should say that they ought to be shared by all of them.[29]

But, as Ladd goes on to point out, the goals in most other health care contexts are not this simply defined. And when the goals of patients, physicians, and nurses do not clearly converge, both the need and the justification for authoritarian structures are considerably weakened.

In situations in which authoritarian relationships between physicians and nurses cannot be justified, we agree with Ladd's suggestion that "we try to find more 'democratic' procedures, procedures involving mutual counseling, consultation, and collaboration. Mutual accommodation and persuasion should take the place of one person issuing commands to others below."[30] If such procedures had been in effect in the Bering case, it is highly likely that further efforts would have been undertaken to involve Bering or his family in the decision as to whether to increase the dosage of his morphine. And if they had been in effect in the Jane Jones case, her postpartum hemorrhage probably would have been detected and treated much sooner.

Conflict, Compromise, and Integrity

CASE 4: "LACK OF AGREEMENT"

Susan Cory is a twenty-nine-year-old critical care staff nurse who enjoys the nursing challenges of a medical intensive care unit (ICU) in a large medical center. Her reputation among nursing and medical staffs is that of a caring and exceptionally competent nurse. At present, though, she is at odds with most persons working in the ICU over whether aggressive treatment should be continued for Marsha Hocking, a severely brain damaged young single woman her own age, a victim of viral encephalitis. Marsha's parents are so overwhelmed by the situation that they are relying completely on the judgment of the care providers. Susan and the medical and nursing staffs are in agreement as to the medical details of the case—that is, the extent of brain damage and the very poor prognosis. After careful deliberation, Susan decided that aggressive treatment in Marsha's case should be reduced sharply because no hope remains for recovery. Susan based her decision on her belief that to continue treating Marsha is morally wrong since no one would want to be kept alive in Marsha's condition. Without aggressive treatment, which includes artificial ventilation, Marsha will die quickly.

Susan has asked the other nurses and the physicians to think about her recommendation. Some nurses agree with Susan. Others agree with most of the physicians, including the one in charge of Marsha's case, that now is not the time to give up. They point to a variety of reasons for continuing aggressive treatment—Marsha's age, the sudden onset of the disease, her previous excellent condition, and their personal belief about the value of life. Throughout the discussion, which has continued for the past two weeks, Susan has not requested of the ICU nurse manager that she be excused from the case, an infrequent request that has been honored in the ICU for other nurses.

Ethical uncertainty and complexity

This case differs in one important respect from cases 2 and 3. In each of those cases, the nurse's ethical position seemed to be more well grounded than that of the physician with whom she disagreed. In this case, however, it is not clear whether those advocating continued aggressive treatment or those advocating much less aggressive treatment have the most defensible position.

Given the complexity of many issues in health care ethics and our limited knowledge and understanding, ethical disagreements are often not the result of simple conflicts over what is right or wrong. As Arthur Kuflik, a philosopher at the University of Vermont, has pointed out:

> Individuals must often base their respective moral judgments on a picture of their situation that is relevantly, but irremediably, incomplete. Their differences of opinion may have less to do with deficiencies of moral sensibility than with uncertainties that are inherent in the situation itself.... [Moreover] even individuals who are adequately informed and acknowledge the same fundamental principles can find themselves in disagreement when an issue engages several morally relevant considerations at the same time. In such cases the sheer complexity of the matter enables reasonable persons to form somewhat different assessments.[31]

Both these factors, uncertainty and complexity, seem to be at the root of the disagreement in this case.

Susan Cory believes that no one would want to be kept alive in Marsha's condition. But how can she be sure of this? Perhaps Susan and many of her acquaintances would not want to be kept alive in this condition. But what about Marsha? Susan would be on much stronger ground if she knew that before Marsha's illness she had shared this view. But Susan lacks such knowledge. Similarly, those who are opting for continued aggressive treatment appeal to factors that are roughly related to possible recovery—the patient's age, the sudden onset of the disease, her previous excellent health—but they have little else to go on in estimating her chances of survival. Perhaps more important, they cannot determine her future level of consciousness and activity even if she were to survive. If they knew whether she would survive and that her ensuing condition would be good, or at least tolerable, they might be on stronger ground. But they do not have such knowledge.

Moreover, apart from empirical uncertainty, each side can appeal to morally relevant considerations to support its view. Susan can appeal (though without full assurance) to the patient's autonomy and, perhaps, to the inefficient use of medical resources. The latter appeal will be considerably strengthened if the ICU is full or if other patients in the ICU are likely to benefit from increased attention if the staff were not doing so much for Marsha Hocking. Those taking the opposing view, however, can invoke the value of each human life and the importance of their roles as protectors and preservers of life. Each side, then, may invoke ethical considerations on its behalf.

In this case and in others similarly clouded by empirical uncertainty and moral complexity, what is someone like Susan to do?

Compromise and integrity

If the parties to this and similar disagreements can recognize the nature of their situation, they may be able to reach some sort of compromise. Moreover, they may be able to do so in a way that does not compromise anyone's moral integrity.

First, they should see to it that subsequent deliberations are carried out in a spirit of mutual respect. As Kuflik indicates, "if they carefully hear each other out and earnestly try to see matters from one another's perspective, people will often find themselves traveling some distance from their original positions and meeting each other part-way."[32] In many cases, for example, one will not only come to appreciate the strength of an opposing position but one will also come to recognize that one's own motives include self-interested as well as ethical considerations. Thus, it is not unlikely that Susan Cory's concern for the patient's autonomy and the efficient use of resources is supplemented by her frustration with the nursing problems presented by patients in this condition. And the desire of most of the physicians to continue treatment may be attributed in part to their desire to practice and refine certain technical skills. As University of Maryland philosopher Samuel Gorovitz has pointed out:

> Skills that have been acquired at substantial personal cost are skills that people like to use. People who can do sophisticated things like to do them. There is an intrinsic payoff in satisfaction. State-of-the-art medicine is very sophisticated, and people who can do it often find it a very beautiful thing to be doing. We should bear that in mind when we think about the motivation behind a lot of medical care.[33]

If such possible motivations are identified and discussed, there may be less self-certainty and more willingness to reach a mutually satisfactory accommodation.

Such accommodation may take the form of each party relinquishing his or her original view and agreeing on a third position, or it may take the form of each party retaining her or his original view but agreeing, in the interest of obtaining a speedy, practical, and mutually respectful solution, on a compromise position. In the first instance there is no problem of moral integrity. In autonomously replacing one's original position with a new or revised one, one's subsequent actions can be consistent with one's rational deliberation and moral reflection. It is, however, more difficult to see how one can retain moral integrity while holding one's original position and yet acting in accord with a compromise position. Doesn't this amount to compromising one's integrity?

In this regard, Kuflik is helpful in distinguishing:

> (1) what one judges ought to be done about a matter that happens to be in dispute, leaving aside any consideration of the fact that there is a dispute; (2) what one judges ought to be done, *all things considered*. When an issue is in dispute there is more to be considered than the issue itself—for example, the importance of peace, the presumption against settling matters by force, the intrinsic good of participating in a process in which

each side must hear the other side out and try to see matters from the other's point of view, the extent to which the matter does admit reasonable differences of opinion, the significance of a settlement in which each party feels assured of the other's respect for its own seriousness and sincerity in the matter.

Taking *all* this into account, a person of goodwill might well decide that compromise is the wisest course. But to judge, all things considered, that there ought to be compromise and to act accordingly, is hardly to compromise one's moral integrity. On the contrary, integrity is compromised, not when one acts, but when one elects *not* to act, on what one can clearly judge ought to be done, all things considered.[34]

Thus, if Susan Cory and those wanting to continue aggressive treatment could find a compromise position that, all things considered, would provide a workable solution, they could do so without compromising their integrity. That is, such mutual accommodation would allow them to work together and respect one another while not requiring them to relinquish their original views.

In this case, an acceptable compromise might take the form of an agreement to continue treatment for a specified amount of time and then review the patient's condition and prognosis together with considerations regarding the effective use of resources. If after this period of time certain changes make continued aggressive treatment appear a significantly more favorable option than it is at present, it will continue. But if there are no such changes, treatment will become less aggressive.

If Susan Cory agreed to such a compromise either because she thought it was more plausible than her original position or, while not relinquishing her original view, she thought that, all things considered, it provided a mutually acceptable accommodation of the differing positions, she would do so while fully preserving her ethical autonomy and personal integrity.

Conscience and integrity

Sometimes health care providers will be unable to agree on a compromise position. At such times a nurse may believe that she cannot be party to the disputed procedures or treatments because for her to do so would violate her sense of herself. To preserve her integrity, a nurse may in some instances, after exploring all other options, conscientiously refuse to participate.[35]

Suppose, for example, that a nurse who counsels women about

amniocentesis[36] is asked to meet with a couple interested only in determining the sex of their child-to-be. Suppose, too, that the nurse has good reason to believe that the couple will want an abortion if the fetus is not of the preferred sex. Although the nurse may not be opposed to abortion as such, she is opposed to abortion for this reason; she would feel a loss of integrity if she were to participate in a test that might lead to the death of a healthy fetus. Under such circumstances a nurse who refuses, on the basis of conscience, to be a party to such a use of amniocentesis acts within her rights and should not be reprimanded.

Nursing supervisors and fellow workers can distinguish conscientious refusal from self-serving pleas such as refusing to cooperate because of petty dislikes or inconvenience by using criteria developed by James F. Childress, professor of religious studies and medical education at the University of Virginia.[37] According to Childress, an appeal to conscience is (1) personal and subjective, in that it is based on standards that one does not necessarily apply to others, (2) founded on a prior judgment of rightness or wrongness, and (3) motivated by personal sanction rather than external control. If a nurse's refusal to perform a particular act meets these three conditions, as does the nurse involved in the amniocentesis example, the nurse's supervisors should provide some latitude in their response to her, both for the sake of the nurse's personal integrity and for the welfare of future patients.

An important reason for respecting appeals to conscience in nursing is the recognition that a nurse who conscientiously chooses to refuse to participate is often representative of the more effective and thoughtful nurses in an institution. An institution needs to keep such valuable nurses in order to provide the best nursing care possible. In addition, a nursing organization will not collapse if it allows some room for the exercise of conscience. But most important, coercing a nurse to act against her deepest convictions may not only have a brutalizing effect on her, but it may also have a "chilling effect" on independent thought and judgment among the nursing staff.

One final note: conscientious refusal in nursing is not obstructive. In an appeal to conscience, one aims primarily to preserve his or her own integrity. Thus, a nurse who conscientiously refuses to participate in amniocentesis for sex selection cannot, on these grounds, coercively prevent others from doing what she cannot in good conscience do herself.[38]

Institutional and Public Policy

CASE 5: HOSPITAL AND PUBLIC POLICY VERSUS THE PATIENT'S WISHES

Joan O'Brien is evening charge nurse on a small, busy, cardiac care unit. Joseph Mesick, age eighty-one, has been hospitalized for four days following a severe episode of angina. Mesick, a retired lawyer who is much respected in the community, plans to return to his daughter's home in the morning.

Although Mesick passively accepted treatment (including nasal oxygen and IV therapy during the first twenty-four hours), he later told Joan that he did not want to be treated again with "tubes and machines" and that he "had made his peace and was ready to die."

Upon responding immediately to his roommate's urgent cry for help, Joan found Mesick slumped in his bed. She could not detect a pulse, and he did not respond when she called his name. She believed that if she did not start cardiopulmonary resuscitation immediately, death was imminent. Joan also knew that usual hospital policy in such cases was to initiate resuscitation and call immediately for help. But she believed, too, that she should honor Mesick's wishes not to be treated with "tubes and machines." Mesick's physician had made no comment or notation about whether to withhold aggressive treatment in an emergency. And since Mesick was pain-free after the first day and planned to return home very soon, Joan had not discussed the question of withholding resuscitation with other persons involved in his care or in detail with Mesick.[39]

Making the best of a bad situation

Joan O'Brien's dilemma in this case is clearly drawn. If she is to respect the patient's autonomy and respond to what she believes are his overriding wishes, it appears that she should not start cardiopulmonary resuscitation. But if she is to act according to hospital policy, it appears that she must start it. Given the facts of the case, there is no clear way of resolving this dilemma. The situation is a bad one, and Joan must quickly determine which alternative is, all things considered, best.

Although we agree that patients in Mesick's position have a right to refuse being treated with "tubes and machines," we believe it important that health care providers and others make certain that such refusals are genuinely autonomous.[40] Perhaps Mesick's decision was genuinely autonomous. But Joan has not determined that it was; and even if she had, the hospital's policy to initiate immediate resuscitative measures and the questionable legal status of such decisions in cases like this one are troublesome. For although a conscious, competent adult may legally refuse life-saving medical treatment, the legal standing of a previously expressed refusal is unclear in a situation in which, because of illness or injury, the patient can no longer express his desires. Moreover, Joan's not having specifically discussed this type of situation with Mesick, his daughter, his physician, and others involved in his care further complicates an already complicated problem.

Thus, even though it is possible that Mesick does (or would) not want to be resuscitated in these circumstances, on balance it seems that Joan must proceed with cardiopulmonary resuscitation and immediately call for help. Resuscitation is, under the circumstances, the best thing to do. Where the stakes are so high, it is better to err on the side of continued life whenever the competence and resolve of a patient are as problematic as this one.

Making bad situations better

But if this is the best that Joan O'Brien can do in these circumstances she can, nonetheless, take steps to help ensure that similar situations do not recur. For example, the first time Mesick told Joan that he did not want to be treated again with "tubes and machines" and that he "had made his peace and was ready to die," she could have discussed this matter with him further. She could have tried to determine exactly what he meant and together with his physician and daughter tried to determine whether his request was autonomous, that is, freely made, in accord with his long-standing character traits and values, and based on a clear-headed understanding of his prognosis and the probable consequences of further treatment. Had Joan made such an assessment, had all parties agreed both that Mesick's decision was autonomous and that cardiopulmonary resuscitation in the circumstances described in the case came under the heading of what he meant by "tubes and machines," then a decision not to resuscitate would have been more defensible.

Nonetheless, the questions of hospital policy and the law would have remained. Even if Mesick, his daughter, Joan O'Brien, and the physician had agreed that resuscitation in such circumstances should not be undertaken, hospital policy and state law might have limited their ethical autonomy by restricting their free action. That is, considerations of institutional and public policies may have coerced Joan and the physician into resuscitating Mesick even though the results of their rational deliberation and moral reflection pointed the other way.

In such an event, we believe that both Joan and the physician would have an obligation to make reasonable efforts to alter both hospital policy and the law. Generally, obligations we have to others entail as a corollary a requirement that we take steps to ensure that conditions exist for fulfilling these obligations. In this case, this line of reasoning implies that Joan's obligation to respect the rights and wishes of patients like Mesick entails a further obligation to do what she can to alter institutional and public policies that may restrict her freedom to do what she morally ought to do. Since the grounds of this obligation are not limited to nurses like Joan, however, it is important to note that the responsibility does not fall solely on her shoulders. Nursing supervisors, physicians, and others are also obligated in various, and in some cases greater, degrees to attend to this problem. But if other persons do not appear to be fulfilling their responsibilities, Joan's responsibility, though perhaps not increased, is not thereby diminished. She remains obligated to patients like Mesick to make reasonable efforts to alter institutional and public policies that limit her freedom to act in ways that respect their rights. In making such efforts she may increase her effectiveness if she enlists the support of other nurses, physicians, or her professional nursing association.

In dealing with legal restrictions, Joan will probably work for the adoption of legislation to ensure that a patient's desire, expressed while conscious and competent, not to be resuscitated under certain circumstances would retain its legal standing even when, because of illness or injury, the patient is no longer able to express it. Legislation of this sort has been passed in various forms in various states. And in Michigan, where such legislation has been introduced but not passed, individual nurses have been active participants in a Legislative Task Force on Death and Dying that is addressing the problem.

Inquiry into issues like those raised in the Joan O'Brien case demonstrates that the obligations of an ethically autonomous nurse are social and political as well as owed to particular individuals. If, as we assume, altering institutional and public policy would allow nurses (and physicians) more freedom to respect the rights of their patients, and if there are ways in which they *can* help alter such policies, then nurses (and physicians) *ought* to do so. That they ought is a mere, and often demanding, corollary of their ethical obligations to respect patients' rights.

Conclusions

FURTHER QUESTIONS

Much remains to be said about the topics raised in this chapter and we hope that readers will pursue them in greater detail. In particular, three further topics merit extensive consideration. First, interesting and important questions arise in attempting to understand and determine responsibility for the actions of health care teams. The complexity of modern medicine and nursing seems to require that interdisciplinary teams rather than particular individuals administer certain treatments and forms of care. How, then, we must ask, are ethical autonomy and moral responsibility to be understood within the context of health care teams?[41] Second, to what extent, if any, and for what reasons, if any, may or should a nurse "blow the whistle" on substandard or dangerous conduct or policies? There are strong psychological and sociological barriers to making a public accusation against a colleague or employer. Yet sometimes it seems that there is no other way to protect members of the public from an existing or imminent threat. "At what point," we might ask, "should a nurse resolve that allegiance to the public safety supersedes allegiance to the organizational policies and then act on that resolve by informing outsiders?"[42] Third, in attempting to alter institutional policy, nurses may determine that only a strike or the threat of a strike will bring about the desired change. To what extent, then, if any, and for what reasons, if any, may nurses collectively withdraw their services from patients in order to achieve a morally justifiable end?[43]

SUMMARY

We have argued here that nurses, in their capacity as nurses, should be permitted and encouraged to think and act for themselves on matters involving questions of health care ethics. Nonetheless, because the traditional conception of nursing remains deeply embedded in the health care system, nurses will often find ethical autonomy problematic and sometimes personally hazardous. The main question is whether nurses, as nurses, should be free to act in accord with the results of their own rational deliberation and moral reflection and, if they exercise this freedom, whether they should risk punitive responses from physicians, nursing supervisors, and administrators. Answers to this question must be determined on a case-by-case basis. But given the intrinsic and extrinsic value of ethical autonomy, together with the fact that decision points in a hospital are located on a wide spectrum of urgency, there are strong reasons for shifting from authoritarian to more collaborative relationships among health care professionals. When mutual consultation, accommodation, and persuasion take the place of some persons exercising extensive power over others, nurses no longer find the price of ethical autonomy so unreasonably high.

This is not, however, to say that ethical conflict will disappear when collaboration becomes the rule rather than the exception. The factual uncertainty and moral complexity that characterize many problems in health care ethics will often require compromise solutions that, for the reasons given, do not compromise the integrity and autonomy of those who reach them. And when satisfactory compromise cannot be achieved, efforts must be made to accommodate those who cannot in good conscience participate in procedures that go against their deepest conviction. Finally, inasmuch as a nurse's freedom of action is restricted by faulty institutional or public policies, she should, in the interests of ethical autonomy, take reasonable steps to alter them. It is in this sense that the obligations of an ethically autonomous nurse are social and political as well as interpersonal.

Notes

Acknowledgments: We are grateful to Laurie Eagle, Ann Seagren, Judy Leatherwood Smith, and Thomas S. Tomlinson for helpful comments on an earlier draft of this chapter.

1. George Rosen, *From Medical Police to Social Medicine: Essays on the History of Health Care* (New York: Science History Publications, 1974), 296; Joann Ashley, *Hospitals, Paternalism, and the Role of the Nurse* (New York: Columbia University Teachers College Press, 1976), 76.

2. Barbara Ehrenreich, "The Purview of Political Action," in National League of Nursing, *The Emergence of Nursing as a Political Force* (New York, 1979), 13.

3. Sarah Dock, "The Relation of the Nurse to the Doctor and the Doctor to the Nurse," *American Journal of Nursing* 17 (1917); 394. Cited in Marjorie J. Stenberg, "The Search for a Conceptual Framework as a Philosophic Basis for Nursing Ethics: An Examination of Code, Context, and Covenant," *Military Medicine* 44 (January 1979): 10.

4. Philip A. Kalisch and Beatrice J. Kalisch, "The Image of Nurses in Novels," *American Journal of Nursing* 82 (August 1982): 1,220–1,024; Janet

Muff, "Handmaiden, Battle-ax, Whore: An Exploration into the Fantasies, Myths, and Stereotypes about Nurses," in *Socialization, Sexism, and Stereotyping: Women's Issues in Nursing*, ed. Janet Muff (St. Louis: C. V. Mosby, 1982), 113–156.

5. This case has been adapted from one discussed in Charles M. Culver and Bernard Gert, *Philosophy in Medicine: Conceptual and Ethical Issues in Medicine and Psychiatry* (New York: Oxford University Press, 1982), 157–163.

6. To say that a person is ethically autonomous is not to say that there are no constraints on what he or she may consider or do. For example, well-grounded appeals to the rights or well-being of a patient justifiably limit the options of both nurses and physicians. But within such constraints they may still be confronted with choices of an ethical nature and the opportunity to exercise ethical autonomy.

7. For an illuminating account of the elements of *patient* autonomy see Bruce L. Miller, "Autonomy and the Refusal of Lifesaving Treatment," *Hastings Center Report* 11 (August 1981): 22–28. Most accounts of autonomy in biomedical ethics focus on patient autonomy. We have benefited from Miller's analysis and have drawn on parts of it in developing our account of ethical autonomy as it applies to health care professionals.

8. S. I. Benn, "Freedom, Autonomy and the Concept of a Person," *Proceedings of the Aristotelian Society* 66 (1976): 127.

9. For a deeper account of the nature and importance of moral reflection see Gerald Dworkin, "Moral Autonomy," in *Morals, Science and Society*, ed. H. Tristram Engelhardt, Jr., and Daniel Callahan (Hastings-on-Hudson: Hastings Center, 1978), 156–171; Harry G. Frankfurt, "Freedom of the Will and the Concept of a Person," *Journal of Philosophy* 68 (January 14, 1971): 5–20; and Charles Taylor, "Responsibility for Self," in *The Identities of Persons*, ed. Amelie Rorty (Berkeley: University of California Press, 1976), 281–299.

10. Martin Benjamin and Joy Curtis, *Ethics in Nursing*, 2nd ed. (New York: Oxford University Press, 1986), 126.

11. This account of the value of autonomy draws on Robert Young, "The Value of Autonomy," *Philosophical Quarterly* 32, NO. 126 (1982): 35–44.

12. Lisa H. Newton, "In Defense of the Traditional Nurse," *Nursing Outlook* 29 (June 1981): 348–354.

13. Newton, 353.

14. Newton.

15. Adina Schwartz, "Meaningful Work," *Ethics* 92 (July 1982): 634–646.

16. Schwartz, 638.

17. See Christine Mitchell, "Integrity in Interprofessional Relationships," in *Responsibility in Health Care*, ed. George J. Agich (Dordrecht, Holland: D. Reidel Publishing, 1981), 163–184.

18. Ann M. McElroy, "Burnout—A Review of the Literature with Application to Cancer Nursing," *Cancer Nursing* 5 (June 1982): 211–217.

19. Mitchell, "Integrity in Interprofessional Relationships," 175ff.

20. For one physician's defense of an outlook similar to that attributed here to Dr. Rhodes, see Richard C. Bates, "It's *Our* Right to Pull the Plug," *Medical Economics* 54 (May 16, 1977): 163–166.

21. See Miller, "Autonomy," and David L. Jackson and Stuart Youngner, "Patient Autonomy and 'Death with Dignity,'" *New England Journal of Medicine* 301 (August 23, 1979): 404–408.

22. Jolene L. Tuma, "Professional Misconduct" (Letter), *Nursing Outlook* 25 (September 1977): 546; Benjamin and Curtis, *Ethics in Nursing*, 98–101.

23. This case was prepared by Marjorie C. Keller, MSN, School of Nursing, East Carolina University.

24. Newton, "In Defense of the Traditional Nurse," 350.

25. Newton, 351.

26. Benjamin and Curtis, *Ethics in Nursing*, 92–94.

27. Benjamin and Curtis, 93.

28. For an encouraging account of recent changes along these lines, see Mila Ann Aroskar, "Establishing Limits to Professional Autonomy: Whose Responsibility?" in *Who Decides? Conflicts of Rights in Health Care*, ed. Nora K. Bell (Clifton, N.J.: Humana Press, 1982), 67–78.

29. John Ladd, "Some Reflections on Authority and the Nurse," in *Nursing: Images and Ideals*, ed. Stuart F. Spicker and Sally Gadow (New York: Springer, 1980), 171ff.

30. Ladd, 172.

31. Arthur Kuflik, "Morality and Compromise," in *Compromise in Ethics, Law, and Politics: Nomos XXI*, ed. J. Roland Pennock and John W. Chapman (New York: New York University Press, 1979), 49.

32. Kuflik, 50.

33. Samuel Gorovitz, "Can Physicians Mind Their Own Business and Still Practice Medicine?," in *Who Decides?*, 89ff.

34. Kuflik, "Morality and Compromise," 51.

35. Benjamin and Curtis, *Ethics in Nursing*, 108–115.

36. Amniocentesis is a procedure to obtain cells from the fetus that may then be used to detect genetic disorders. In some cases parents will decide on abortion if it is determined that the fetus has certain genetic disease.

37. Jamed F. Childress, " Appeals to Conscience," *Ethics* 89 (July 1979): 316ff.

38. In other cases, however, when a nurse is unable to compromise her ethical position, a personal exemption from participating in a wrongful action may not be sufficient. For if the act in question is clearly wrong, not only should she not participate in it, but neither should anyone else. Thus the nurse may have to do whatever she can to prevent the act from occurring. See Benjamin and Curtis, *Ethics in Nursing*, 92–94.

39. This case has been adapted from one reported in Janice Olson, "To Treat or to Allow to Die: An Ethical Dilemma in Gerontological Nursing," *Journal of Gerontological Nursing* 7 (March 1981): 141–147.

40. See Miller, "Autonomy," and Jackson and Youngner, "Patient Autonomy."

41. Richard Hull, "Responsibility and Accountability, Analyzed," *Nursing Outlook* 29 (December 1981): 707–712; George J. Agich, ed., *Responsibility in Health Care* (Dordrecht, Holland: D. Reidel Publishing, 1982).
42. Patricia Murphy, "Deciding to Blow the Whistle," *American Journal of Nursing* 81, no. 9 (September 1981): 1,691–1,692.
43. James L. Muyskens, "Nurses' Collective Responsibility and the Strike Weapon," *Journal of Medicine and Philosophy* 7 (1982): 101–112.

Suggestions for Further Reading

Benjamin, Martin, and Curtis, Joy. "Nursing." In *1986 Medical and Health Annual.* Chicago: Encyclopaedia Britannica, 1985, 282–285.
_____. "Virtue and the Practice of Nursing." In Shelp, Earl E., ed. *Virtue and Medicine.* Dordrecht, Holland: D. Reidel, 1985, 257–273.
_____. *Ethics in Nursing,* 2nd ed. New York: Oxford University Press, 1986.
Curtin, Leah, and Flaherty, M. Josephine. *Nursing Ethics: Theories and Pragmatics.* Bowie, Md.: Robert J. Brady, 1982.
Davis, Anne J., and Aroskar, Mila A. *Ethical Dilemmas and Nursing Practice,* 2nd ed. Norwalk, Ct.: Appleton-Century-Crofts, 1983.
Jameton, Andrew. *Nursing Practice: The Ethical Issue.* Englewood Cliffs, NJ: Prentice-Hall, 1984.
Mappes, E. Joy Kroeger. "Ethical Dilemmas for Nurses: Physician's Orders vs. Patients' Rights." In Mappes, Thomas A., and Zembaty, Jane S., eds. *Biomedical Ethics,* 2nd ed. New York: McGraw-Hill, 1986, 127–134.
Mitchell, Christine. "Integrity in Interprofessional Relationships." In *Responsibility in Health Care,* ed. George J. Agich. Dordrecht, Holland: D. Reidel, 1982, 163–184.
Miya, Pamela A. "Do Not Resuscitate: When Nurses' Duties Conflict with Patients' Rights." *Dimensions of Critical Care Nursing* 3 (September–October, 1984): 293–298.
Murphy, Catherine P., and Hunter, Howard, eds. *Ethical Problems in the Nurse-Patient Relationship.* Boston: Allyn and Bacon, 1983.
Muyskens, James L. *Moral Problems in Nursing: A Philosophical Investigation.* Totowa, N.J.: Rowman and Littlefield, 1982.
Pence, Terry. *Ethics in Nursing: An Annotated Bibliography.* New York: National League for Nursing, 1983.
Spicker, Stuart F., and Gadow, Sally, eds. *Nursing: Images and Ideals.* New York: Springer, 1980.
Winslow, Gerald R. "From Loyalty to Advocacy: A New Metaphor for Nursing," *Hastings Center Report* 14 (June 1984): 32–40.

CHAPTER XII

Health Care Institutions

H. Tristram Engelhardt, Jr.

Introduction

Health care institutions reflect the goals and purposes that fashion them and distinguish them from their sibling institutions such as the law and religion. In terms of these goals and purposes and their social articulation, different societal institutions construe circumstances as diseased, criminal, or sinful. There are major consequences, as a result, depending on whether an event is brought within the institutions of health care, law, or religion. Such choices affect the ways in which the individuals involved are treated. For example, there are major differences between a homosexual or an alcoholic being treated as a criminal, a sinful person, or a person who is ill and in need of treatment. Indeed, many homosexuals, and perhaps even some who engage in hearty drinking, might protest that not only are they neither criminals nor sinful, but that they are healthy and free of disease. They would be protesting views with regard to norms for psychological or physiological functions, accepted by some members of the health care professions. Their protest would also likely reflect their realization that the environment of social reactions in which they live depends in part on whether their behaviors are understood as crimes, diseases, or sins. These issues do not attend only those circumstances with major psychological valences such as alcoholism. They exist as well for other diseases. Consider, for example, syphilis or cancer of the lung, each of which could be construed as the outcome of a criminal or sinful act, such as fornication or the willful smoking of cancer-causing cigarettes. It is therefore important to understand the relationship that the health care institutions have with the institutions of law, religion, and education, in order to appreciate the social role into which patients (as opposed to criminals and penitents) are cast when they come into socially structured relationships with physicians, nurses, and other health care practitioners. These understandings will illuminate as well the nature of health care institutions.

At the onset it is important to be clear about the term "institution." The term is ambiguous. It may mean *general* institutions, in the sense of general ways of structuring social organizations. Examples are the institution of law or the institution of courts of equity or of hospitals. Or it may focus on *particular* institutions such as the probate court of Galveston County, Texas, or the Charity Hospital of Louisiana in New Orleans. This essay will sketch what is embraced in the notion of health care institutions in general. However, some examination will be provided of particular health care institutions. One might think here of medicine or nursing, hospitals or clinics. By taking this approach, we can explore the extent to which institutions embrace numerous, often incompatible, goals.[1] Or at least we can disclose the ways in which these diverse, often competing, goals display themselves in tensions that both characterize and structure major social institutions.

One might think, for example, of the institution of law, which has as its goal the preservation of both public safety and individual rights. One finds as a result lawyers assuming two quite different social roles, those of officers of the court and advocates of a client's rights. Thus on the one hand, a lawyer is charged with the task of aiding the court in acquiring sufficient information for the processes of justice, while on the other hand, as a defense lawyer, a lawyer is charged with the duty of defending a client's position, even if this may impede an adequate appreciation of the truth.[2] One finds, in short, a strategic tension in Anglo-American law, which is in fact considered a virtue in allowing for the beneficial balance of competing interests. Such tensions can be found as well in the competing roles of health care practitioners as defenders of the public health, versus health care practitioners as defenders of the health of a particular individual.[3] An example is the reporting of venereal diseases: should one maintain the character and confidentiality of the physician-patient relationship as a relationship directed primarily to the care of the individual patient, or should one alter its character and compromise confidentiality in order to secure the goals of public health? Or consider clinics for homosexuals, which are purported to exist in some large cities, guaranteeing complete confidentiality for individuals coming to them for the treatment of sexually transmitted diseases. They are tolerated by the local authorities, even though they fail to report reportable diseases.

Not only will we need to map with care the conflicts indigenous to the institutions of health care, but we also need to recognize the ambiguities of the term 'health care.' Under the rubric of health care and medicine, a wide range of variously related practices exists.[4] These include the activities of internists, surgeons, psychoanalysts, cosmetic surgeons, nurses, occupational therapists, physical therapists, occupational physicians, and epidemiologists. The roles played by particular health care practitioners are as much the result of historical accidents and social distributions of authority and perquisites as they are reflections of basic conceptual differences. Much of what physicians do and have done is found, only in a more specialized form, in the profession of nursing. In fact, it is very difficult at times to draw the line between obstetrics and the endeavors of nurse-midwives or anesthesiologists and nurse-anesthetists. The lines between nursing and medicine are created much more by legal restraints than by differences in scientific viewpoints or in expertise. Similarly artificial is the distinction between nurse-practitioners and physician assistants, at least in many circumstances. Lines are difficult to draw. The medical specialty of physical medicine grades imperceptibly into physical therapy. The boundary between physicians working in oral surgery and the activities of dentists in oral surgery is equally artificial. Nevertheless, within any particular medical profession or health care profession, one finds what, at first blush, might appear to be conceptually quite different undertakings—for example, those endeavors aimed primarily at curing disease versus those aimed at preserving health. Both undertakings are embraced by most health care professionals—dentists, physicians, and nurses.

When I use the term 'health care' here, I mean it broadly, including the various enterprises aimed at the care, cure, and amelioration of disease, as well as the preservation and restoration of health and well-being. One should note that among the undertakings directed to the psychological and physioanatomical bases of well-being one must include abortion, contraception, artificial insemination, genetic counseling, as well as crisis counseling.

Health Care Versus Other Institutions

Major social institutions in part describe the world and evaluate it, as well as provide explanations of its character.

They also fashion social reality. Legal institutions, for example, approach reality with an extensive descriptive vocabulary. In describing grounds for recovery, tort law discriminates among various occurrences by describing those occurrences and placing them within a classification. The classification itself is tied to value judgments concerning harms and injuries, and these are tied to theories of causation, accountability, and duty that allow the institution of law to give a construal of events for its purposes. If a physician is found negligent (a value-infected judgment) because of performing a sterilization operation poorly (a judgment dependent on accounts of causation), the world is being described, evaluated, and explained. In addition, social reality is being fashioned. In finding that the physician is liable for damages, the physician has been cast into a social role, just as when the sheriff, in stating "You are under arrest," fashions social reality.[5]

In drawing lines of authority among the various social institutions, society attempts to balance interests in blaming and praising, educating, redeeming, punishing, and curing. A "single" event can, for example, be cast within the province of more than one major social institution. The phenomenon of excessive alcohol use will be used as an example to illustrate the competing responses of social institutions. The competition among religious, legal, educational, and medical accounts of alcoholism conceptually places the position of health care among these other social institutions by placing the "medical facts" within the conceptual terms that constitute the explanatory frameworks employed by these institutions.

THE INSTITUTIONS OF RELIGION

Excessive alcohol use traditionally has been regarded in the West as a major vice that can lead to damnation. It invokes religious responses such as praying for grace and providing absolution for sin. Social roles such as that of a penitent are available for the individual drinker. The social institutions of religion, in short, place excessive alcohol use within a comprehensive account of reality. Such behavior is understood within an explanatory account that presumes the existence of God, grace, sin, and the need for divine forgiveness. Moreover, individuals play special functions as gatekeepers of various religious social roles: priests, rabbis, and ministers in different fashions certify the penitent sinner's status as fallen or repentant.

The significance of facts, events, and actions is thus found within a complex web of presumptions about the reality of the world. Religion, with its heavily metaphysical commitments, offers deep interpretations of the meaning and the purposes of ordinary happenings. What otherwise might appear to be of no enduring moment is shown to be a revelation of divine grace, an indication of the care of the gods, a token of divine providence, a reward of the deity, or an act of divine punishment and wrath. Indeed, because of its tie to the ultimate, and its claims regarding final, often infinite powers of God, religion has the capacity to give one of the most, if not the most, encompassing and elaborate interpretations of everyday reality. Partly for this reason, religious explanations are a balm for many. For example, in illness, when patients often ask for the meaning of their suffering, pain, and death, religion enters with a complementary, if not competing, interpretation to medicine. Where medicine often is able to disclose events only as the surd happenings of natural chance, without enduring meaning or purpose, religion is able to offer a metaphysical account of the cosmic economics of pain, suffering, and death. Religion in such cases can satisfy an emotional and intellectual need for a sense of purpose.

In their alternative interpretations of alcoholism, there is opportunity for religion and medicine to compete, though there need in principle be nothing more than complementarity between them. To see alcoholism as a sin does not exclude, in principle, interpreting it as well as a disease, or as a problem to be treated by medicine. An approach that emphasizes that an event can be interpreted as one of both religious and medical significance often captures better what is at stake. The competition, when it does exist, is more of a competition for funds or a sense of pre-eminence in resolving the problem at hand. The more medicine is able to "cure" sins, the less seriously religious concerns may be taken. Such circumstances may illicitly lead to the conclusion that the choice is one either of accepting a religious or a medical interpretation of the event in question. However, one can, for example, see the phenomenon of drunkenness to be a habit that can be cured by medicine but that springs from an initial series of culpable and hence sinful acts, just as one can hold both that someone is suffering from lung cancer and that he is responsible because of smoking for having developed the cancer. Religious and medical interpretations can be rendered complementary.

Yet insofar as medicine, for example, offers cheap and effective cures for important "sins," medicine's interpretations will with good reason be given special priority. Further, in many cases the medical interpretation of reality will make religious interpretations highly implausible. One might think here of Hippocrates' treatment of epilepsy, the so-called sacred disease of Greece. In holding that "it is not any more divine or sacred than other diseases," Hippocrates was surely offering a competing interpretation.[6] The same, no doubt, could be said of the New Testament accounts of Jesus curing individuals possessed by devils. Often a complementary interpretation is not possible, or is difficult, and it becomes more plausible to choose a medical rather than a religious account of an event.

In order to understand the relations between medical and religious or other institutions, one will need to determine with care the extent to which they are complementary or competing with respect to particular issues. Since there tends to be a single paradigm for scientific medicine, while there remain numerous mutually competing paradigms regarding what will count as proper religious institutions, the areas for competition and complementarity will be diverse. The thoughtful care of patients by physicians will thus require a detailed understanding of the geography of religious interpretations of reality in order to understand when a particular medical event or intervention is seen to carry religious significance. Moreover, an actual examination of current health care institutions reveals that complex accommodations between religious and medical institutions have in fact taken place. It is not simply because of the religious origins of many hospitals that chaplains are found in most, regardless of their historical origins. In fact, patients see themselves as subjects of events bearing both religious and medical significance. The consequence is that there is an ongoing and unavoidable need to integrate the encounters of these two major clusters of social institutions.

Given the predominance of the scientific model, however, the religious perspective is often, up to a point, medicalized. This occurs, for example, when the minister is regarded as a member of the health care team. As such, he or she is seen as performing a service that is not simply complementary to the enterprises of medicine but also supportive of them. That is, the activities of the chaplain can be construed in secular medical terms as lowering the morbidity of the patient, if not in fact having a beneficial impact on mortality statistics by helping control stress and anxiety. In all of this, the chaplain's contributions need not be understood in a particularly religious, magical, or metaphysical sense, but as a form of psychological therapy. Much, for example, of clinical pastoral education can be interpreted as a partial medicalization of traditional religious institutions. This transformation should, after all, not be unexpected, given the vast success of scientific medicine and the predominance of the scientific model.

THE LAW

The law for its part addresses excess alcohol consumption under the rubrics of criminal and civil law. Public drunkenness and drunk and disorderly conduct are grounds for criminal prosecution. So, too, is driving while intoxicated a special crime with special sanctions. Though secular law does not characterize the guilty individual as sinful, it incorporates elements of moral judgments in holding the individual to be guilty and worthy of punishment for retributive, deterrent, or reformative reasons.[7] In short, the law, as religion, describes the world in categories that import value judgments and explanatory interests, while casting individuals in social roles. The drunk thus receives a place in a legal framework, which in part includes categories for description erected in statutory and in case law. Views of criminal and civil liability are tied to legal theories of accountability and of causation that justify the ways in which the law responds to the acts of drunks. In imposing a role for punishment, an evaluation is passed. Moreover, a social role is created.

In the law one finds descriptions and explanations of reality, which are nearly on a par with the accounts offered by medicine and religion. Because events are placed by the law within a special language with its own rules of evidence and inference, the law fashions a competing view of reality. It differs from religion and medicine in being more clearly acknowledged as an artificial construal. Religions, after all, usually claim to describe and explain the world from a divinely inspired, if not infallible, perspective. Their construal is thus rarely seen to be merely the work of humans, at least by the adherents of the religion in question. Similarly, physicians often purport to speak from a timeless, scientific standpoint. The law, in contrast, more clearly acknowledges that its equivalent of the medicalization of reality is a human artifice. Yet in order to appreciate its power and intrusiveness, one must acknowledge the extent to which its deliverances become taken for granted as elements of reality. Certain events come to be appreciated as crimes, as behaviors to be punished, rather than as conditions to be treated. Current disputes, for example, regarding the legitimacy of the insanity defense, reflect competing, deeply felt judgments regarding whether certain events should be seen as crimes justifying retribution, or illnesses requiring psychiatric intervention.[8] Such competing judgments underlie the tensions in the geography of major social institutions. For example, the world of social practices changes appreciably as different crimes are seen as diseases, or different diseases regarded as crimes. Recall Samuel Butler's *Erewhon*, in which larceny was treated as a disease and diseases were visited with punishments.[9] By drawing lines among competing social institutions, and interpreting events as primarily objects of religious, legal, medical, or educational concerns, one fashions a world out of a universe of possible social realities.

EDUCATION

Education, as religion and law, can address the problem of excess alcohol consumption from its own perspective. For the educator, the problem is teaching individuals how to control their drinking. The model of the educator presumes that at least some excess drinking comes from ignorance concerning the effects of alcohol or the ways to control one's inclinations toward, or interest in, using alcohol. The individual who drinks to excess is thus not so much sinful or criminal, or in fact guilty, as ignorant and in need of instruction.

Though educational institutions do not fashion as encompassing an interpretation of reality as do the medical, legal, and religious, they must be borne in mind in appreciating the significance of health care institutions. They share similarities with medicine, religion, and law. Like medicine, the object of educational intervention (i.e., ignorance) is understood as an undesirable circumstance. Like religion and law, there is often the imputation of culpability to the person who remains ignorant. Like medicine, educational institutions hold the states they address to be beyond the immediate control of persons. One cannot simply will away either ignorance or diseases. Also, educational institutions compete with health care institutions for funds and social resources, even when they do not possess the same tradition of competition that marks the interrelations of law, medicine, and religion. The place of educational institutions on the terrain of social institutions characterizes and defines, in part at least, the place and significance of health care institutions.

MEDICINE

Medicine, of course, addresses the problem of alcoholism as well. For medicine, excess alcohol consumption is not a sin or a crime, nor an issue of ignorance, but a category of disease or disorder. The

Diagnostic and Statistical Manual of the American Psychiatric Association places excess alcohol consumption within categories such as "alcohol abuse" and "alcohol dependence."[10] Its diagnostic criteria for alcohol abuse are:

> *Pattern of pathological alcohol use*: need for daily use of alcohol for adequate functioning; inability to cut down on or stop drinking; repeated efforts to control or reduce excess drinking by "going on the wagon" (periods of temporary abstinence) or restricting drinking to certain times of the day; binges (remaining intoxicated throughout the day for at least two days); occasional consumption of a fifth of spirits (or its equivalent in wine or beer); amnesic periods for events occurring while intoxicated (blackouts); continuation of drinking despite a serious physical disorder that the individual knows is exacerbated by alcohol using; drinking of non-beverage alcohol.[11]

The problem of excess alcohol consumption is thus translated into the language of medicine so that the factual situation is appreciated within a theoretical framework, which attends to physiological and psychological determinants, and which will allow one to predict the development and course of such a disease, as well as direct health care practitioners in treating the disorder. Excess alcohol consumption in being treated as a disease is also evaluated as the failure to meet a minimal level of psychological and physiological excellence. It therefore justifies the imposition of a therapy role, converting the excess drinker into a patient to be treated. Unlike the priest who prays for the excess drinker, the police officer who might arrest him, or the educator who might give pointers on moderation in drinking, the physician will attempt to secure psychological and physiological approaches to treat the individual. An example is the excess drinker who as a patient may be treated with disulfiram (Antabuse).

In terming excess drinking a disease, there is a shift in the values that frame the description. If drinking is considered a sin, or a legal infraction, or an act out of ignorance, each of these carries with it particular value judgments regarding acting in a way worthy of divine or civil punishment or public reproach. Problems are brought to health care institutions insofar as they involve pain, suffering, deformity, or disability that are held to have a physiological or psychological basis beyond the immediate control of the patient, and not the result, or a part of, sinful or criminal behavior or ignorance (though they may have aspects that allow them *also* to be construed as criminal, sinful, etc.). Although diseases exempt the bearer from moral culpability for being ill (as opposed to becoming ill or remaining ill through the patient's own fault), value judgments still play a role. To be diseased, disabled, or deformed is to fail to realize an anatomical, physiological, or psychological minimal standard of excellence. To be diseased is to be anatomically, physiologically, or psychologically abnormal where "abnormality" is not simply statistical deviance (individuals with high IQ's are statistically deviant). It involves reference to a set of values and expectations that define the health care professions. Judgments such as "You are a sinner," "You are a lawbreaker," or "You are ignorant" are now replaced by health care statements that are equivalent to "You are deviant," where deviance implies a negative nonmoral judgment. The more such deviances involve important ideals of psychological or physiological function, anatomical form or freedom from pain or anxiety, the stronger the social power of the value judgments involved. Judgments regarding insanity or deformities have powerful negative connotations. These connotations exist even when it is clear that the disease or deformity is not contagious or directly threatening to others. However, even judgments of physical diseases grade the individual as falling short of a biological or psychological norm. When a set of circumstances is brought across the border that demarcates health care institutions from other social institutions, the context of evaluation changes. Value judgments are not abandoned. To be sick is to be in a state that is undesirable and found to be wanting.[12]

The same event is differently assessed given the different purposes of major social institutions. In drawing the boundaries between such institutions, one is allocating major social powers amongst these social institutions. The more that medicine has the opportunity to medicalize excessive drinking, the more difficult it becomes to criminalize it, or to see it as a problem for religion or education. The priority of a particular institution's intervention is established partly in terms of straightforward considerations of efficiency. For example, if medicine were able easily and definitively to cure alcoholism, the medicalization of the problem would likely meet with little challenge. However, one may become concerned about the medicalization of excessive drinking if the treatments employed lend themselves to being misused as instruments of political oppression. By way of illustration, few individuals object either to the treatment of transient mental disturbances in diabetics who inadvertently take more insulin than required or to the treatment of the psychological problems of hyperthyroidism through medical and surgical intervention. There is, however, concern about the use of psychiatry to treat political deviants.[13]

Here historical examples may help. Consider the nineteenth-century "disease" of masturbation. In order to prevent the supposed serious complications of masturbation, which were thought to include death, the clitorises of female masturbators were cauterized, at times excised, and in some cases men were castrated. The medicalization of masturbation clearly led to some rather serious harmful consequences.[14] However, individuals from the period were able to recognize the attempt by both religious and medical institutions to appropriate the problem of masturbation.

> Now it happens in a large number of cases, that these young masturbators sooner or later become alarmed at their practices, in consequence of some information they receive. Often this latter is of a most mischievous character. Occasionally too, the religious element is predominant, and the mental condition of these young men becomes truly pitiable.... The facts are nearly these: Masturbation is not a crime nor a sin, but a vice.[15]

Though the history of the "disease of masturbation" is a complex one, it serves to recall the fact that the border between religious institutions and health care institutions has been frequently crossed. Many phenomena have been imported into the domain of health care from the domains of religion and morals. Though many of these inclusions have proved justified, others have produced more costs than benefits.

The nineteenth century provides further examples of disputes regarding the boundary between political institutions and institutions of health care. Consider, for instance, the special diseases for slaves "identified" by Samuel Cartwright. Cartwright argued that slaves who fled the plantations of the South were in fact suffering from a disease he termed drapetomania, "the disease causing slaves to run away." In so doing he attempted to medicalize the political acts of southern blacks seeking refuge in the North. Similarly, he proposed the disease of "dysaesthesia aethiopis" to account for what slave plantation overseers called "rascality."[16] Though most commentators have interpreted Cartwright as attempting to support the southern establishment,[17] one might also, more against the general facts concerning Cartwright, view him as an individual arguing for more humane treatment of blacks who were caught as runaway slaves or who would not cooperate on plantations. Rather than having them punished as lawbreakers, Cartwright was suggesting that they be treated medically. This suggestion provided a humane alternative under the circumstances. However one interprets the actual facts of this particular case, the general point is that construing problems within one social institution rather than another has consequences for all parties who have an interest in the state of affairs. As one moves phenomena such as masturbation, the flight of a refugee, or homosexual activities, from a circumstance with religious significance to one with political or medical significance, one radically changes the social and personal appreciation of the phenomena. Since all human behavior has underlying physiological and psychological causes, it can all in principle be medicalized. The justification for medicalization requires an assessment of individual and social costs, as well as the ability of science actually to explain and manipulate biological and psychological processes. Here the warnings of social critics such as Ivan Illich[18] and Thomas Szasz[19] regarding the overmedicalization of problems are relevant.

Competing and Complementary Institutions—Competing and Complementary Realities

To understand health care institutions is to see their relationship with competing institutions, and to understand why and how the lines are drawn among those institutions. As has been suggested, these lines can in part be understood as sociohistorical outcomes. They can also be justified or brought into question in terms of general rational arguments regarding the costs and benefits of competing construals of reality. To appreciate these construals of reality as the outcome of social and historical forces is to introduce the question of the theory-ladenness and value-ladenness of facts. A great deal of recent literature supports the claim that pictures of reality should be understood in sociohistorical terms.[20] In this view, there are no naked, brute, or uninterpreted facts. Facts appear always within theoretical understandings and metaphysical presuppositions about the world. Facts are always irradicably theory-dependent. To classify something is already to see that something in terms of basic assumptions, or within one or another interpretation of reality. To have a naked or theory-free fact would be to have an uninterpreted experience.

With regard to medicine, this argument is made by Ludwik Fleck in *Genesis and Development of a Scientific Fact*.[21] Because of its influence on Thomas Kuhn's *The Structure of Scientific Revolutions*,[22] Fleck's work has had a major impact on modern understandings of the philosophy of science. Fleck uses the example of syphilis to indicate that there is no concept of syphilis independent of a social historical context. There is no timeless fact of syphilis. Syphilis, as Fleck argues, changes in meaning from the first classical descriptions by Fracastoro[23] through the descriptions by Sydenham,[24] to the descriptions by Wassermann,[25] until today. A similar point was made by Kuhn regarding oxygen. Who discovered oxygen? Was it Priestley, who thought that he had identified dephlogisticated air, or Lavoisier, who held that he had discovered a necessary condition for acids?[26] The term *oxygen* thus does not identify a noninterpreted fact. The meaning of oxygen is as much discovered as it is interpreted through scientific theories that are the inventions of human minds.

Kuhn and Fleck both argue that even the epistemic endeavors of scientists must be seen within a sociohistorical context. Further, as Fleck notes, medical facts are not influenced simply by an abstract desire for knowledge. Applied bodies of knowledge have special goals that direct the use of knowledge, as well as views regarding costs of applications. This point is central to understanding the role not only of medical institutions but also of religion, law, and to some extent, education. Facts are not simply described, they are evaluated. They are graded in terms of evaluative norms. Events may be sinful for religious, criminal for the law, and psychologically or physiologically deviant for medicine. Moreover, in being practical enterprises without access to divine knowledge, medicine and law classify reality in terms that are useful to their special goals. They fashion pragmatically oriented artificial classifications. Deciding what will count as a normal level of blood pressure versus a level that will count as mild hypertension depends on judgments regarding the usefulness of treating versus not treating certain elevations. Events or states are categorized and described in terms of evaluations regarding when a condition should be seen as providing a warrant for medical or legal interventions.[27]

Because different institutions may assign different costs and benefits to outcomes, their interpretation of alcoholism, drug abuse, violent behavior, or social instability can be in competition or incompatible. At times such competition can have major social consequences. In addition to the examples already mentioned, consider also abortion, artificial insemination by donor, and contraception. With regard to such issues, secular medicine's interpretations of the balance of costs and benefits can be quite different from those of medicine practiced in the context of a particular moral viewpoint. The same holds for civil versus canon law. As a result, there is competition not only among types of social institutions but also within institutions of one type (e.g., medical). To judge that an abortion is "medically indicated" is to appeal to a set of costs and benefits measured in mundane mortalities and morbidities. Such a judgment is not a value-free judgment. Rather, it is a judgment made in terms of the general secular goals that shape secular health care institutions: avoiding death and suffering. These presuppose general secular assumptions, such as: the pains or discomforts of a woman are of greater significance than the pains or discomforts of a fetus.

Health Care in Secular, Pluralist Societies

In peaceable secular pluralist societies, such as those that characterize the West, and the developed open societies of the East, judgments concerning costs and benefits can be justified only in terms generally accessible to all. Moral judgments that presuppose particular forms of grace or special metaphysical insights cannot carry general moral authority. The moral calculi that direct institutions in such societies must therefore be framed in secular terms appealing to those kinds of arguments that one may reasonably expect to cut across the boundaries of particular moral communities. Since a justified basis or moral authority in such circumstances cannot be a simple appeal to force, nor an appeal to a special moral viewpoint to which all are not likely to convert, one is left with establishing the moral bases of secular institutions through an appeal to general rational arguments or to common agreement. However, since it is difficult, if not impossible, to establish by rational argument alone the moral authority of a particular concrete view of the good life (e.g., such will require an appeal to a particular moral sense, and one will need to presuppose a particular moral sense to know to which moral sense one ought to appeal), a greater proportion of the authority of moral communities will depend on the explicit or implicit mutual agreement of their members. As a consequence, rights to privacy and self-determination loom large in such societies. Educational systems tend to retreat from teaching particular religious moral values, and medicine comes to acknowl-

edge free and informed consent as central to the moral conduct of
the profession. If it cannot be established what the patient must do
from a moral point of view, one must treat the patient as the free
person, and let the patient make the final choice. Social institutions
in secular societies tend to have a recognizable libertarian theme,
especially if one contrasts them with communist dictatorships or
the Christian kingdoms of the Middle Ages, which presumed to be
able to identify, and have the moral right to enforce, a particular
view of the good life for everyone.

Contemporary health care institutions have been affected by the
retreat of the law from regulating major elements of sexual activity
tangential to health care. Here in particular one should note the Supreme Court's ruling in *Griswold v. State of Connecticut* (1965)
which held unconstitutional a $100 fine levied against a Dr. Gris-
wold for having given information and medical advice to married
people regarding the prevention of conception.[28] The decriminali-
zation of the provision of contraceptive information, including the
requirement that physicians be the providers, was made complete
with *Eisenstadt v. Baird* (1972), which gave unmarried individuals
the same right of access to contraceptive information and material
as married individuals.[29] In fact, *Roe v. Wade* (1973) can be seen in a
similar light.[30] Abortion was moved by that ruling into an area to
be determined by physicians and patients, except after the fetus's vi-
ability. In so doing, the prerogatives of health care institutions and
legal institutions were redrawn.

These changes reflect major shifts in the views regarding the
proper role of legal institutions in directing human conduct and in
defining what will count as proper or unnatural acts. This shift receives a particular emphasis on the 1980 holding of New York (*People v. Onofre*) that sodomy statutes are unconstitutional:

We express no view as to any theological, moral or psychological evaluation of consensual sodomy. These are aspects of the
issue on which informed, competent authorities and individuals may and do differ. Contrary to the view expressed by the dis-
sent, although on occasion it does serve such ends, it is not the
function of the Penal Law in our governmental policy to provide
either a medium for the articulation or the apparatus for the intended enforcement of moral or theological values. Thus, it has
been deemed irrelevant by the United States Supreme Court
that the purchase and use of contraceptives by unmarried persons would arouse moral indignation among broad segments of

our community or that the viewing of pornographic materials even within the privacy of one's home would not evoke general approbation. . . . The community and its members are entirely free to employ theological teaching, moral suasion, parental advice, psychological and psychiatric counseling and other non-coercive means to condemn the practice of consensual sodomy. The narrow question before us is whether the Federal Constitution permits the use of the criminal law for that purpose.[31]

This ruling marks a major shift in the role of legal institutions in defining what is unnatural in a fashion warranting legal intervention, including often, as part of reformatory punishment, psychiatric treatment.

As a consequence, social institutions tend to exist on two levels: one, that of the general secular society, and second, that of a particular moral community. Thus, within the law it becomes quite proper to hold that "access to abortion on request should be an element of the basic right of privacy in a secular pluralist society," although it is totally consistent to hold it to be an offense at canon law punishable by excommunication. So, too, secular health care institutions will treat many procedures such as abortion, artificial insemination by donors, and contraception to be proper goals of health care, though medical institutions with religious commitments may disagree on these points. These two frameworks, dimensions, or tiers of moral understanding both create and relieve tension in fashioning places for beliefs to flourish and to be tolerated. However, in that very toleration, they guarantee that there will be numerous conflicting moral viewpoints existing side by side, often entering into dispute. This contrast between the secular pluralist society, and the particular moral communities it embraces, marks the character of contemporary social institutions in large-scale states. Such large-scale states and their institutions are amoral in the sense that they do not embrace a particular view of the good life. Or rather, they are forced to affirm a minimalist articulation of what the good life entails, emphasizing whenever possible the rights of individuals to fashion freely their own understandings of the good life.

An appreciation of contemporary social institutions must, therefore, start with the recognition that they exist in states spanning numerous moral and religious communities. One must at the same time recognize as well that the classical roots of Western political thought are framed not in terms of large-scale states but rather in terms of the city-state and its institutions. Aristotle and Plato, who

were extremely influential in fashioning Western political understandings, took the city-state as their paradigm political institution.
The city-state, as Aristotle argued in the *Nicomachean Ethics*,
should include fewer than 100,000 people (*Nicomachean Ethics*
10.1170, 631–632) and be able to be taken in at a single view (*Politics* vii.4 1326, 618–625). Only under such circumstances could citizens and those elected to office know each other well enough for the
government to function effectively (*Politics* vii.4 1326, 310–318). It
is one of the ironies of history that Aristotle, the tutor of Alexander
the Great, framed this understanding of the state as a community of
individuals who were not strangers in the same era that Alexander
the Great was fashioning a large-scale state spanning numerous
moral communities. Unlike the Greek city-state, individuals in
modern large-scale states often, if not usually, meet as strangers.
Physician and patient, lawyer and client, cannot presume that they
belong to the same moral community. In modern states, one is continually surrounded by what Aristotle would have recognized as
metics and foreigners. There is not a single moral community with a
concrete view of the good life spanning modern large-scale states.

Health care institutions, as well as other secular institutions such
as the law, must be understood within the context of large-scale
states and those values and presuppositions that underlie them.
This circumstance is acknowledged in *People v. Onofre* quoted earlier. *Onofre's* use of "moral" is best interpreted as identifying the
mores of particular moral communities, rather than the presuppositions for peaceable secular societies spanning numerous communities. The moral commitment of the medical and legal professions in
a secular society will include a commitment to the peaceful negotiation of common endeavors in which the character of the good life is
as much to be created as discovered. As a consequence, the moral
propriety or impropriety of abortion, contraception, the refusal of
life-saving treatment, or artificial insemination are left to resolution
within the context of particular moral communities. Physicians and
lawyers, working within the framework of a secular state, can at
best commit themselves to laying out the alternatives in as much
detail as possible. It is not accidental, then, that free and informed
consent becomes the moral linchpin of bioethical discussions.
When a physician's activities do not involve the use of uncon-
sented-to force against the innocent, or when public funds are not
employed in areas in which a group of citizens effectively vetoes
such use, there tend to be few restrictions on what physicians and
patients may consent to do together. A consequence of this circum-

stance is that much of the authority of physicians is undermined. Indeed, the law is slowly retreating from cases that support a professional standard for disclosure to patients[32] and is moving toward a patient-oriented standard,[33] a phenomenon that is refashioning the authority of physicians and signaling some of the major consequences of health care institutions existing in a secular pluralist society. Health care institutions are as much in control of citizens generally as in the control of the health care professions.

Bioethical Issues and Health Care Institutions

Problems are always problems of a particular sort, interpreted within a theoretical and evaluational framework and as a result can be adequately appreciated only if the context is well specified. This circumstance is often underappreciated in the assessment of bioethical issues. In addressing the problem of euthanasia, for instance, one will need to appeal to ideas of good and bad lives and deaths to understand when, in fact, within health care institutions euthanasia can be a policy to be supported rationally. So, too, for issues of experimentation on humans. Insofar as these involve calculations of possible benefits and risks, such assessments appeal to schedules of costs and benefits in which one must decide regarding the comparative significance of possible benefits versus possible risks of death, however remote. The same is true for any meaningful appreciation of informed consent. One will need to have an understanding of what actual persons, and what reasonably prudent persons, would hold to be significant benefits or risks in order to determine the proper content of disclosures.

In short, bioethical problems, since they exist in particular social contexts, presuppose a rich web of taken-for-granted understandings and hierarchies of risks and benefits. These frame the contexts within which physicians, nurses, or hospitals are judged to be acting correctly, or to be negligent and liable for damages to patients or clients. It is only against such social backgrounds that one can appreciate what the duties of nurses or physicians or hospitals should be, what will count as significant harms, and to what causal connections one should attend. As H. L. A. Hart and A. M. Honore indicated in a classic discussion of causation and the law, it is only in terms of such social understandings that one can identify causal connections in the law as opposed to background conditions.[34]

They give an example of flowers that wither in a garden *because* a gardener fails to water them. It is the gardener who *caused* the flowers to wither, though many individuals passing by could have watered them as well, and though the death of the flowers was caused as much, in one sense of cause, by the absence of sufficient rain. The gardener's social role with its expectations mark him as responsible. Bioethical problems are embedded within such sets of expectations that define the roles of physicians and nurses within health care institutions.

Physicians and nurses function not simply as dispassionate scientists, nor simply as individuals interested in curing or ameliorating disease, but as special gatekeepers for social rights, privileges, and opportunities. Thus, tension exists between the roles of health care professionals as curers and carers on the one hand, and individuals engaged in diagnoses for administrative purposes on the other. As commentators have indicated, this is a root of bioethical problems in that physicians are cast, because of their institutional positions, in the role of double agents.[35] One should note that this occurs not simply when the physician is a member of two distinct institutions, as for example when the physician is also an officer in the military or an employee of a corporation, other than a health care facility. Rather, it is a function of the institutionalized significance of therapy roles or sick roles themselves.

Further, health care as a general social institution embodies sometimes explicit, sometimes implicit, judgments concerning the proper uses of resources in health care. As a consequence, accepted grounds or indications for making a diagnosis, instituting a particular form of treatment, or using a preventive medical intervention reflect cost-benefit and cost-effectiveness judgments. These judgments in part are made on the basis of the likely consequences with respect to patient morbidity and mortality from following a particular rule for diagnosis and treatment. With regard to diagnoses, there must always be risks of false positive or false negative diagnoses. The significance of such risks will then be measured in terms of what health care professionals consider to be the comparative costs of going without treatment for the disease in question, or being treated when one does not have the disease, and as a consequence being pointlessly exposed to the side effects of the treatment. Judgments will vary in terms of the seriousness of the disease, the efficaciousness of the treatment, and the possible side effects of treatment. A classical example of such standards for diagnosis is the criteria for the diagnosis of rheumatic fever, in which the presence of two major manifestations of the disease, or one major manifestation and two minor manifestations, is taken to justify the diagnosis.[36] Given a different view of either the seriousness of the disease if left untreated, the efficaciousness of the treatment, or the risks of the treatment itself, one can imagine revising the grounds for establishing the diagnosis so that they require three major manifestations or two minor manifestations and a major manifestation; in such a fashion one would avoid more false positive diagnoses than at present. However, if one were more concerned with undertreatment than overtreatment—that is, more concerned with false negative diagnoses than with false positive diagnoses—one might require less certainty for establishing the diagnoses.

In short, medicine, like the law, establishes tests of truth that reflect a set of important nonepistemic considerations regarding costs of choosing the wrong description of a state of affairs. Indications for diagnoses in medicine have their parallel with tests of truth in the law, where, for example, one must show that an accused is guilty beyond a reasonable doubt in a criminal case, in contrast to a civil case, in which a suit is determined on the preponderance of evidence. The law presumes that loss of life or liberty with the imputation of criminality is so serious a matter that one would rather have the system exposed to the possibility of making a large number of false negative judgments (acquittal of guilty individuals) in order to avoid any significant number of false positive judgments (conviction of innocent individuals). The fact of guilt, or the fact of a particular patient having a particular disease, is thus understood within a set of institutionalized calculations regarding the relative seriousness of possible costs and benefits of accepting particular knowledge claims.

Diagnoses must be made in terms of their consequences because they are tied to therapeutic imperatives. To be found to be suffering from a particular disease invites a particular set of therapeutic responses. The initiation of particular therapeutic responses is itself placed within a set of cost-benefit justifications. Arguments as to when and under what circumstances one should perform a radical versus a simple mastectomy, or provide coronary bypass surgery, reflect a set of often institutionalized assumptions regarding proper exchanges of morbidities and mortalities. Further, insofar as the provision of health care occurs through societal programs or third-party payers, financial considerations will also play a large role. This explains why coronary bypass surgery is not usually seen as an indicated form of treatment within the British National Health Service, where more stringent criteria for "effectiveness" are employed.[37] Similar decisions are made in the United States. One might also think of the recent controversy regarding whether women over thirty should receive Pap smears every three years, as has been recommended by the American Cancer Society, or every year, as had been past practice. Some calculations have been made indicating that the costs involved in yearly Pap smears amount to $50,000 per woman saved as a result of the early diagnosis of cervical cancer.[38] The point is that judgments regarding which health care procedures should be seen as a routine part of good health care reflect a complex web of cost-benefit judgments.

Of course, not all individuals would come to the same judgment regarding the proper comparison of the costs and benefits involved in establishing diagnoses, initiating treatments, or engaging in preventive health measures. As a consequence, questions arise regarding the proper modes of gaining the consent of individuals and of society to the standards established by health care institutions. A wide range of otherwise isolated bioethical issues are found to be integrated in such controversies, in that such judgments regarding indications for treatments or grounds for a diagnosis require comparing years of life, while often making assessments of the quality of life afforded. Quality of life judgments, problems of consent, and the comparison of particular costs in utilitarian calculi converge in the institutionalized conventions that direct health care.

What might appear to be straightforward factual judgments regarding the diagnoses of a particular patient's problem or the choice of treatment thus turn out in the end to be strongly influenced by the various explanatory, evaluative, and social assumptions that frame the character of a health care institution. As has been noted, such assumptions frame all social institutions. To place a problem within any particular institution is indirectly to select a certain constellation of background assumptions. Such a selection involves a commitment to a particular view of authority and of rights to constrain choices within particular institutional settings. Thus, insofar as diagnostic and therapeutic choices are seen to be purely factual choices by health care providers, they will rarely be acknowledged as open to the consent of, or emendation by, patients or clients. That is, it may seem plausible that patients have a right to refuse a treatment outright, but not to refuse a particular diagnosis, or to choose a mode of treatment considered by health care practitioners as less than optimal. A recent and well-discussed exception has been the reclassification of homosexuality as "ego-dystonic," making the appropriateness of the diagnosis of the disorder dependent on whether the individual involved sees him- or herself as disordered.[39] Insofar as diagnoses and treatments are not necessary to the protection of third parties, and insofar as the independent authority of health care professionals is brought into question, it becomes more plausible that patients may participate, should they have the interest, in setting the thresholds of certainty for making a diagnosis or in setting the balance of benefits and risks in choosing a mode of therapy.

There are limitations on the roles of individual patients. Medicine is a social endeavor, often paid for by third parties who have a vested interest in establishing the ways in which their funds will be expended in the control, treatment, or prevention of disease, disability, or defect. To the role of health care professionals who have a view of the standards established through the good practice of their profession, and individuals who have views as to what would maximize their advantage, one must add the role of communities (e.g., members of a third-party insurance group) and society in general, in choosing the level of expenditures and the distribution of common resources. Health care institutions set at least *pro tempore* balances among the interests and rights of these parties. In addition to easily recognized areas in which such balances must be established, these problems of balancing arise as well in terms of who should control the social constitution of reality within the domain of a particular profession. Since "facts" receive a social standing as they move from one professional context to another, the issue is then not only who controls these border crossings (e.g., the transformation of a legal problem to a medical problem) but also who should control, and in what way, the interpretation of such problems for the health care professions. There is, in short, a wide array of hidden bioethical problems of consent and control, problems that are often unacknowledged because they are addressed in a language that appears to involve a factual presentation of medical indications and medical data.

Conclusion:
Medicalization Problems and the Social
Control of Reality

To understand the ethical problems that arise in health care, one must attend to the context in which they appear. As

I have argued in this chapter, this will require providing a conceptual geography of the boundaries among the various major societal institutions, noting the explanatory and evaluative assumptions that distinguish problems as health care problems, as opposed to legal or religious problems. Such a geography is a philosophical task. It is the endeavor of analyzing or drawing out the role of major conceptual commitments. Such a geography can help individuals appreciate the costs and benefits of border crossings, importations of problems from law into medicine, or the exportation of those problems from medicine into law. Such trade between institutions has costs and benefits that can be assessed only if one weighs the consequences for society in general, as well as for the standing of individual persons. Moreover, one must acknowledge that there are numerous alternative ways in which problems can be appreciated within health care institutions themselves. Though as social institutions they are committed to developing general conventions for making diagnoses and instituting treatment in terms of background judgments regarding proper cost-benefit calculations and proper ways of acknowledging the authority and prerogatives of the participants, the character of such cost-benefit analyses can be brought into question, and lines of authority redrawn under challenge. This element of the social reconstruction of reality is unavoidable. Acknowledging its character affords an educated appreciation of the ways in which medical facts are not simply facts but are fashioned in terms of the complex nonepistemic goals and interests that direct health care.

Notes

1. One might think here of the Tuma case, in which a nurse was charged with unprofessional conduct for informing a patient with cancer about the use of Laetrile. See Tuma v. Board of Nursing, 593 P. 2d 711 S. Ct. Idaho 1979.

2. See, for example, the discussion of the conflicting roles of lawyers in Monroe H. Freedman, *Lawyers' Ethics in an Adversary System* (Indianapolis, Ind.: Bobbs-Merrill, 1975). A discussion of this book and its implication for physicians is provided by Stephen Toulmin, "The Meaning of Professionalism: Doctors' Ethics and Biomedical Science," *Knowledge, Value, and Belief*, ed. H. T. Engelhardt, Jr., and Daniel Calahan (Hastings-on-Hudson, N.Y.: Hastings Center, 1977), 254–278.

3. H. Tristram Engelhardt, Jr., "Goals of Medical Care," in *Who Decides: Conflicts of Rights in Health Care*, ed. N. Bell (Clifton, N.J.: Humana Press, 1982), 49–66.

4. ————. "Clinical Judgment," *Metamedicine* 2 (October 1981): 301–

317; "Doctoring the Disease, Treating the Complaint, Helping the Patient: Some of the Works of Hygeia and Panacea," in *Knowing and Valuing: The Search for Common Roots*, ed. H. Tristram Engelhardt, Jr., and Daniel Callahan (Hastings-on-Hudson, N.Y.: Hastings Center, 1980), 225–249.

5. What happens to the physician in such a circumstance is similar to what occurs when a patient is cast into a sick role.

6. Hippocrates, "The Sacred Disease", *Hippocrates*, vol. 2, trans. W. H. S. Jones (Cambridge, Mass.: Harvard University Press, 1959), 139.

7. The law requires, it should be noted, *mens rea*, or evil intent, in order to justify criminal punishment.

8. See Baruch Brody and H. Tristram Engelhardt, Jr., eds., *Mental Health: Law and Public Policy* (Dordrecht, Holland: D. Reidel Publishing, 1980); and Stuart F. Spicker, Joseph M. Healy, and H. Tristram Engelhardt, Jr., eds., *The Law-Medicine Relation: A Philosophical Exploration* (Dordrecht, Holland: D. Reidel Publishing, 1981).

9. Samuel Butler, *Erewhon* (New York: Dutton, 1959).

10. American Psychiatric Association, *Diagnostic and Statistical Manual of Mental Disorders*, 3d. ed. (*DSM-III*) (Washington, D.C., 1980), 169–170.

11. *DSM-III*, 170.

12. "Illnesses, Diseases, and Sicknesses," in *The Humanity of the Ill*, ed. Victor Kestenbaum (Knoxville: The University of Tennessee Press, 1982), 142–156.

13. See, for example, Harvey Fireside, *Soviet Psychoprisons* (New York: Norton, 1979); and U.S. Senate, "Abuse of Psychiatry for Political Repression in the Soviet Union," *Hearing before the Subcommittee to Investigate the Administration of the Internal Security Act and Other Internal Security Laws*, September 26, 1972 (Washington, D.C.: U.S. Government Printing Office, 1972).

14. H. Tristram Engelhardt, Jr., "The Disease of Masturbation: Values and the Concept of Disease," *Bulletin of the History of Medicine* 48 (Summer 1974): 234–248.

15. James Nevins Hyde, "On the Masturbation, Spermatorrhoea and Impotence of Adolescence," *Chicago Medical Journal & Examiner* 38 (1979): 451–452.

16. Cartwright, Samuel, "Report on the Diseases and Physical Peculiarities of the Negro Race," *The New Orleans Medical and Surgical Journal* 4 (May 1851): 691–715.

17. Thomas S. Szasz, "The Sane Slave," *American Journal of Psychotherapy* 25 (1971): 228–239.

18. Ivan Illich, *Medical Nemesis* (New York: Pantheon Books, 1976).

19. Szasz, Thomas, *The Myth of Mental Illness* (New York: Hoeber-Harper, 1961).

20. See, for example, N. R. Hanson, *Patterns of Discovery* (Cambridge: Cambridge University Press, 1961); and I. Lakatos and A. Musgrave, eds., *Criticism and the Growth of Knowledge* (Cambridge: Cambridge University Press, 1970).

452 · H. TRISTRAM ENGELHARDT, JR.

21. Ludwik Fleck, *Entstehung und Entwicklung einer wissenschaftlichen Tatsache* (Basel: Benno Schwabe, 1935); English version, *Genesis and Development of a Scientific Fact*, ed. T. J. Trenn and R. K. Menton, trans. F. Bradley and T. J. Trenn (Chicago: University of Chicago Press, 1979).

22. Thomas S. Kuhn, *The Structure of Scientific Revolutions* (Chicago: University of Chicago Press, 1962).

23. Girolamo Fracastoro, *Syphilis, sive morbi Gallici* (Venice, 1735).

24. Thomas Sydenham, *Observationes medicae circa morborum acutorum historiam et curationem* (London: G. Kettilby, 1676).

25. A. von Wassermann, et al., "Eine sero-diagnostische Reaktion bei Syphilis," *Deutshe Medizinische Wochenschrift* 32 (1906): 745–746.

26. Kuhn, *The Structure of Scientific Revolutions*, 52–56.

27. Peter Achinstein, "The Problem of Theoretical Terms," *American Philosophical Quarterly* 2 (July 1965): 193–203. The failure to draw distinctions among the various ways in which medical facts are dependent on or independent of theories, values, and social roles may lie at the root of some of the arguments that have surfaced regarding the status of medical findings. See, for example, Ernan McMullin, "A Clinician's Quest for Certainty," and John L. Gedye, "Simulating Clinical Judgment: An Essay in Technological Psychology," *Clinical Judgment: A Critical Appraisal*, ed. H. Tristram Engelhardt, Jr., et al. (Dordrecht, Holland: D. Reidel Publishing, 1979), 115–129, 93–113. In any event, the reader should note that the degree of independence of facts from theories and expectations is a matter of considerable controversy.

28. Griswold v. State of Connecticut, 381 U.S. 479, 85 S.Ct. 1678, 14 L. Ed. 2d 510 (1965).

29. Eisenstadt v. Baird, 405 U.S. 438, 92 S.Ct. 1029, 31 L. Ed. 349 (1972).

30. Roe v. Wade, 410 U.S. 113, 93 S.Ct. 705, 35 L.Ed. 2d 147 (1973).

31. People v. Onofre, 415 N.W. 2d at 940 n.3, 434 N.Y.S. 2d at 951 n.3 (1980).

32. Natanson v. Kline, 186 Kan. 393, 350 P.2d 1093 (1960).

33. Canterbury v. Spence, 464 F.2d 772 (1972).

34. H. L. A. Hart and A. M. Honore, *Causation in the Law*, (Oxford: Clarendon Press, 1959).

35. H. D. Lomas and J. D. Berman, "Diagnosing for Administrative Purposes: Some Ethical Problems," *Social Science and Medicine* 17 (1983): 241–244.

36. T. Duckett-Jones, M.D., "The Diagnosis of Rheumatic Fever," *Journal of the American Medical Association* 126 (1944): 481–484.

37. Barry Newman, "Socialized Care: Frugal Medical Service Keeps Britons Healthy and Patiently Waiting," *Wall Street Journal*, February 9, 1983.

38. "Less Frequent Paps Called Sheer Idiocy," *Ob. Gyn. News*, December 1–14, 1982, 4.

39. *DSM-III*, 281–283.

Suggestions for Further Reading

The social construction of medical reality and the role of explanatory and evaluative judgments in framing problems for health care have to date been explored primarily in the literature bearing on medical decision making and cost-benefit analysis. In addition to the readings suggested here, there are various useful articles available in such journals as *Medical Decision Making* and the *Journal of Medicine and Philosophy*.

Engelhardt, H. Tristram, Jr.; Spicker, Stuart F.; and Towers, Bernard, eds. *Clinical Judgment: A Critical Appraisal.* Dordrecht, Holland: D. Reidel Publishing, 1979.

Feinstein, Alvan. *Clinical Judgment.* Baltimore: Williams and Wilkins, 1967.

Luke, Roice D., and Bauer, Jeffery C., eds. *Issues in Health Economics.* Rockville, Md.: Aspen, 1982.

Nordenfelt, Lennart, and Lindahl, Ingemar, eds. *Causality and Health: Essays in the Philosophy of Medicine.* Dordrecht, Holland: D. Reidel Publishing, 1984.

Office of Technology Assessment. *The Implications of Cost-Effectiveness Analysis of Medical Technology.* Washington, D.C.: U.S. Government Printing Office, 1980.

Warner, Kenneth E., and Luce, Bryan R. *Cost-Benefit and Cost-Effectiveness Analysis in Health Care.* Ann Arbor, Mich.: Health Administration Press, 1982.

Wulff, Henrik. *Rational Diagnosis and Treatment.* Oxford: Blackwell Scientific, 1976.

About the Contributors

Margaret Pabst Battin, who received her Ph.D. from the University of California at Irvine, is now Associate Professor of Philosophy at the University of Utah. She is the editor, with David Mayo, of *Suicide: The Philosophical Issues;* the author of *Ethical Issues in Suicide,* a volume in the Prentice-Hall series on Philosophy and Medicine; and editor, with Michael Rudick, of a scholarly edition of John Donne's treatise on suicide, *Biathanatos.* She also publishes short fiction, much of it on issues in bioethics.

Michael D. Bayles received an M.A. from the University of Missouri, and a Ph.D. from Indiana University. He has previously taught at the University of Idaho, Brooklyn College, and the University of Kentucky, and held fellowships at Harvard Law School and The Hastings Center. Until recently he was Director of the Westminster Institute for Ethics and Human Values in London, Canada, and a Professor of Philosophy at the University of Western Ontario. Currently, he is Professor of Philosophy at the University of Florida. He is the author of *Principles of Legislation, Morality and Population Policy,* and *Professional Ethics,* as well as numerous articles.

Martin Benjamin received an M.A. and a Ph.D. in philosophy from the University of Chicago. Between his undergraduate and graduate years he served as a secondary school teacher with the Peace Corps in Ethiopia. He has taught at Miami University in Ohio and is presently a member of the Philosophy Department at Michigan State University. He is co-author with Joy Curtis of *Ethics in Nursing* and has written a number of articles on ethics and social philosophy. During the 1983–84 academic year he was an NEH Fellow at the Hastings Center.

Christopher Boorse received his Ph.D. from Princeton in 1972. Since then his research interests have been in the area of philosophy of medicine, psychiatry, and law. His most recent essay is on premenstrual syndrome as a criminal defense.

Dan W. Brock received his Ph.D. in philosophy in 1970 from Columbia University. In 1969 he joined the Brown University philosophy department where he is now Professor and Chairman of Philosophy, and is past Chairman of the Brown Program in Biomedical Ethics. During the 1981–82 academic year, he served as Staff Philosopher on the President's Commission for the Study of Ethical Problems in Medicine and Biomedical and Behavioral Research. He has published many papers in moral and political philosophy, and in biomedical ethics.

Allen Buchanan is Professor of Philosophy at the University of Arizona, Tucson. He received a Ph.D. in philosophy from the University of North Carolina at Chapel Hill in 1975. He has taught at the University of Minnesota at Minneapolis and at the University of Pittsburgh. In 1982 he served as Staff Philosopher for the President's Commission for the Study of Ethical Problems in Medicine and Biomedical and Behavioral Research in Washington, D.C. His publications include *Marx and Justice: The Radical Critique of Liberalism* and articles on epistemology, ethics, political philosophy, and medical ethics.

Joy Curtis is an Associate Professor in the College of Nursing and a member of the Medical Humanities Program at Michigan State University. Her nursing career includes five years each as a staff nurse, clinical nursing instructor, nurse–writer of multimedia materials, and director of a federally funded project for minority nursing students. For the past eight years her primary responsibilities have been in nursing school administration. She and Martin Benjamin have team-taught undergraduate courses in nursing ethics, presented workshops on ethical analysis and inquiry, and are co-authors of *Ethics in Nursing*.

Norman Daniels received degrees from Balliol College, Oxford, and Harvard. He is chairman of the Tufts University Philosophy Department and author of *Thomas Reid's 'Inquiry' Search of Equity*, and has recently published *Just Health Care*. He has written on topics in the history and philosophy of science, philosophy of psychology, ethics, and social philosophy, and with support from the NEH and the Retirement Research Foundation, he is currently working on a book on justice between age groups.

H. Tristram Engelhardt, Jr., is Professor in the Departments of Medicine and Community Medicine of Baylor College of Medicine and Member of the Center for Ethics, Medicine, and Public Issues in Houston, Texas. He holds doctoral degrees in philosophy and in medicine. He is the author of *Mind-Body* and co-editor with Stuart Spicker of the book series *Philosophy and Medicine*. He has edited or coedited over 16 volumes in the field of philosophy of medicine and is the author of over 90 articles.

Bruce Miller is Professor and Chairperson of the Department of Philosophy at Michigan State University. He is also Assistant Coordinator of the Medical Humanities Program in the College of Human Medicine at the University. His research and teaching interests are in philosophy of law and medical ethics. He has published essays on judicial decision making, autonomy of patients and research subjects, rights of infants, informed consent, and law and medicine.

Tom Regan was awarded the M.A. and Ph.D. degrees from the University of Virginia. Since 1967 he has taught philosophy at North Carolina State University, where he has twice been elected Outstanding Teacher and, in 1977, was named Alumni Distinguished Professor. He is sole editor of *Matters of Life and Death: New Introductory Essays in Moral Philosophy, Just Business: New Introductory Essays in Business Ethics,* and *Earthbound: New Introductory Essays in Environmental Ethics.* His other books include *Understanding Philosophy, All that Dwell Therein: Essays on Animal Rights and Environmental Ethics, The Case for Animal Rights,* and, most recently, *Bloomsbury's Prophet: G. E. Moore and the Development of His Moral Philosophy.*

L. W. Sumner was born in Toronto and educated at the University of Toronto and Princeton University. In 1965 he joined the faculty of the University of Toronto, where he is now Professor of Philosophy. He is the author of *Abortion and Moral Theory* and of numerous articles in moral and political philosophy.

Donald VanDeVeer is Professor of Philosophy at North Carolina State University. He received a Ph.D. in philosophy at the University of Chicago. His published essays are in health-care ethics, political philosophy, and environmental ethics. He is co-editor with Tom Regan of *And Justice for All* and co-editor with Christine Pierce of *People, Penguins, and Plastic Trees: Issues in Environmental Ethics.* He is the author of *Paternalistic Intervention: The Moral Bounds on Benevolence.*

Mary Anne Warren received her Ph.D. from the University of California at Berkeley and currently teaches philosophy at San Francisco State University. She has published articles on abortion, affirmative action, the feminist concept of androgyny, and other topics, and is author of an encyclopedia, *The Nature of Woman.*

Daniel Wikler is Professor in the Department of Philosophy and the School of Medicine's Program in Medical Ethics at the University of Wisconsin. He has published scholarly articles on several issues in medical ethics and health policy, ranging from allocation of health care resources to ethical issues in psychiatry. In 1980 and 1981 he served as Staff Philosopher with the President's Commission for the Study of Ethical Problems in Medicine and Biomedical and Behavioral Research, and has been a member of several committees and advisory boards in both national and state governments.

A Guide to Research

In addition to the Suggestions for Further Reading at the end of each chapter, we provide here some suggestions concerning how to engage in further research. One source frequently leads to another. A number of journals focus especially on issues in health care ethics. We list a few:

Bioethics (an Australian journal)
Bioethics Quarterly
Hastings Center Reports
Journal of Medical Ethics
Journal of Medical Humanities and Bioethics
The Journal of Medicine and Philosophy
Theoretical Medicine

Certain philosophical journals have a significant to high proportion of articles on ethical issues, e.g.:

Canadian Journal of Philosophy
Ethics
Philosophy and Public Affairs
Philosophical Quarterly (a British journal)
Social Theory and Practice

On occasion, important related essays may be found in journals focusing primarily on health care or medical (or scientific) research, e.g.:

American Journal of Nursing
Journal of the American Medical Association
Lancet
New England Journal of Medicine
Nursing Research

Two useful sources that usually can be found in university libraries are the *Encyclopedia of Bioethics* and *The Philosopher's Index*. The latter can be used to locate philosophical articles in the journals by topic or author. On certain issues (for example, informed consent or decision-making for incompetents), it may be useful to consult law journals such as the *Harvard Law Review*, the *Yale Law Journal*, or the *Columbia Law Review*, among others. There are also more specialized journals, e.g.:

American Journal of Law and Medicine

Typically, one also can find bibliographical help by examining some of the other available texts in the field. Here are some:

Natalie Abrams and Michael Buckner, *Medical Ethics.* Cambridge: MIT Press, 1983.

Elsie Bandman and Bertram Bandman, eds., *Bioethics and Human Rights.* Boston: Little, Brown, and Company, 1978.

Vincent Barry, *Moral Aspects of Health Care.* Belmont, Calif.: Wadsworth, 1982.

Tom Beauchamp and James F. Childress, *Principles of Biomedical Ethics.* New York: Oxford University Press, 1979.

Tom Beauchamp and LeRoy Walters, eds., *Contemporary Issues in Bioethics.* Belmont, Calif.: Wadsworth, 1982.

Martin Benjamin and Joy Curtis, *Ethics In Nursing.* New York: Oxford University Press, 1981.

Samuel Gorovitz et al., eds., *Moral Problems in Medicine.* Englewood Cliffs, N.J: Prentice-Hall, 1983.

Robert Hunt and John Arras, eds., *Ethical Issues in Modern Medicine.* Palo Alto, Calif.: Mayfield, 1977.

Thomas Mappes and Jane Zembaty, *Biomedical Ethics.* New York: McGraw-Hill, 1981.

Terrance McConnell, *Moral Issues in Health Care.* Belmont, Calif.: Wadsworth, 1982.

Ronald Munson, ed., *Intervention and Reflection.* Belmont, Calif.: Wadsworth, 1979.

Robert Veatch, ed., *Case Studies in Medical Ethics.* Cambridge, Mass.: Harvard University Press, 1977.

Richard Wertz, ed., *Readings on Ethical and Social Issues in Biomedicine.* Englewood Cliffs, N.J.: Prentice-Hall, 1973.

Index